Biotherapy

Jones and Bartlett Series in Oncology

Biotherapy

A Comprehensive Overview

Edited by

Paula Trahan Rieger, RN, MSN, OCN
Oncology Nurse Specialist
Clinical Immunology and Biological Therapy
The University of Texas M.D. Anderson Cancer Center
Houston, Texas

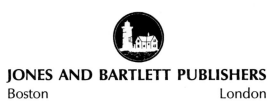

JONES AND BARTLETT PUBLISHERS
Boston   London

To my husband, Marty, without whose love, support, patience, and
understanding this dream would not have been possible.

Editorial, Sales, and Customer Service Offices
Jones and Bartlett Publishers
One Exeter Plaza
Boston, MA 02116
1-800-832-0034
617-859-3900

Jones and Bartlett Publishers International
7 Melrose Terrace
London W67RL
England

Library of Congress Cataloging-in-Publication Data

Biotherapy : a comprehensive overview / edited by Paula Trahan Rieger.
     p.   cm.
   Includes bibliographical references and index.
   ISBN 0-86720-707-8
   1. Cancer—Immunotherapy.   2. Biological products—Therapeutic use. I. Rieger, Paula Trahan.
   RC271.I45B54 1994
   616.99'406—dc20   94-19780
                                                CIP

Printed in the United States of America
98 97 96 95 94   10 9 8 7 6 5 4 3 2 1

Contents

CHAPTER 5   **The Interleukins   93**

Eileen Sharp, RN, BSN, OCN

CHAPTER 6   **Hematopoietic Growth Factors   113**

Debra Wujcik, RN, MSN, OCN

CHAPTER 11   **Fatigue   221**

Karen A. Skalla, RN, MSN
Paula Trahan Rieger, RN, MSN, OCN

CHAPTER 12   **The Flu-Like Syndrome   243**

Douglas Haeuber, RN, MSN, MA, OCN

Foreword

Dr. Paul Ehrlich, in the 1900 article, "On immunity with special reference to cell life," states "we are brought more and more to the conviction that the blood serum is the *carrier of substances innumerable as yet little known or conceived of*" (Ehrlich, 1900, p. 445). Dr. William B. Coley published a review that included four long-term survivors of sarcoma and noted that each developed high fevers and postoperative infections, which he felt contributed to their success (Coley, 1891). He noted, "nature often gives us hints to her profoundest secrets, and it is possible that she has given us a hint which, if we will but follow, may lead us on to the solution of this difficult problem" (p. 210). As a result he developed Coley's toxin, which was used as one of the first forms of nonspecific immunotherapy. Bacillus Calmette Guérin (BCG) and *Corynebacterium Parvum (C. Parvum)* were other immunotherapy agents commonly used later in the 1960s and 1970s. Over the last century, the identification and manipulation of these "substances" have been the focus of many researchers. These have been used in addition to the more traditional cancer treatments: surgery, chemotherapy, and radiation therapy.

Over the last 25 years, technologic advances, such as genetic engineering and hybridoma techniques, have allowed for the identification and production of large amounts of biologic agents for study and clinical testing. These advances have expedited and expanded our understanding of biologic responses and their modifiers. Biotherapy is the therapeutic use of biologic response modifiers (BRM). These agents may restore, augment, or modify biologic responses as well as have direct antitumor effects. As a result of these advances, the Food and Drug Administration approved interferon-alpha in 1986, granulocyte and granulocyte-macrophage colony-stimulating factors in 1991, interleukin-2 in 1992, OncoScint® for monoclonal imaging of colon and ovarian cancer in 1992, and BCG for bladder cancer in 1990. Many more BRM agents are in various stages of development and testing and include growth and maturation factors, tumor vaccines, and gene therapy.

Nurses have been significant contributors to the development of this fourth modality of cancer treatment, both in the conduct of clinical trials and the care of individuals receiving biotherapy. The history and science of BRM development is presented along with information about specific agents. Administration and nursing management of BRM side effects are delineated along with areas for future nursing research. This timely and important book, a result of the "coming of age" of biotherapy, is a reflection of the nursing experiences in this field.

Deborah K. Mayer, MSN, OCN, FAAN
Oncology Clinical Nurse Specialist
Ontario Cancer Institute/Princess Margaret
  Hospital
Toronto, Ontario
Canada

References

Coley, W. 1891. Contribution to the knowledge of sarcoma. *Annals of Surgery* 14: 199–220.

Ehrlich, P. 1900. On immunity with special reference to cell life. *Proceedings of the Royal Society of London* 66: 424–448.

Preface

It has been many years since Coley's toxins were used as the first form of nonspecific immunotherapy. The progress of science and technology since that era has provided the means to make biotherapy the fourth modality of cancer therapy. Today, many cancer patients will receive some form of biotherapy during treatment for their disease. This integration of new forms of therapy into cancer care mandates that oncology nurses become knowledgeable about this therapeutic modality so that they can provide quality care. The challenge for the authors of this text was to synthesize a rapidly changing field of knowledge into a text that is both up-to-date and understandable to those unfamiliar with this field.

The inspiration to create this text grew out of a need expressed by many nurses for a comprehensive resource on biotherapy. Although much has been written in the nursing literature over the last ten years, no one text completely addresses this need. In addition, because of its sometimes complex nature, many nurses feel that biotherapy is too "difficult" to understand. A text that provides the foundation to understand and apply this therapeutic modality in patients and the skills to care for patients who receive it was essential. Conversely, those with a strong background in biotherapy needed a text that could provide further insight into the field and a perspective of the knowledge acquired so far.

This text is primarily intended for oncology nurses, but many others may find it interesting and useful. The use of biotherapy is expanding to patients with other medical conditions, such as hepatitis, sepsis, and autoimmune diseases. Nurses in a medical/surgical setting may find this text of use in their unit reference library. The text could also be used as a resource for curriculum development in schools of nursing or as a reference text. Other health care professionals involved in the care of patients, such as pharmacists, medical students, and physician's assistants, will find this text useful in gaining a general understanding of the field.

Part 1 provides an overview of the field of biotherapy: historical perspectives, technological changes that have fueled the development of this field, a framework to define and classify biotherapy, and an overview of the major agents in clinical use or under investigation. Chapters on the immune system and on the dosing and scheduling of biological agents provide a foundation for understanding material presented in Part 2, a review of the major categories of biological agents. These chapters review the definition and biological actions, important clinical studies, regulatory approvals, side effects profile, and future directions for the interferons, interleukins, hematopoietic growth factors, monoclonal antibodies, tumor necrosis factor, immunomodulators, differentiation agents, and vaccines.

Part 3 addresses nursing management of patients who are receiving biotherapy, with special chapters highlighting the challenging side effects of fatigue, the flu-like syndrome, and mental status changes. Because educating patients to become self-sufficient in their care is of such importance in today's health care environment, a chapter has been devoted to this subject. Issues related to reimbursement for biological agents are also reviewed in recognition of the prevalence of this problem in clinical practice. The text ends with a view toward the future: Where will biotherapy be in the next ten years? Issues that remain to be addressed before the full therapeutic possibilities of biotherapy can be realized, current investigational trials, as well as new approaches for treatment are reviewed.

References are provided throughout the text to guide the reader in pursuing further information on clinical studies, biological actions of the major agents, and nursing care. Words included in the glossary are set in bold type throughout the text to assist the reader in developing the "new" vocabulary needed to understand this therapeutic modality.

The rapid integration of biotherapy into the cancer armamentarium represents the speed with which technology is changing the way we both treat and provide care to patients with cancer. Although many biological agents remain at an investigational stage, numerous agents have received regulatory approval over the last five years. Nurses and other health care professionals must make a commitment to expand their knowledge base to be aware of these trends. In daily practice, this text can serve as an information resource in providing quality care for patients who are receiving biological agents. Although many skills used in caring for patients who are receiving radiation therapy or chemotherapy can be transferred to caring for patients who are receiving biotherapy, the side effect profile for biological agents differs, requiring that new skills be mastered.

This text represents an assimilation of the knowledge gained by those who have worked in the field of biotherapy for many years. The benefit of their understanding of this field, their insights into the problems that need to be overcome and the future directions of research, as well as their expertise in the management of patients, are presented for the welfare of those new to the field.

Because discoveries in this area occur rapidly, some of the content may be incomplete or outdated. However, it is our desire that the information presented in this text will provide a beginning for understanding biotherapy and will assist in providing answers to the numerous questions generated in managing patients who are receiving this exciting, yet challenging, therapeutic modality.

ACKNOWLEDGMENTS

My sincere thanks to the many reviewers who assisted in assuring the quality of this text: Patricia Jassak, RN (Chapters 1 and 3), Kimberly Rumsey, RN (Chapters 1, 2, and 10), Dr. Saroj Vadhan-Raj (Chapters 3, 5, and 6), Dr. James Lee Murray (Chapter 7), Michael Rosenblum, PhD (Chapter 3), Dr. Richard Pazdur (Chapter 3), Dr. Avi Markowitz (Chapter 5), Barbara St. Pierre, PhD (Chapter 8), Dr. Waun Kee Hong (Chapter 9), Paula Shackelford, RN, and Patricia Corcoran Buchsel, RN (Chapter 10), Maryl Winningham, PhD (Chapter 11), Jim Sergi, RN (Chapter 12), Deborah Volker (Chapter 14), and Dr. Gabriel Lopez-Berestein (Chapter 16).

To the physicians and staff members at the University of Texas M.D. Anderson Cancer Center, especially the Department of Clinical Immunology and Biological Therapy, who have fostered my interest in biotherapy over the years and have answered the many questions generated as I developed my knowledge base and clinical expertise. A special thank you to the many patients who were the inspiration to learn more so that I could become a better care giver.

To the staff nurses of the CIBT clinic and those throughout M.D. Anderson whose interest, support, and desire to learn more have helped me to remember why this book is so important. To Cecil Brewer, RN, for his vision and support during the early stages of development of this project. To Dr. James Lee Murray and Dr. Saroj Vadhan-Raj for their encouragement in pursuing professional endeavors, understanding of the importance of this project, and tolerance of absences necessary during critical developmental stages.

To the members of the Scientific Publications Department at the University of Texas M.D. Anderson Cancer Center, especially Walter Pagel, Katie Hale, Lisa Matthews, and Dianne Rivera, whose editorial assistance in the development of this text was indispensable. To the M.D. Anderson library staff whose helpful assistance with computer searches and locating difficult-to-find references was invaluable. To Bambi Grilley, RPh, in the Investigational Pharmacy, for her assistance in tracking drug information. And to Dianna Fredericks, for her expert editorial and secretarial assistance, and giving of her time so generously over the Christmas holidays.

To Margaret Barton Burke, RN, and Marie Bakitas Whedon, RN, who helped me to realize that this dream could become reality. To my professional colleagues both at the University of Texas M.D. Anderson and across the country who supported and encouraged me through this, at times, difficult task. A special thank you to Kimberly Rumsey and Paula Shackelford for their patience, counsel, and insight. To the remarkable people at Jones and Bartlett, especially Jan Wall, whose guidance, assistance, and belief in my ability made this text possible.

And lastly, to several very special people. To the authors, who shared their knowledge and expertise and worked hard to achieve the excellence I requested of them. To my husband, who accepted the many hours this project demanded from me and supported me by being the wonderful man that he is. And to my parents, who raised me to believe in myself and that I could achieve any goal I set my mind to.

Contributors

Lynne Brophy, RN, MSN, OCN
Oncology Clinical Nurse Specialist
Rex Hospital
Raleigh, North Carolina
Clinical Instructor
Department of Adult and Geriatric Health
School of Nursing
University of North Carolina
Chapel Hill, North Carolina

Grace E. Dean, RN, MSN
Research Specialist
City of Hope National Medical Center
Duarte, California

Janet E. DiJulio, RN, MSN
Nurse Manager—Oncology Unit
Petersen Cancer Center
Stanford University Hospital
Palo Alto, California

Robert A. Figlin, MD, FACP
Director, Clinical Research Unit
Jonsson Comprehensive Cancer Center
University of California Los Angeles
Medical Center
Los Angeles, California
Associate Professor of Medicine
University of California Los Angeles
School of Medicine
Department of Medicine
Division of Hematology/Oncology
Los Angeles, California

Betty Bierut Gallucci, PhD
Associate Professor–Physiological Nursing
University of Washington
School of Nursing
Seattle, Washington

Douglas Haeuber, RN, MSN, MA, OCN
Formerly: Staff Nurse Medical Oncology
Massachusetts General Hospital
Boston, Massachusetts

Patricia F. Jassak, RN, MS, OCN
Manager, Cancer Center Clinical Services
Loyola University Medical Center
Maywood, Illinois
Clinical Assistant Professor
Department of Medical-Surgical Nursing
Marcella Neihoff School of Nursing
Loyola University Medical Center
Maywood, Illinois

Tina Marie Liles, RN, BSN
Research Nurse Oncology Division
Stanford University Hospital
Palo Alto, California

Mary McCabe, RN, BA, BS
Clinical Trials Specialist
Investigational Drug Branch
Cancer Treatment and Evaluation Program
Division of Cancer Treatment
National Cancer Institute
Bethesda, Maryland

Donna O. McCarthy, PhD
Associate Professor
Adult Medical-Surgical Nursing
School of Nursing
University of Wisconsin-Madison
Madison, Wisconsin

Christina Meyers, PhD
Associate Neuropsychologist
Department of Neuro-Oncology
University of Texas
M.D. Anderson Cancer Center
Houston, Texas

Nancy P. Moldawer, RN, MSN
Research Nurse—Clinical Research Unit
University of California Los Angeles
Department of Medicine
Division of Hematology/Oncology
Los Angeles, California

Paula Trahan Rieger, RN, MSN, OCN
Oncology Nurse Specialist—Division of
  Medicine
Clinical Immunology and Biological Therapy
University of Texas
M.D. Anderson Cancer Center
Houston, Texas
Adjunct Instructor of Nursing
Department of Adult Health
University of Texas Health Science Center
School of Nursing
Houston, Texas

Kimberly A. Rumsey, RN, MSN, OCN
Clinical Instructor III
Division of Nursing
University of Texas
M.D. Anderson Cancer Center
Houston, Texas

Eileen Sharp, RN, BSN, OCN
Oncology Clinical Coordinator
Williamson Medical Center
Franklin, Tennessee

Karen Skalla, RN, MSN
Oncology Clinical Nurse Specialist
Hematology/Oncology Division
University of Pennsylvania
Philadelphia, Pennsylvania

Vera Wheeler, RN, MN, OCN
Consultant: Cancer Nursing and Biotherapy
San Diego, California
Formerly: Clinical Nurse Specialist
Cancer Nursing Service
National Institutes of Health
Bethesda, Maryland

Debra Wujcik, RN, MSN, OCN
Clinical Nurse Specialist/Case Manager
Vanderbilt University Medical Center
Nashville, Tennessee
Adjunct Instructor of Nursing
Department of Adult Health
Vanderbilt University
School of Nursing
Nashville, Tennessee

PART 1

Biotherapy Principles and Foundations

CHAPTER 1 | An Overview of Biotherapy

Patricia Jassak, RN, MS, OCN

The field of biotherapy has undergone alternating periods of excitement and frustration, but scientific interest has remained steadfast. Although we now possess significant knowledge of the intricate workings of the immune system, we also realize that there is much more about biotherapy to learn and integrate into the clinical arena before we can improve its therapeutic efficacy in cancer.

HISTORICAL PERSPECTIVE

The historical foundation for the use of immunotherapy to treat malignant disease can be traced back to the 19th century and even earlier (Oettgen and Old, 1991; Hersh et al., 1973). The current use of cytokines relates to Dr. Coley's initial work with bacterial toxins in solid tumors. Coley's toxins were used to induce an immune response which would, it was hoped, activate the immune system to eliminate or reduce tumor burden. Early experiments in which tumor-specific immunity in the mouse was achieved by lymphocyte transfer laid the groundwork for the current use of cytotoxic T lymphocytes. Whereas the original vaccines were made from crude tumor preparations, today's vaccines contain purified cancer antigens. Modern investigations of monoclonal antibodies are refinements of early studies which used horse and rabbit antisera. A timeline summary of the key events in the development of biotherapy is depicted in Table 1.1.

The basis of the quest to understand and control the relationship of the immune system to cancer is linked to three observations which have withstood the test of time (Oettgen and Old, 1991). These observations are the spontaneous remissions of patients with cancer, the increased incidence of cancer in immunosuppressed patients, and the presence of lymphoid infiltrates in solid tumors. However, Oettgen and Old point out that although these

Table 1.1 Timeline of key events in the development of biotherapy

Late-1800s to mid-1900s
- Impure vaccines
- Coley's toxins
- Interferon discovered, 1957

1960s
- Clinical trials of bacterial agents used

Early-1970s
- Impure agents used
- Variability in experimental procedures
- Incongruence between animal and human studies
- Lack of generalizable results

Late-1970s to mid-1980s
- Major technological advances aided quest
- Increased understanding of immune system
- Advances in genetic engineering
- Continued advances in molecular biology
- Advances in laboratory methods and processes and computer systems
- Single-agent cytokine studies initiated
- First BRM agent (IFN-α) approved by the FDA

Late-1980s to the Present
- Discovery and isolation of a variety of immune system products
- Numerous agents recombinantly produced for clinical trials
- Multi-site clinical trials initiated and ongoing
- Combination cytokine therapy clinical trials initiated
- Combination cytokine and chemotherapy clinical trials initiated
- Six additional BRM agents approved by the FDA

observations are credible when viewed through an immunologic perspective, other explanations exist that are independent of immune system recognition and action. They postulate that these observations provide the impetus for continued scientific inquiry until it is clearly established that the human immune system is capable of recognition and surveillance of malignant cells. Thus, the therapeutic success of biotherapy is dependent on the evolving insight into the physiologic mechanisms of the host-tumor relationship, host relationship, and tumor biology (Creekmore *et al.*, 1991).

In 1894, William B. Coley, a surgeon at New York's Memorial Hospital from 1891 to 1936, began studying the effects of bacterial products in patients with cancer. He pursued his hypothesis, suggested by clinical observation, that infection and subsequent fever accounted for the differences in disease response after surgical resection for cancer. He found that patients who experienced high fevers after surgery were more likely to remain free of tumor recurrences. Coley administered extracts of streptococci and serratia to patients with inoperable sarcomas and observed local and systemic regression of their disease (Coley, 1911; Coley, 1893). Coley's toxins continued to be used until 1975 and provided the rationale for the current explorations of cytokine therapy. They were effective in producing tumor remissions in some cases. However, with the advent of the more predictable and comprehensive treatment options, radiation therapy, and later, chemotherapy, the use of Coley's toxins declined. Oettgen and Old reported that only one clinical trial evaluated the use of Coley's toxins in a rigorous scientific manner. In this trial, patients with non-Hodgkin's lymphoma were given chemotherapy alone or chemotherapy combined with Coley's toxins. At the first five-year analysis, patients treated with Coley's toxins demonstrated a higher rate of complete response, increased duration of response, and longer survival. However, as time passed these differences diminished.

Subsequent work in the field of biotherapy used nonspecific stimulators of the immune system, such as bacillus Calmette-Guérin (BCG), methanol-extracted residue of BCG (MER-BCG), *Coryne bacterium parvum* (*C. parvum*), and levamisole in a variety of tumors. These agents seemed to be clinically effective only when used in patients with minimal tumor burden, and most of these studies failed to demonstrate any benefit from these agents when they were used alone in patients with large tumor burdens. In general, clinical outcomes were poor because of the use of impure agents and variability in experimental procedures. The variability in procedures led to results that were neither generalizable nor, when animal models were used, predictive of human response.

Scientific advances in identifying, isolating, producing, and using biological agents in the 1980s improved tumor responses and positioned biotherapy as a viable cancer treatment modality. Advances in four areas were critical in establishing biotherapy as a recognized treatment entity. These were (1) increased understanding of the intricate complexities of the immune system; (2) refinements in recombinant **deoxyribonucleic acid (DNA)** and hybridoma technology; (3) laboratory success in establishing methods to produce large volumes of effector cells in culture; and (4) isolation and purification of new biological products aided by advances in computer hardware and software (Oldham, 1991; Gallucci, 1987; Oldham, 1984; Oldham and Smalley, 1983).

RECOMBINANT DNA TECHNOLOGY

Clinical use of biological agents was severely limited until the advent of recombinant DNA technology. For recombinant technology to be successful, a system was needed that was able to support the large-scale production of cells that, because their DNA can be manipulated, can be made to express a desired protein. The bacterium *E. coli*, because it had been extensively studied and was well understood, was developed as such an expression system making a critical contribution to the evolution and expansion of the field of molecular biology. *E. coli* is a good choice for an expression system because it is relatively simple genetically, grows rapidly, and is generally well-characterized (Ramel *et al.*, 1983).

E. coli is made up of one large circular thread of chromosomal DNA and several smaller circular units of genetic material called plasmids. Because plasmids replicate independently of the chromosomal DNA, they were quickly singled out as the target of genetic engineering. Recombinant DNA technology involves the use of special enzymes called restriction endonucleases that are used to cut open the plasmid circles at specific locations, allowing for insertion of selected fragments of DNA into the openings. Another enzyme, DNA ligase, is required to close the ends of the open plasmid to the ends of the insert.

The DNA fragment is derived in one of several ways (Ramel *et al.*, 1983). It can be chemically synthesized to code for the known amino acid sequence of a particular protein or excised from the chromosome of interest; alternatively, complementary DNA (cDNA) may be synthesized, by using purified messenger RNA as a template, with the enzyme reverse transcriptase. The new plasmid is called a **vector** and is introduced into the *E. coli* host which in culture grows cells that produce the desired protein. **Cloning** refers to the selection of colonies for optimal growth in culture. This cloning process allows the cells to produce an unlimited supply of the donor DNA. Figure 1.1 depicts this process schematically.

The *E. coli* expression system is somewhat restricted in that its natural structure does not include an enzyme system for adding sugar side chains to proteins (Ramel *et al.*, 1983). This is of little consequence when the substance to be cloned is not a glycoprotein, but when it is, its natural carbohydrate moiety will be missing. Clinical trials must address whether this is an important variable. Other expression systems now in use, such as yeast, have the ability to bind glycosylating proteins.

The protein produced by this recombinant DNA technology is then purified with the goal of 100% homogeneity and the highest possible product yield. Higher levels of homogeneity are accompanied by an unavoidable loss of product. Biological response modifiers are examples of proteins produced by this process.

The production of substances used in biological therapies must meet product quality control regulations and the good manufactur-

Figure 1.1   Recombinant DNA technology

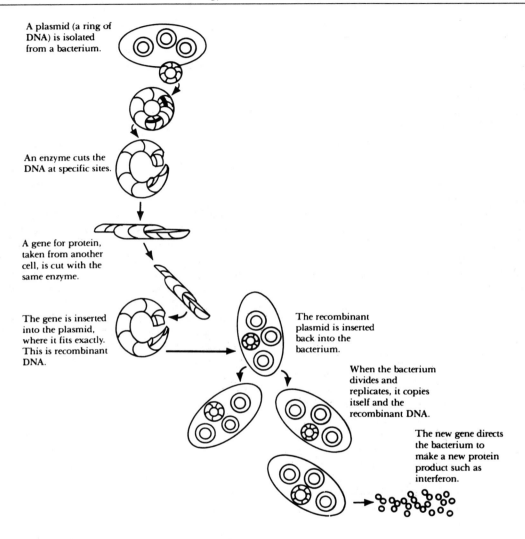

A plasmid (a ring of DNA) is isolated from a bacterium.

An enzyme cuts the DNA at specific sites.

A gene for protein, taken from another cell, is cut with the same enzyme.

The gene is inserted into the plasmid, where it fits exactly. This is recombinant DNA.

The recombinant plasmid is inserted back into the bacterium.

When the bacterium divides and replicates, it copies itself and the recombinant DNA.

The new gene directs the bacterium to make a new protein product such as interferon.

Source: Schindler, L. 1988. *Understanding the Immune System.* NIH publication number 88–529. Bethesda, MD: U.S. Department of Health and Human Services, p. 29.

ing product (GMP) guidelines. Evidence of safety, efficacy, purity, and identity of a product must be presented to the Food and Drug Administration before testing and when appropriate marketing approvals are granted.

DEFINITION AND CLASSIFICATION OF BIOTHERAPY

Biotherapy encompasses the use of agents derived from biological sources or of agents that affect biological responses (Oldham, 1991). In 1983, the National Cancer Institute, Division of Cancer Treatment Subcommittee on Biologic Response Modifiers, defined **biological response modifiers (BRMs)** as "agents or approaches that will modify the relationship between tumor and host by modifying the host's biologic response to tumor cells, with resultant therapeutic benefit" (Mihich and Fefer, 1983, p.3). The terms used to describe these agents and approaches have changed as scientific advances have increased our understanding of them. Historically, the term *immunotherapy* was used as the focus was on modulation of the immune response. Although modulation of the immune response remains a major focus, the term *biotherapy* or *biological therapy* is now used instead of immunotherapy to describe this field as the scope has broadened. Biological agents have pleiotropic effects, that is, they possess multiple actions: agents are capable of producing immunologic actions, other biological effects, or a combination of these activities. *Biotherapy* is generally used as a global term to describe this approach. BRMs, or more commonly now, biological agents, refer to the agents used within this therapeutic modality.

No one classification system exists for biotherapy. In addition, because agents often possess multiple biological actions, it is difficult to classify them. Biological response modifiers exert at least one of the following effects: they augment, modulate, or restore the host's immune response; they have direct cytotoxic

Table 1.2 Biotherapy's effects on the immune system

- *Active* stimulates host's instrinsic function
  nonspecific use of microbial or chemical agents to activate general host defense systems
  specific use of vaccines to augment or induce host response to tumor cells or tumor-associated antigens
- *Adoptive* transfer of immune cells with antitumor properties to tumor bearing host (e.g., LAK cells, TILs)
- *Restorative* restores deficient immunologic subpopulation
- *Passive* transfer of antibodies or short-lived antitumor "factors"
- *Cytomodulatory* agents that cause increased recognition of tumor-associated antigens and histocompatibility (HLA) antigens on the surface of tumor cells

Source: Data from Mitchell, M. 1992. Chemotherapy in combination with biomodulation: A 5-year experience with cyclophosphamide and interleukin-2. Seminars in Oncology 19(2): 80–87 (Suppl. 4, April).

or antiproliferative activity; or they produce other biological effects, for example, differentiation or maturation of cells or interference with tumor cell metastasis or transformation (Dutcher, 1992; Borden and Sondel, 1990; Clark and Longo, 1986). Another approach classifies the biotherapy of cancer into five broad categories described in Table 1.2 (Mitchell, 1992). These categories are based on the principal function of the agent or approach in the immune system.

CLINICAL DEVELOPMENT OF BIOLOGICAL AGENTS

Identification, development and testing of a biological agent requires that specific intricacies of physiologic and pharmacologic parameters be thoroughly investigated. This complete evaluation measures not only the agent's effectiveness but also takes into account the cellular immune response. Thus, the approach to the clinical investigation of a

Table 1.3   Phases of a clinical trial/key elements of biological trial

Characteristics shared by both biological and chemical agents	Specific to biological agents alone
Phase I • Defines toxic effects • Determines MTD & dose limiting toxicity • Uses escalating doses • Determines pharmacokinetics • rage 3–6 patients/dose level • Generally single-institution trials *Endpoint: Unacceptable toxic effects define MTD*	• Determines OBD • Correlates observed clinical responses with biological endpoints • 5–15 patient/dose level • Immunologic monitoring
Phase II • Determines antitumor activity at given dose and schedule in specific disease • Further defines toxicity • Refines toxicity interventions/management • Usually 30 patients at fixed dose • Involves multiple institutions *Endpoint: Substantial information obtained about drug's therapeutic activity related to best dose, route and schedule of administration*	• Given dose and schedule can be at MTD or OBD
Phase III • Compares therapeutic efficacy • Randomized study design • Large numbers of patients • Cooperative study groups	• In multiple disease states, no effective therapy exists, thus most biological agents approved for use after analysis of phase II data

biological agent is different from that of a chemical agent.

The Food and Drug Administration (FDA) requires preclinical and clinical trial evaluation of all chemical and biological agents prior to their commercial approval (Johnson and Temple, 1985). The preclinical development of a new biological agent must encompass three major steps (Creekmore *et al.*, 1991). The first step includes the identification, isolation, recombinant expression, and preclinical production of the new agent, determination of its physiologic role, and development of early therapeutic models. The second step focuses on the clinical development of the drug, including increased production under the GMP guidelines and analysis of the preclinical toxicity profile, pharmacology, and application studies. The third step is directed toward completion and filing of an investigational new drug (IND) application with the

FDA. A phase I protocol accompanied by supporting preclinical toxicology and pharmacology studies is required for IND submission (Collins *et al.*, 1990). Once IND status is granted, the agent enters sequential clinical trials. Clinical trials traditionally consist of three phases. The major characteristics of each phase and specific points that must be addressed when evaluating biological agents are found in Table 1.3.

The underlying hypothesis of cytotoxic drug research is that *more is better*. Thus, a critical first step in evaluating a new drug is to determine the maximum tolerated dose (MTD). This step is also important for biological agents because the agent may exert the best antitumor effect at the MTD. The MTD, however, may not be the same as the optimal biological dose (OBD). Early clinical trials of biological agents demonstrated that immunologic effects occurred at doses lower than the identified MTD. This phenomenon led to the concept of the OBD (Herberman, 1985), which is defined as "that dose which, with a minimum of side effects, produces the optimal desired responses for the parameters deemed important with respect to a particular biological agent" (Creekmore *et al.*, 1991, p. 68). Further discussion of the importance of the OBD and dose response of biological agents can be found in Chapter 3.

Oldham (1985) identified two underlying differences between drugs and biological agents. First, biological agents, unlike drugs, have preprogrammed mechanisms and receptors available for them. Second, biological agents are derivatives of natural products found in mammalian or human genes. It is probably these differences that account for the variance between MTD and OBD. Whereas cytotoxic agents possess one clear clinical outcome, that is, the ability to maximize direct antitumor effects, biological agents are used both for their cytotoxic activity and for the pleiotropic indirect immune effects they mediate to maximize tumor response.

To effectively evaluate a biological agent's activity, clinical trials must routinely incorporate relevant measurements of bioavailability, pharmacokinetics, biological effects, and toxicity (Oldham, 1983). Other issues essential in clinical trials of biological agents include the characteristics of the study population, clinical monitoring (observation, grading of severity, and recording of duration) of toxic effects and the use of immunologic assays (Creekmore *et al.*, 1991).

Nursing has consistently remained in the forefront in the clinical evaluation of biological agents. Many articles were generated in the 1970s and early 1980s that addressed administration and monitoring issues related to BCG, *C. Parvum,* and early trials of human interferon-alpha. Numerous reports have been published in a variety of formats, e.g., journal articles, books, and pharmaceutical sponsored series, that describe the involvement of nursing in identifying and managing the clinical toxic effects of biological agents. Furthermore,

steadily increasing numbers of nurses are undertaking clinical research in the management of symptoms related to biological agents. This research will doubtless have an effect on the well-being of the patient receiving biotherapy and his or her family.

BIOLOGICAL AGENTS

The majority of biological agents are cytokines. **Cytokines** are a broad class of protein cell regulators that share a variety of characteristics. These include low molecular weight and a polypeptide structure, often glycosylated; they act at short range on the cells that produce them or on nearby cells, and they play a role in the extent and interval of immune responses. Cytokines interact with specific high-affinity cell receptors, via mechanisms not yet understood, to alter cellular protein synthesis. These alterations cause deviations in cell behavior, e.g., direction of inhibition of growth, differentiation, or cytotoxicity, stimulation of host defense cells or disruption of the host-tumor relationship by acting on tumor vasculature and nutrient supply. Cytokines for the most part are **pleiotropic** cell regulators, possessing multiple overlapping and sometimes contradictory functions. Thus, production or administration of one cytokine influences production of or response to other cytokines.

Clinical evaluation of biological agents in the mid- to late-1980s enabled investigators to identify several principles of cytokine therapy (Table 1.4). The foundation for the development of these principles was the initial clinical experience with interferon and other cytokines. A brief discussion of the most important biological agents is provided here to familiarize the reader with each agent's investigational status and clinical uses.

Interferons

Virologists in the 1940s noted that under specific conditions exposure to one virus protects against infection by other viruses. In 1957,

Table 1.4 Principles of cytokine therapy

- Simple dose-response relationship may not always occur (less may be better).
- Cytokine-responsive tumors may require longer periods to achieve therapeutic response.
- Stable disease may become accpetable outcome.
- Common constellation of toxic effects—severity may vary by agent, dose, and other cumulative factors.

Isaacs and Lindenmann isolated a protein substance whose presence appeared to interfere with viral activity in cells. They called this substance interferon (IFN). Nearly a decade later other properties of IFN were identified including its antiproliferative capabilities. Because the difficulty of isolating and preparing the natural product precluded obtaining large amounts of the agent, clinical trials were limited until IFN was cloned, allowing it to be produced in large quantities (Pestka, 1983).

It is interesting that IFN-alpha (IFN-α) was the first biological agent to be approved by the FDA (in 1986) and thus is often referred to as the prototypic biological agent. Initially, IFNs were described according to their cell of origin, then according to physical-chemical properties; now they are classified according to their antigenic type (Fischer *et al.*, 1993). Three major types of IFNs have been isolated, recombinantly produced, and approved by the FDA, including IFN-α (Alferon®, Roferon®-A, Intron®-A); IFN gamma (IFN-γ) (Actimmune®); and IFN beta (IFN-β) (Betaseron®). All three types of IFN exhibit antiviral, immunomodulatory, and antiproliferative activity in various degrees.

The FDA has approved IFN-α for use in hairy cell leukemia, Kaposi's sarcoma related to AIDS, condyloma acuminata, and hepatitis B and non-A, non-B, with specific doses and schedules established for each disease. Other cancers demonstrating a response to treatment with IFN-α include chronic myelogenous leukemia and myeloproliferative disorders (Talpaz *et al.*, 1991), cutaneous melanoma (Kirkwood and Ernstoff, 1991) and a variety of other tumors (Kurzrock *et al.*, 1991).

Interferon-β is approved for treatment of multiple sclerosis, and IFN-γ to treat infections associated with chronic granulomatous disease. Currently the IFNs are approved for clinical use as single agents in specific disease states, but their optimal use may be in combination with chemotherapeutic or other biological agents. This may be determined only after continued clinical trials. In-depth discussion of the IFNs is found in Chapter 4.

Interleukins

Interleukins (ILs) can be produced by and regulate many cell types. In 1986, the Sixth International Congress of Immunology decided that new cytokines would be named according to their biological properties but that, on identification of the amino acid sequence, a sequential IL number would be assigned (Dinarello and Mier, 1987). Twelve ILs have so far been identified and isolated, and are undergoing either preclinical or clinical evaluation. Only one, IL–2, has been approved by the FDA; it is indicated for treatment of metastatic renal cell cancer.

Interleukin–2 is an excellent example of the impact of technology on scientific advancement. It was discovered in 1976 by Morgan and his co-workers and was originally called T cell growth factor (Morgan *et al.*, 1976). It entered clinical trials in the early 1980s and was approved by the FDA in 1992, a speedy record for the development of an agent from the scientific laboratory to use in the clinical arena. The biological effects of IL–2 are numerous and include the production of two cell subsets, lymphokine-activated killer cells and tumor-infiltrating lymphocytes. Clinical trials continue to evaluate IL–2 alone at various doses, schedules, and routes of administration as well as in combination with chemotherapeutic and other biotherapeutic agents. Chapter 5 discusses the interleukins in depth.

Hematopoietic Growth Factors

Hematopoietic growth factors (HGFs) are a complex network of glycoprotein hormones responsible for the differentiation, proliferation, maturation, and functional activity of hematopoietic cells (Turner, 1992). These factors are classified as either lineage restricted (affect only one cell type) or multilineage (affect several different cell types) (Crosier and Clark, 1992). Three HGFs have been approved by the FDA including granulocyte-CSF (G-CSF), yeast-derived granulocyte-macrophage CSF (GM-CSF), and erythropoietin (EPO). Three others, IL–3 (multi-CSF), PIXY–321 (a combination of GM-CSF and IL–3 fused together), and stem cell factor, are in clinical trials. A detailed description of HGFs and their role in cancer therapy can be found in Chapter 6.

Monoclonal Antibodies

The use of antibodies as carriers to deliver drugs and toxins to tumor cells was proposed as early as the 1900s by Paul Ehrlich (1910). He termed these antibodies "magic bullets". In 1975, the development of hybridoma technology by Köhler and Milstein, allowed for the production of large volumes of antibodies produced from a single clone of cells. These antibodies are termed monoclonal antibodies (MABs).

Over the last ten years, MABs have been investigated in clinical trials for the diagnosis of cancer and in both unconjugated and conjugated forms for the treatment of cancer. In addition, they have been evaluated in bone marrow transplantation to prevent the development of graft-versus-host disease or to purge autologous marrow of lingering malignant cells prior to transplantation. They are used extensively by pathologists to classify leukemias and lymphomas or to aid in the differential diagnosis of tumors that look alike on routinely processed light microscope specimens.

Two MABs have received regulatory approval: Orthoclone® OKT–3 (muromonab-CD3), a murine MAB targeted to the CD3 receptor of human T cells, for the treatment of acute allograft rejection in renal transplant patients; and OncoScint® CR/OV (satumomab

pendetide) for the detection of colorectal and ovarian cancer. More approvals can be expected as future investigations explore and refine this area. See Chapter 7 for a detailed discussion of this area.

Tumor Necrosis Factor

Tumor necrosis factor (TNF) was discovered in 1975 and subsequently found to be the same molecule as cachectin (Tracey *et al.*, 1989). This factor is a protein that selectively targets and destroys malignant cells. Two distinct types of TNF have been isolated: TNF-α is produced primarily by activated macrophages, whereas TNF-β, also known as lymphotoxin, is produced primarily by lymphocytes. The preclinical and clinical trials that have evaluated the efficacy of this agent have yielded only minimal and inconspicuous therapeutic responses. The potential clinical impact of TNF depends on an increased understanding of its cellular mechanisms and tumor cell resistance (Frei and Spriggs, 1989). Further discussion of clinical trials and toxicity experienced by patients who receive TNF can be found in Chapter 8.

SUMMARY

Biotherapy is established with surgery, chemotherapy, and radiotherapy as a treatment modality for cancer. Clearly, much has been achieved in a very short period of time, but a vast amount about these agents and their uses remains to be discovered, understood, and evaluated in preclinical and clinical trials. These agents or approaches cannot be viewed as independent factors, but instead as critical elements of a complex, intricate network that produces many positive and negative interactions. Although incomplete, our current understanding of biotherapy rests on the following observations: the majority of biological agents are produced by more than one type of cell; each biological agent has its own distinct receptors but produces striking, overlapping biological effects; most biological agents possess pleiotropic effects; a single stimulus can induce responses from multiple cytokines; and biological agents interact within the cytokine network through a variety of actions, including stimulating production of other agents, modulating receptor sites, and enhancing or inhibiting the biological activity of other cytokines.

References

Borden, E., and Sondel, P. 1990. Lymphokines and cytokines as cancer treatment: Immunotherapy realized. *Cancer* 65: 800–814.

Clark, J., and Longo, D. 1986. Biological response modifiers. *Mediguide to Oncology* 6(2): 1–4.

Coley, W. 1911. A report of recent cases of inoperable sarcoma successfully treated with mixed toxins of erysipelas and *Bacillus prodigious*. *Surgical Gynecology and Obstetrics* 13: 174–190.

Coley, W. 1893. The treatment of malignant tumors by repeated inoculations of erysipelas: With a report of ten original cases. *American Journal of Medical Science* 105: 487.

Collins, J., Grieshaber, C., and Chabner, B. 1990. Pharmacologically guided phase I clinical trials based upon preclinical drug development. *Journal of the National Cancer Institute* 80: 1321–1326.

Creekmore, S., Urba, W., and Longo, D. 1991. Principles of the clinical evaluation of biologic agents. In DeVita, V., Hellman, S., and Rosenberg, S. (eds). *Biologic Therapy of Cancer*. Philadelphia: J.B. Lippincott, pp. 67–86.

Crosier, P., and Clark, S. 1992. Basic biology of the hematopoietic growth factors. *Seminars in Oncology* 19: 349–361.

Dinarello, C., and Mier, J. 1987. Current concepts: Lymphokines. *New England Journal of Medicine* 317(15): 940–945.

Dutcher, J. 1992. Future directions in biologic therapy of cancer. *Hospital Formulary* 27: 694–707.

Ehrlich, P. 1910. *Studies in Immunity* 2nd ed. New York: Wiley.

Fischer, D., Knobf, M., and Durivage, H. 1993. *The Cancer Chemotherapy Handbook*, 4th ed. St. Louis: Mosby-Year Book, pp. 217–246.

Frei, E. and Spriggs, D. 1989. Tumor necrosis factor: Still a promising agent. *Journal of Clinical Oncology* 7(3): 291–294.

Gallucci, B. 1987. The immune system and cancer. *Oncology Nursing Forum* 14(6 Suppl): 3–7.

Herberman, R. 1985. Design of clinical trials with biological response modifiers. *Cancer Treatment Reports* 69: 1161–1164.

Hersh, E., Gutterman, J., and Mavligit, G. 1973. *Immunotherapy of Cancer in Man: Scientific Basis and Current Status*. Springfield, IL: Charles C. Thomas, Publisher.

Isaacs, A., and Lindenmann, J. 1957. Virus interference. I. The interferon. *Proceedings of the Royal Society of London* (series B): 259–267.

Johnson, J., and Temple R. 1985. Food and Drug Administration requirements for approval of anticancer drugs. *Cancer Treatment Reports* 69: 1155–1159.

Kirkwood, J., and Ernstoff, M. 1991. Interferons: Clinical applications—cutaneous melanoma. In DeVita, V., Hellman, S., and Rosenberg, S. (eds). *Biologic Therapy of Cancer*. Philadelphia: J.B. Lippincott, pp. 311–333.

Kurzrock, R., Talpaz, M., and Gutterman, J. 1991. Interferons: Clinical applications—other tumors. In DeVita, V., Hellman, S., and Rosenberg, S. (eds). *Biologic Therapy of Cancer*. Philadelphia: J.B. Lippincott, pp. 334–345.

Mihich, E. and Fefer, A. (eds.) 1983. *National Cancer Institute Monograph*, 63. U.S. Department of Health and Human Services, Public Health Service, National Institutes of Health: NIH Publication No. 83–2606, pp. 3–31.

Mitchell, M. 1992. Chemotherapy in combination with biomodulation: A 5-year experience with cyclophosphamide and interleukin–2. *Seminars in Oncology* 19(2): 80–87.

Morgan, D., Ruscetti, F., and Gallo, R. 1976. Selective in vitro growth of T lymphocytes from normal human bone marrow. *Science* 193: 1007–1008.

Oettgen, H., and Old, L. 1991. The history of cancer immunotherapy. In DeVita, V., Hellman, S., and Rosenberg, S. (eds). *Biologic Therapy of Cancer*. Philadelphia: W.B. Saunders, pp. 87–119.

Oldham, R. 1991. Biotherapy: General principles. In Oldham, R. (ed). *Principles of Cancer Biotherapy*. 2nd ed. New York: Marcel Dekker, pp. 1–22.

Oldham, R. 1985. Biologicals and biological response modifiers: Design of clinical trials. *Journal of Biological Response Modifiers* 4: 117–128.

Oldham, R. 1984. Biologicals and biological response modifiers: Fourth treatment modality of cancer treatment. *Cancer Treatment Reports* 68(1): 221–232.

Oldham, R. 1983. Biologicals: New horizons in pharmaceutical development. *Journal of Biological Response Modifiers* 2: 199–206.

Oldham, R., and Smalley R. 1983. Immunotherapy: The old and the new. *Journal of Biological Response Modifiers* 2: 1–37.

Pestka, S. 1983. The purification and manufacture of human interferons. *Scientific American* 249(2): 37–43.

Ramel, A., McGregor, W., and Dziewanowska, Z. 1983. Methods of preparation. In Sikora, K. (ed.). *Interferon and Cancer*. New York: Plenum Press, pp. 17–32.

Talpaz, M., Kurzrock, R., Kantarjian, H., *et al.*, 1991. Interferons: Clinical applications—chronic myelogenous leukemia and myeloproliferative disorders. In DeVita, V., Hellman, S., and Rosenberg, S. (eds). *Biologic Therapy of Cancer*. Philadelphia: J.B. Lippincott, pp. 289–297.

Tracey, K., Vlassara, H., and Cerami, A. 1989. Cachectin/tumor necrosis factor. *Lancet* 1:1122–1126.

Turner, S. 1992. Colony-stimulating factors: An understandable approach. *Pharmacy and Therapeutics* 17: 1423–1428.

CHAPTER 2 | The Immune System

Betty Bierut Gallucci, PHD

Donna McCarthy, PHD

Modern biotherapy has been in use for some 30 years. The first types of biotherapy were nonspecific stimulators of the immune response, but advances in genetic engineering are allowing the mass production of pure biological products which are now being tested as pharmaceutical agents. Biotherapy connotes the administration of products (1) that are coded by the mammalian genome; (2) that modify the expression of mammalian genes; or (3) that stimulate the immune system. In this chapter the discussion of the immune system will be limited primarily to topics relevant to cancer or autoimmune diseases.

Because understanding the new biological agents requires an understanding of both the immune response and the molecular basis of oncogenesis, this chapter first presents a summary of the structure and function of the immune system. Following a discussion of immune responses, and the cells involved in these responses, will be a discussion on the

current concepts of oncogenesis, particularly oncogenes and growth factors. Because research efforts are beginning to identify many biological proteins as having a role in autoimmune and other diseases, a brief introduction to autoimmune diseases is also included at the end of the chapter.

THE IMMUNE SYSTEM

Overview of the Immune Response

The immune system is a complex, dynamic system which evolved to protect the individual against pathogenic organisms (Figure 2.1). In addition to recognizing and destroying foreign substances or **antigens**, immune responses can also destroy altered and malignant cells. This latter function of the immune system is called **immune surveillance.** The destruction of microorganisms and the de-

Figure 2.1   The humoral branch and cell-mediated branches of the immune system. The humoral response involves interaction of B lymphocytes with antigen and their differentiation into antibody-secreting plasma cells. The secreted antibody binds to the antigen and facilitates its clearance from the body. The cell-mediated response involves various subpopulations of T lymphocytes that recognize antigen presented on self-cells. T_H-cells respond to antigen with the production of lymphokines and cytotoxic T lymphocytes (CTL) mediate killing of cells that have been altered by antigen *(e.g., virus-infected cells).*

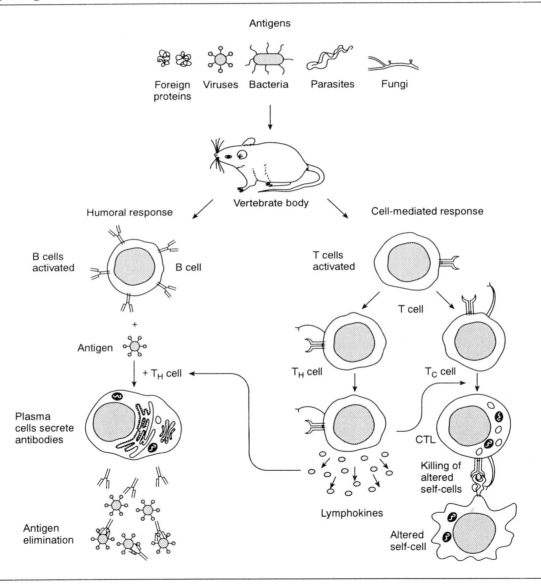

Table 2.1 Functions of the Immune System

Protection	Recognition and destruction of pathogenic microorganisms
Surveillance	Destruction of malignant cells
Homeostasis	Destruction of worn and damaged cells
Tolerance	Recognition of self components
Regulation	Augmentation and depression of immune responses

struction of tumor cells involve the same immunologic mechanisms. The mechanisms used to fight viral diseases are particularly important in immune responses to tumors. See Table 2.1 for a summary of functions of the immune system.

Immune responses involve a number of different cell types and their products. Because it is impossible to discuss or study all the responses at the same time, they are divided into two types, innate and adaptive. **Innate immunity** is also called natural or nonspecific immunity and includes the inflammatory response. **Adaptive immunity** is also known as specific or acquired immunity. For a review of innate and adaptive immune responses, see Table 2.2.

Innate immunity is the first line of defense against pathogenic organisms; adaptive immunity involves the recognition of specific foreign determinants and a memory response. To recognize and destroy what is foreign also implies that the immune system must be able to tolerate self, that is, to tolerate its own cells and their products. If the molecules on the microorganism or tumor cell are recognized as foreign (nonself or altered self) and stimulate a specific immune response, they are called antigens. The small area of the antigen that binds to the lymphocyte receptor is the **antigenic determinant** or **epitope.**

The cells and products of innate and adaptive immune responses act in concert and are all responsible for resistance to pathogens and surveillance. For instance, the first line of defense against pathogenic organisms (e.g. *Pseudomonas)* are mechanical barriers such as intact skin and mucous membranes. If these physical barriers are breached, an inflammatory response attempts to limit the colonization of the microbe. The acute inflammatory response involves the physiological processes of capillary dilatation, exudation of fluid and plasma protein into the tissues, and accumulation of neutrophils at the site of infection. These responses are manifested clinically as the five cardinal signs of inflammation: heat, redness, swelling, pain, and loss of function. The invading organism is then killed through **phagocytosis** by neutrophils or soluble chemical factors generated during the inflammatory response (Figure 2.2). The influx of neutrophils is replaced by monocytes, which continue to migrate to the inflamed area. The activation of monocytes is the bridge between innate and adaptive immunity. Monocytes are capable of processing the antigen they phagocytize and presenting it to other white blood cells involved in adaptive or specific immunity.

Thus, if this innate response fails and the organism colonizes the body, the adaptive immune system is stimulated and responds. The specific immune response on the next exposure to the same antigen will be heightened and more rapid. This secondary response is called **memory** or **anamnestic response.**

Generally speaking, the white blood cells are responsible for immune responses; granulocytes (neutrophils, eosinophils, and basophils), monocytes and their tissue counterparts macrophages are involved in innate immunity, whereas lymphocytes are responsible for specific immune responses. Lymphocytes have two different ways of recognizing antigenic determinants. The first is by antibodies located on the membrane of B lymphocytes and the second is by T-lymphocyte (or T-cell) receptors. For the T-cell receptors to recognize the antigenic determinants the antigen must be present along with self molecules or **major histocompatibility (MHC) molecules.** Typically, both the innate and adaptive systems (both B and T lymphocytes) are needed to effect a response sufficient to contain and eliminate pathogens.

Table 2.2 Features of innate and adaptive immunity

System	Hallmarks	Features and Functions

Innate Immunity	Primary line of defense
	Non-specific
	No memory
		Mechanical Barriers
		  Intact Skin
		    Mucous Membranes
		Chemical Barriers
		Inflammatory response
		Fever
		Phagocytic Cells
		Soluble Factors
		Protects against pathogens

Adaptive Immunity	Secondary line of defense
	Specificity
	Memory
		Lymphocytes
		  T-cells: Provide cell mediated
		  immunity
		Primarily protects against intracellular
		organisms, immune surveillance,
		responsible for rejection of transplanted
		organs and modulation of immune
		response
		  B-cells: Provide humoral immunity
		Primarily protects against viruses and
		bacteria

ANTIGENS

The major function of the immune system is to distinguish between self molecules and non-self or altered-self molecules. Molecules that induce a specific immune response are called **immunogens.** All immunogens are also antigens. Allergens are antigens that induce allergic responses. The epitope or antigenic determinant is that specific part of an antigen, allergen, or immunogen that binds directly with the immunoglobulin or T-cell receptor. For example, an antigenic protein may consist of hundreds of amino acids, but only six or seven of these bind directly with an immunoglobulin. The binding area of the antigen is the epitope. **Tolergens** are molecules that induce a state of immunologic unresponsiveness. Most times antigens are exogenous molecules such as bacterial or viral proteins. Rarely, immune responses are generated to self molecules, that is autoantigens or autologous antigens, resulting in serious pathologic states called autoimmune diseases. **Alloantigens** are endogenous molecules that

distinguish one individual from another individual of the same species. The A, B, and O blood-type molecules and the histocompatibility antigens are examples of alloantigens. A bone marrow transplant between siblings is called an allogeneic transplant.

The distinction between self molecules and foreign molecules is a learned response. Exposure of the immune system to molecules *in utero* will generate tolerance to these molecules: the immune system will not respond to these molecules, rather they will be considered self molecules (self antigens). The greater the difference between self molecules and exogenous or foreign molecules, the more likely it is that an immune response will be generated. Also, the greater the evolutionary divergence between two species, the greater the likelihood that an immune reaction will occur. In humans, for instance, an immune response to avian albumin is more likely than a response to primate albumin. There are, however, some proteins that are phylogenetically

Figure 2.2   The inflammatory response. A bacterial infection causes tissue damage with release of various vasoactive and chemotactic factors. These factors induce increased blood flow to the area, increased capillary permeability, and the influx of white blood cells, including phagocytes and lymphocytes, from the blood into the tissues. The serum proteins contained in the exudate have anti-bacterial properties and the phagocyte will begin to engulf the bacteria.

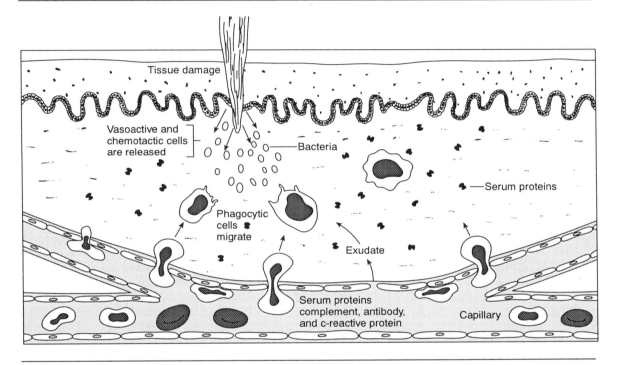

Source: IMMUNOLOGY by Janis Kuby. Copyright (c) 1992 by W.H. Freeman and Company. Reprinted with permission.

conserved, such as collagen; these proteins will not generate immune responses even if transplanted across species lines.

Besides the degree of foreignness, the size and the chemical nature of the molecules will determine if a specific immune response is generated. In general, proteins are more efficient immunogens than other compounds; complex carbohydrates are also good immunogens. Lipids and nucleic acids are poor immunogens unless they are bound to proteins. A complex molecule is likely to generate an immune response, whereas polymers composed of a single amino acid are unlikely to generate a response. The B and T lymphocytes

will recognize different epitopes on the same molecule. For the T cell to recognize a molecule as foreign, the molecule first must be phagocytized and processed, and then small segments of the molecule must be linked to MHC molecules on the surface of the accessory cell. Molecules that resist digestion by phagocytes are less likely to stimulate a T-helper cell response. If the T-helper response is limited, then neither a B-cell response nor a T-cell response is likely. The route by which the antigen is presented to the immune system and the dosage will affect the type and degree of immune responses. Antigens present in the mucosa are much more likely to generate immunoglobulin A or E than immunoglobulin G. A systemically administered antigen is likely to produce an immunoglobulin G response. If the antigen is administered in very high quantities or in very low quantities, the host may come to tolerate the antigen.

Mitogens are molecules that can induce nonspecific division and activation of lymphocytes; mitogens will also stimulate many clones of lymphocytes. This contrasts with the specific stimulation of a single lymphocyte clone by an antigenic epitope. Mitogens are used in laboratory situations to test the functional ability of lymphocytes. Some common mitogens used in testing of lymphocytes are phytohemagglutinin (PHA), concanavalin A (Con A), and pokeweed mitogen (PWM). Both PHA and Con A are proteins derived from plants and are T-cell mitogens; PWM stimulates both T and B cells. These protein mitogens are also known as **lectins.** Some bacterial toxins act like mitogens in that they nonspecifically stimulate multiple colonies of lymphocytes. **Super antigens** are very potent T-cell mitogens and stimulate T-helper cells, an example of a super antigen is the toxic shock syndrome toxin. This stimulation may lead to a massive release of cytokines and to shock and death. The lipopolysaccharide in bacterial endotoxin is another example of a super antigen.

CYTOKINES

Cytokines and lymphokines are discussed here because these molecules are a part of a network of mediators released in inflammatory and specific immune responses. These compounds are produced primarily by T cells, but they can be produced by other types of cells such as monocytes, or their mature counterpart, macrophages. The term *cytokine* describes a soluble protein produced by cells, and includes polypeptide molecules such as interleukins, lymphokines, monokines, interferons, tumor necrosis factor, and transforming growth factor. They are biologically very

active, have short half lives, and are functional at low concentrations. Cytokines bind to plasma membrane receptors; they affect the growth and differentiation of white blood cells, and regulate immune and inflammatory responses.

Cytokines act as signals between cells and can exert their effect in the same cell from which they were secreted, that is, in an **autocrine** action. Cytokines can affect cells in the immediate area, a **paracrine** action, or they can exhibit **endocrine** actions, that is, on distant cells. A cytokine can have different effects in different target cells, that is, they are **pleiotropic.** Cytokines can also act in concert: one cytokine may potentiate (or inhibit) the action of another cytokine. This effect is known as the **cytokine cascade.**

When a T-helper cell is activated by an antigen, for instance, the cell can secrete a variety of cytokines, which in turn activate B cells, NK cells, other T cells, macrophages, or stem cells. The target cells secrete the same cytokine or another cytokine which can either amplify or inhibit the immune response. Often more than one cytokine is needed for cellular activation, and the sequence of exposure to the cytokines may also be important. It is best to consider cytokines as a system or a network in which the cytokines can act in a **redundant, synergistic, antagonistic** or **pleiotropic** fashion. (See Figure 2.3.)

When cytokines were first studied, their chemical structures were not known, so functional assays were developed for each one. Each cytokine was studied and named by the action it produced. For instance, investigators who studied a substance that destroyed tumor cells named it tumor necrosis factor (or lymphotoxin). Other investigators who studied a substance that caused weight loss called it cachectin. When the chemical natures of these compounds were described, it was discovered that tumor necrosis factor, lymphotoxin, and cachectin were really the same compound. More than one name exists for many of the cytokines. In 1986 an international system was established to try to stan-

Figure 2.3   Examples of the cytokine attributes of pleiotropy, redundancy, synergism, and antagonism.

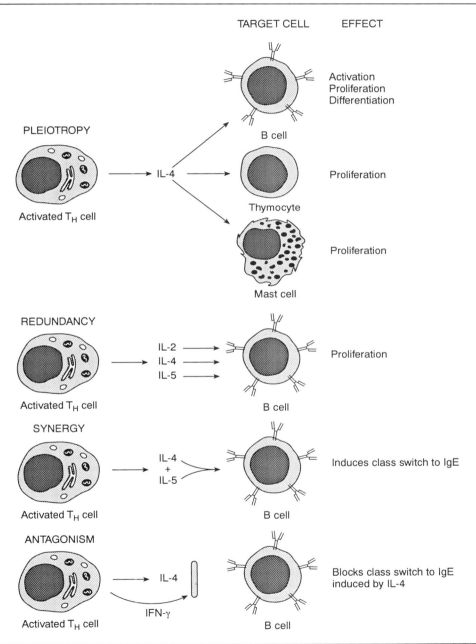

dardize the cytokine nomenclature. (See Chapter 5.) When the DNA sequence coding for a protein has been discovered, it is now given an interleukin designation. The term **interleukin** literally means "between white cells," however, some of these protein molecules are made by, or act on, cells other than white blood cells.

An example is interleukin–6 (See chapter 16). Previously it was called B-cell differentiation factor, B-cell stimulation factor, hepatocyte-stimulating factor and interferon–β2, depending on the assay used. Interleukin–6 stimulates T-cell proliferation and differentiation in addition to the production of IL–2 and IL–2 receptors by the T-cell. Interleukin–6 also stimulates plasma cells to secrete immunoglobulins and hepatocytes to secrete acute phase response proteins such as C reactive protein. Interleukin–6 is also important in hematopoiesis. It is produced not only by T-helper cells but also by macrophages and fibroblasts. Therefore, it acts in a pleiotropic, redundant, and synergistic fashion. Since it can also be manufactured by and influence cells other than white blood cells, the term cytokine may be better than interleukin.

Cytokines may also play a role in bidirectional communication between the neuroendocrine and immune systems. For example, interferon–α can increase the levels of circulating cortisol. Interleukin–2 infused in pharmacologic doses can cause fatigue and depression. Some of the cytokines induce fever by affecting the temperature-regulating center in the hypothalamus. Thus, cytokines may be important for integrating the immune response within the total person, not just within the immune system. Likewise, changes in the neuroendocrine system can heighten or diminish immune responses. Hormones such as cortisol and the sex hormones generally depress the immune responses, whereas growth hormone and thymosin enhance T-cell responses. This communication between systems is possible because there are receptors on the surfaces of lymphocytes and other white blood cells for hormones such as cortisol and epinephrine, while the nervous system has receptors for cytokines such as interferon–α and IL–2.

MAJOR HISTOCOMPATIBILITY COMPLEX

Regulation of immune responses occurs at many levels: by antigens, cytokines (between cells), and the neuroendocrine system. The ability to respond to an antigen is determined not only by the factors listed above but also by the genetic constitution of the individual. The part of the genome that we know the most about with respect to immune responses is called the **major histocompatibility complex (MHC)**. This area was first studied in relationship to transplantation of tissue. Because the first cells used for testing the compatibility of tissues between individuals were lymphocytes, in humans the MHC is called the **human leukocyte antigen (HLA) complex.** Here the term antigen is used, because lymphocytes from one person or donor, would be foreign to another person, or recipient, and would stimulate an immune response to the donor cells in the recipient. Much of the research done in this area has used rodent models. In the mouse, the MHC is called the H2 complex (H for histocompatibility and 2 for the second erythrocyte antigen of the mouse).

The MHC or HLA genes are located on chromosome 6 and code for molecules on the cell membrane needed for the presentation of the antigen to T lymphocytes. These genes also code for some soluble molecules, including those of the complement system and tumor necrosis factor. The MHC comprises about 40 to 50 genes and, although the functions of many are understood, others are not. The HLA is further divided into class I, II, and III regions; the genes code for class I, II, and III molecules. These MHC molecules are often referred to as MHC antigens.

Class I genes are located at the HLA-A, HLA-B, HLA-C, -E, -F and -G loci. The **locus** is the position on the chromosome where a gene is positioned. The HLA genes are located on the short arm of chromosome 6. The class I genes code for molecules that are present on most nucleated cells. For a cytotoxic T cell to recognize an antigen, the antigen must be complexed with a MHC class I molecule. Considering that a virus can infect any cell in the body and that the cytotoxic T cell is responsible for killing cells infected with viruses, it makes sense that class I molecules are ubiquitous. Class I molecules are absent in sperm and in trophoblasts. Some cells of the body, such as liver cells, fibroblasts, and neurons, express very low levels of these genes. Perhaps the reason for the success of liver transplantation and the acceptance of the fetal tissues as grafts is the low numbers of class I molecules on the membranes of these cells. Cytokines such as tumor necrosis factor and interferons can increase (up-regulate) the expression of these genes, increasing the numbers of class I molecules on the surfaces of these cells.

Class II molecules are found on cells of the immune system: **B lymphocytes,** antigen-presenting cells, accessory cells, **macrophages,** Langerhans cells, and dendritic cells. The major role of class II molecules involves the presentation of the antigen to T-helper cells. The antigen is first processed, then it binds to the class II molecule; it is this complex that binds to and stimulates the T-helper cell. The class II genes are located at the DO, DP, DQ, DR, DV, DX, and DZ loci. The class II genes are also known as the immune response genes and determine the level of response to an antigen. Certain animal strains that tend to respond quantitatively more to an antigen than other strains are called high responders. The existence of high and low responder strains is due to differences in the MHC class II genes. Because both class I and II molecules have some structural similarity to the immunoglobulin molecules, they are considered to belong to the immunoglobulin superfamily.

Class III genes code for some of the proteins involved in the complement pathway, tumor necrosis factor, and steroid hydroxylase enzymes. These molecules are soluble, diverse, and have no role in presentation of the antigen. The class III genes lie between the class II and class I genes on the chromosome.

Haplotypes

There are many variants or **alleles** of each of the MHC genes, allowing many variants in each of the class I and class II molecules. This leads to the great diversity seen in humans and accounts for the difficulties in transplantation among unrelated donors. The MHC genes are tightly linked. Usually, one copy of the entire MHC gene (a **haplotype)** is inherited as a unit from the mother and another copy is inherited from the father. Twenty-three different alleles are known for the HLA-A locus of MHC class I, 49 for the HLA-B locus, and eight for the HLA-C locus. If there are 50 genes in the MHC and there are many variants of these genes; it is easy to see why it is difficult to match for histocompatibility. Theoretically, the number of possible MHC genotypes in the human population would be the number of alleles for each gene multiplied by every other possibility, i.e. 23(A) × 49(B) × 8(C) and so on for the 50 genes. In actuality, the total number of possibilities is less than the theory predicts because certain of these genes are tightly linked to each other making their recombination with other genes highly unlikely. Certain haplotypes are found more frequently than would be expected, so that in isolated populations a greater frequency of certain alleles of the MHC will be found. Because of the tight linkage, there is one chance in four that siblings will share the same haplotypes. In an individual cell both the maternal and paternal genes are expressed, that is, the genes are codominant.

TISSUES AND CELLS OF THE IMMUNE SYSTEM
The Lymphoid System

The cells responsible for the immune response are organized into tissues and organs collectively known as the lymphoid system. Lymphoid tissue can be designated as primary or secondary. The primary organs include the bone marrow and the thymus, and are the sites where lymphocytes develop and mature. Secondary lymphoid organs include the lymph nodes, lymph vessels, spleen, tonsils, and unencapsulated lymphoid tissue lining the respiratory, alimentary and genito-urinary tract. Lymphocytes are stored and activated in the secondary organs. Lymph nodes are chains of encapsulated lymphoid tissue housing B- and T-lymphocytes. They are found throughout the body and are located primarily at the junctions of lymphatic vessels, a network that drains and filters tissue fluid. In sum, lymph nodes filter material draining from body tissues, the spleen filters antigens in the blood, and the unencapsulated lymph tissue monitor mucosal surfaces.

Cells of the Immune System

The white blood cells (granulocytes, monocytes, lymphocytes) responsible for immune responses are derived from bone marrow stem cells in children and adults and the yolk sack, spleen, and liver in the fetus. The stem cells are pluripotent, that is, capable of producing all the formed elements of the blood, including erythrocytes (red blood cells) and platelets. This process of differentiation or maturation is called **hematopoiesis.** Numerous growth and differentiation factors that support hematopoiesis have been identified. (See chapter 6.)

Many of the hematopoietic growth factors were identified by culturing bone marrow stem cells *in vitro*. Since each cluster of cells that grew in culture was derived from a single cell, these growth factors were called colony-stimulating factors. There are four main types of colony-stimulating factors: multilineage colony-stimulating factor, also called interleukin–3 (IL–3), granulocyte-macrophage colony-stimulating factor (GM-CSF), granulocyte colony-stimulating factor (G-CSF), and macrophage colony-stimulating factor (M-CSF). Other cytokines secreted by T-helper lympho-

cytes and macrophages that support hematopoiesis include such factors as interleukins–1, –4, –5, –7, –8, and –9 (IL–1, IL–4, IL–5, IL–7, IL–8 and IL–9). Different growth factors are necessary at different stages of maturation. Multilineage colony-stimulating factor is important early in the differentiation of the myeloid line of blood cells (erythrocytes, monocytes, and granulocytes), whereas G-CSF is important in a later stage of differentiation of the neutrophil line. (See Figure 2.4.)

Granulocytes

Neutrophils, or polymorphonuclear leukocytes, are important early in the inflammatory process and in acute infections. They are the most numerous of all the leukocytes, accounting for approximately 50% to 70% of circulating white blood cells. Neutrophils migrate from the blood stream into the tissue, where they phagocytize pathogens and cellular debris. The ability of these cells to recognize what is antigen (and should be destroyed) is poorly understood but is thought to involve the chemical structure of the antigen. For example, the cell wall of some bacteria contain complex polysaccharides that are not seen in the cell wall of humans. Antibodies, produced by B lymphocytes, may bind to the antigen and mark it for destruction by neutrophils or monocytes. Other circulating proteins known as opsonins may bind to the antigen, also marking it for phagocytosis by neutrophils or monocytes. Basophils contain granules, and have mediators such as histamine, which are important in allergic reactions. In tissues, cells similar to basophils are called mast cells. Eosinophils are phagocytes and play a role in immune responses to parasitic worms. They are present in small numbers in blood: they constitute about 1% to 3% of circulating white blood cells.

Monocytes and the Mononuclear Phagocyte System

Monocytes are large phagocytic cells that comprise approximately 3% to 7% of the circu-

Figure 2.4   Cells of the immune system.

Overview of the Immune System

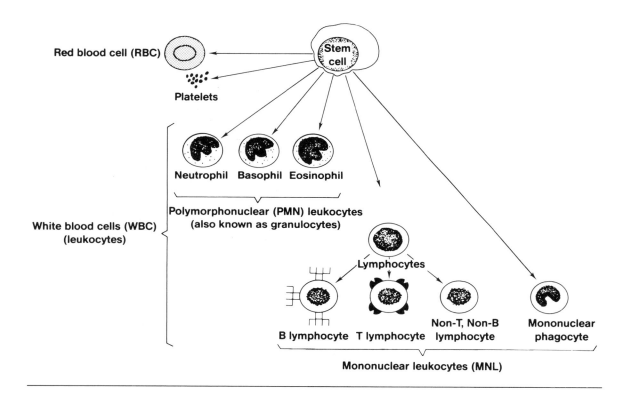

lating white blood cells. They are present late in the inflammatory process and in chronic infections. Tissue monocytes (also called macrophages), when present along with lymphocytes, are often designated as a monocytic infiltrate on **histologic examination.** Macrophages contain many granules and lysosomes and are very effective in removing cellular debris, which is why they are often called the "mop up troops." Many tissues contain resident macrophages, which are called different names in different tissues. For instance, macrophages in the liver are called Kupffer cells; in the skin, Langerhans cells; and in the brain, glial cells. This system of macrophages has been renamed the mononuclear phagocytic system; it was previously termed the reticuloendothelial system.

Macrophages are not only important in innate responses, but also they play a vital role in adaptive immune responses. Macrophages are often involved in the first stage of processing antigens and presenting them to lymphocyte populations. Foreign microorganisms are phagocytized by the macrophage and then digested in the **phagosomes.** Parts of the digested foreign molecule are further processed inside the cytoplasm; these eventually bind to the macrophage cell-surface proteins and are expressed on the cell surface. The antigen, in combination with these cell-surface proteins or class II MHC markers, are presented to the lymphocyte. The lymphocyte specific for that antigen then binds to the antigenic determinant and is activated. The cells responsible for processing antigens are also known as **antigen processing cells** or accessory cells. Macrophages can also bind antibodies on their cell surfaces, which will permit them to more readily phagocytize specific antigens. When the antigen and antibody bind, the macrophage is thus activated and becomes more efficient in destroying invading microorganisms.

Lymphocytes

Lymphocytes constitute about 20% to 40% of circulating white blood cells and are responsible for the recognition of antigens and induction of adaptive (specific) immune responses. Lymphocytes also reside in lymphatic tissues throughout the body, which include such structures as the tonsils, adenoids, lymph nodes, thymus, spleen, appendix, Peyer's patches, and bone marrow. The lymphatic tissue underlining the mucous membranes, MALT (mucosa-associated lymphatic tissue), BALT (bronchus-associated lymphatic tissue), and GALT (gut-associated lymphatic tissue), is not **encapsulated**, nor is it as well organized as that of the lymph nodes. In the mucosa, these loose clusters of lymphocytes can interact with antigens at the lumenal surface and prevent antigens from gaining access to the systemic circulation.

Lymphocytes recirculate throughout the body by leaving the vasculature or lymphatic tissue and infiltrating tissues. They then re-enter the circulation via lymphatic vessels and once again take up residence in the lymphatic tissue. Lymphocytes possess adhesion and homing receptors on their surfaces, which permit them to bind to the vascular endothelial cells in general and endothelial cells in specific tissues. The venule endothelial cells possess vascular adhesion molecules which in turn bind with the lymphocyte homing recep-

tors. This recirculation of lymphocytes ensures that antigens come in contact with responsive lymphocytes. It is thought that only 1 in 1,000 to 1 in 100,000 lymphocytes have the ability to respond to a specific antigen.

Although all lymphocytes look similar in a routine blood smear, there are subpopulations. The current method to distinguish cell populations and subpopulations is by staining cell surface molecules with monoclonal antibodies linked to fluorescent dyes. Monoclonal antibodies are highly specific antibodies produced from a single clone of cells. (See Chapter 7.) These surface molecules are called **cluster of differentiation (CD) antigens** (or **CD markers**). The monoclonal antibodies that are attached to the cell markers and the markers themselves have been assigned CD numbers by an international workshop. Of the three major populations of lymphocytes, T lymphocytes, B lymphocytes, and natural killer (NK) cells, T and B lymphocytes are responsible for specific immune responses and natural killer cells are involved in innate immune reactions to viruses and tumors cells. Although CD5 is a marker for both T and B cells, CD1, CD3, and CD7 are markers only for T cells; CD21, CD22, CD37, and CD40 are a few of the antigens associated with B cells. CD56 is a marker for NK cells. In many cases the function of the cell surface molecule is known. For instance CD21 on B cells is a receptor for a complement molecule and is also the Epstein-Barr virus receptor.

B Lymphocytes   In humans, the stem cells for B lymphocytes are located in the bone marrow. In the bird, however, B cells mature in a lymphoid organ called the bursa of Fabricius, which is similar in structure to the human appendix. Since it was in the bird that the function of B cells was first determined, now all lymphocytes that secrete antibodies are called B cells. The molecules on the surface of B cells that are responsible for binding antigen are called membrane-bound immunoglobulins (Ig). On the surface of any one B cell, all the immunoglobulin receptors are identical in structure and thus bind to only one particular antigen. The most mature form of the B lymphocyte is the **plasma cell**, whose function is to secrete immunoglobulins (i.e., antibodies). All the daughter cells derived from a single B cell will produce the same antibody, therefore the name **monoclonal antibody** is given to the immunoglobulin secreted from a particular clone of B cells. Antibodies or immunoglobulins are found in the plasma, the fluid portion of blood; therefore the historical name associated with the specific immunity produced by B cells is **humoral immunity.** Other names associated with B cell immunity are antibody-mediated immunity and immediate hypersensitivity reactions. (See Figure 2.5).

The B lymphocytes constitute approximately 5% to 15% of circulating lymphocytes; plasma cells, however, do not circulate but remain fixed in the lymphoid tissue. Collections of B cells in lymphoid tissue stain intensely. These collections of B cells are called primary and secondary follicles (or germinal centers). Because B cells predominate, the collections are also called T-independent areas in the lymph nodes. Small amounts of T cells and macrophages are present even in the T-independent areas. Many B cells require the presence of T cells and accessory cells to manufacture antibodies.

T Lymphocytes T lymphocytes are derived from a population of lymphocytes that mature in the thymus. Lymphocyte stem cells migrate from the bone marrow to the thymus in the fetus and in childhood. In the thymus, lymphocyte populations that will react to self molecules (or self antigens) are eliminated and the other T cells differentiate. As the T cells mature, they leave the thymus and migrate to the lymphatic tissue, populating the areas surrounding the germinal centers, paracortical areas. The T lymphocytes constitute about 70% to 80% of circulating lymphocytes. They are responsible for immune reactions such as graft rejection, **graft-versus-host disease**, contact skin sensitivity, and delayed hypersensitivity reactions.

Much of what we know about the T cells was discovered in the nude (hairless) mouse. Because these mice are born without a thymus, they are unable to reject transplanted tissue even if the tissue is from another species. **Nude mice** are often used as incubators of human tumor cell lines because they are unable to reject the foreign tissue. The T lymphocytes are also important regulators of immune responses. As with all physiological responses, regulation of the immune response is necessary to either stimulate or inhibit the reactions.

Like B cells, T cells can recognize and bind to specific antigens. It is the T-cell receptor that binds the antigen. There are two types of T-cell receptors, TCR1 and TCR2; and a particular T cell possesses only one of these types. In the T-cell membrane, the T-cell receptor is linked to a molecule called CD3. The T cell can recognize a foreign antigen only if it is linked to a self molecule (also known as MHC antigens) on the surface of another cell. The T-cell immune responses are particularly effective in eliminating intracellular pathogens, for instance, cells that are infected with a virus and express viral antigens on their cell surfaces. This is in contrast to the immunoglobulins, which can bind to soluble antigens and help eliminate extracellular microorganisms.

The T-lymphocyte population can be further divided into several subpopulations that can be distinguished by the CD4 and CD8 markers. The T4 cells (which express CD4 markers) are called **helper/inducer T-cells.** For the T-helper cells to recognize an antigen, the antigen must be present on another cell that has MHC class II molecules. Thus, T-helper lymphocytes are called class II–restricted cells. These cells secrete cytokines called **lymphokines**, some of which stimulate the growth and differentiation of B lymphocytes and others of which activate macrophages. The T-helper lymphocytes also induce the generation of cytotoxic T lymphocytes. It

Figure 2.5   Differentiation and maturation of T lymphocytes and B lymphocytes. T cells develop in the thymus from cells that originate in the bone marrow. Mature T cells interact with antigen in peripheral tissues and then divide and differentiate into effector T cells. B cells develop in the bone marrow in humans and when mature migrate to peripheral tissues. When stimulated with antigen, they differentiate into antibody-secreting plasma cells and memory cells.

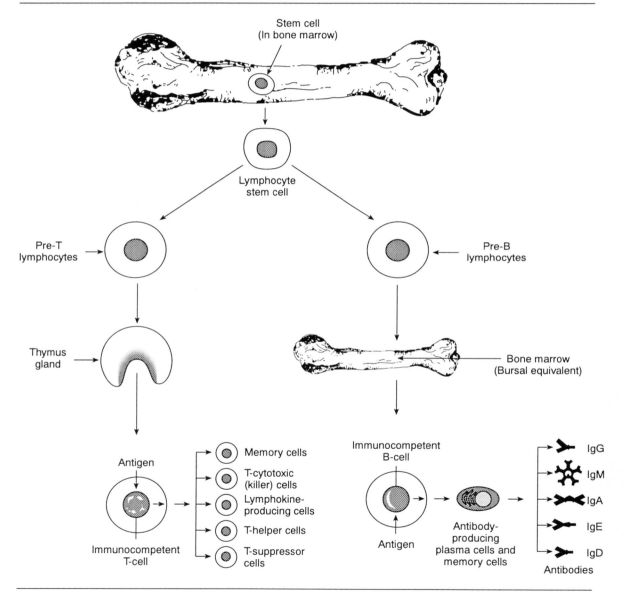

should be noted that the human immunodeficiency virus (HIV) appears to bind to the CD4 molecule on T-helper lymphocytes. The selective infection, and ultimate demise of T-helper lymphocytes, explains the amazing severity with which the HIV virus disables the immune system.

The **cytotoxic T cells**, on the other hand, express CD8 markers and can recognize only antigens associated with MHC class I molecules, that is, they are MHC class I–restricted. Cytotoxic T cells can recognize and bind to cells with altered self antigens or viral antigens bound to MHC class I molecules. They release a variety of mediators that cause the altered cell to lyse, or kill, the target cell. The **suppressor T-cells** also have the CD8 markers on their surfaces. They inhibit, or down-regulate, both T and B cell immune reactions and are responsible for tolerance to self. Various monoclonal antibodies are now being developed that would distinguish the cytotoxic T from the T-suppressor subsets and the helper-inducer from the suppressor-inducer subsets. Both helper and suppressor T lymphocytes are necessary for maintaining an appropriate level of immune responsiveness. (See Figure 2.5.)

Other Lymphocytes   Other lymphocytes that are neither B or T lymphocytes include null, natural killer, killer, lymphokine activated killer (LAK), and tumor infiltrating lymphocytes (TIL) cells. **Null cells** are lymphocytes that lack both T and B cell markers; whereas the NK cells and other killer cells carry some T-cell markers or both T-cell and macrophage markers. At one time it was believed that null, NK, and other killer cells were separate and distinct lymphocyte lineages. We now know, however, that as lymphocytes differentiate or become activated, they lose certain markers and gain others. Thus, some subsets may be simply more mature (differentiated) forms of the same line of lymphocytes. Although the exact lineage has not been worked out for all the subsets of lymphocytes, they can be distinguished from each other by their functional properties and cytoplasmic characteristics.

Natural killer cells are large lymphocytes that possess membrane-bound granules that contain **hydrolytic enzymes.** They constitute about 15% of the circulating lymphocytes. These large granular lymphocytes can in culture spontaneously destroy malignant cell lines. Functionally, NK cells can recognize and destroy tumor cells without having prior exposure and are not MHC restricted. Natural killer cells can destroy tumor cells by direct contact and release of perforins, molecules that form doughnut-shaped pores in the target cell membrane. The other process by which killer cells destroy target cells is by **antibody-dependent cell-mediated cytotoxicity (ADCC).** In the process, killer cells bind antibodies to their surfaces. When these antibodies bind to the tumor cell antigens, cytotoxic enzymes are released, resulting in tumor cell destruction. In laboratory studies, NK cells have potent antitumor activity early in tumor development and prevent the metastatic spread of tumors.

Recent biotherapy clinical trials have identified two other subsets of lymphocytes. When lymphocytes are incubated with large concentrations of the lymphokine interleukin–2 (IL–2), they are able to lyse tumor cell lines and fresh tumor cells. These **lymphokine activated killer (LAK) cells** are able to destroy tumor cells more efficiently than normal lymphocytes. **Tumor-infiltrating lymphocytes (TIL)**, are isolated from excised tumors. These lymphocytes, when grown in culture with lower concentrates of IL–2 than LAK cells, appear to be more specific for killing tumor cells derived from the host. Natural killer, LAK, and TIL cells may all be related to each other and derived from the same lymphocyte cell line. Only future studies will determine this. See Table 2.3 for a summary of immune cell functions.

SPECIFIC IMMUNE RESPONSES

The type and the strength of an immune response is dependent on the properties of the

Table 2.3   Immune system cells and their functions

Innate Immunity	
Neutrophils	Phagocytosis; present in acute infections
Basophils	Release of local mediators (histamine); allergic reactions
Eosinophils	Present in allergic reactions
Monocytes	Phagocytosis; present in chronic infections
Natural Killer Cells	Natural immunity to viruses and tumors; expansion of T-cell responses
Adaptive Immunity	
Lymphocytes	
B lymphocytes	Membrane bound Ig binds to antigen
Plasma Cells	Most mature form of B cell, produces Ig
Memory Cell	Responsible for memory effect
T lymphocytes	Membrane bound receptors bind to antigen
T helper	Initiation of immune response, secretion of lymphokines, assist B cell production of antibody
T cytotoxic	Kills cells by lysis
T suppressor	Decreases the immune response of other T- or B-cells
T memory	Responsible for memory effect

antigen, which lymphocyte populations are activated, and the genetic and hormonal characteristics of the individual. The way the antigen is recognized will determine which types of immune responses occur. Each individual produces both B-cell and T-cell responses as well as the innate immune responses to an antigen. In fact, all these responses are interlinked; all are constituents of an integrated defense system. The responses to a microorganism colonizing the host can not always be predicted, however; even the simplest of microbes are very complex and have many molecules that can activate immune cells. Nor is there any guarantee that the immune responses will be beneficial. Indeed, if one type of immune response prevents another more effective response, then the effect is detrimental.

B-Cell Responses

Activation of B Lymphocytes

Resting B lymphocytes are in the G_0 (resting) phase of the cell cycle. When a lymphocyte is activated, it enters the cell cycle and moves through the G_1, S, G_2, and division phases. In the S phase of the cell cycle, DNA is synthesized, whereas in the G (gap) phases, no DNA

is synthesized but RNA, proteins, and other compounds are synthesized. Cytokines act in concert at each of these phases to drive the cell along its cycle, which ends with mitosis or cell division.

The B lymphocytes have on their cell surfaces immunoglobulins that act as receptors for the antigen. The binding of the antigen is a random process. If an antigen binds tightly (fits) with the immunoglobulin receptor, then the activation process starts. The B cell internalizes the antigen and presents it along with a class II MHC molecule to the T cell. The T and B lymphocytes then form a tight bond with each other, a T-B conjugate. The activated T cell secretes cytokines such as IL–2. Thus, the process of B-cell activation requires (1) membrane changes that induce secondary changes within the cytoplasm and nucleus and (2) the presence of cytokines such as IL–1 and IL–4, in the early and IL–2, IL–4, and IL–5 in the later differentiation events. When a B lymphocyte becomes fully differentiated, the antibody is no longer present on the cell surface acting as a receptor but is in the cytoplasm of a plasma cell that is producing large quantities of a specific antibody. (See Figure 2.6.) The process of clonal selection of responding B cells is the basis of the memory response to that antigen.

Figure 2.6   Activation of B cells to produce antibody. Receptors on the surface of B cells bind matching antigen which is then engulfed and processed by the B cell. A piece of the antigen, bound to a class II protein, is then presented on the surface of the B cell. This complex binds to a mature helper T cell, which releases interleukins that transform B cells into antibody-secreting plasma cells. When released into the bloodstream, antibodies lock onto matching antigens and are eliminated by the complement cascade or by the liver and the spleen.

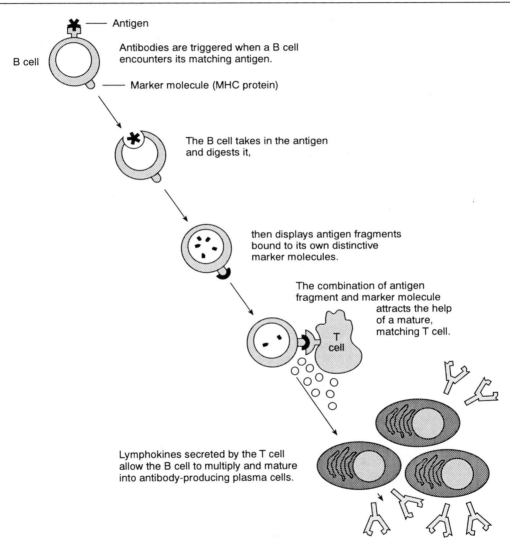

Source: Schindler, L. 1992. *Understanding the Immune System.* NIH pub. no. 90–3229. Bethesda, MD: U.S. Department of Health and Human Services, June 1992, p. 12.

Immunoglobulins

Antibodies are proteins whose function it is to bind the antigen, causing the antigen to lyse, precipitate out, or be more easily phagocytized. The antigen-antibody complex can activate the complement system, or prevent viruses from reacting with receptor sites on cells. When the chemical nature of these proteins are referred to, they are called immunoglobulins. The five main classes of immunoglobulins are IgG, IgM, IgA, IgD, and IgE.

Immunoglobulins are composed of four polypeptide chains. Two of the chains are called the heavy chains and two are called the light chains. This unit of four is also called a monomer. Greek letters have been assigned to the various chains. The light chains are either kappa (κ) or lambda (λ) no matter what the class of the immunoglobulin. The heavy chains take their name from the immunoglobulin class. The heavy chains for IgG, for instance, are called gamma (γ), for IgA, alpha (α), for IgM, mu (μ). Immunoglobulins are bifunctional proteins in that one end of the molecule structure comprises a highly variable region, that is, the amino acid sequence differs greatly from one antibody to another. This is the region which binds to or is complementary to the antigen. The other end of the molecule can bind to membrane receptors and is known as the constant region, or Fc fragment. Macrophages, killer cells, mast cells, and placental cells all have Fc receptors that can bind to immunoglobulins. The fragment that binds to the antigen is composed of one end of the heavy chain and the light chain. The Fc fragment consists of the other end of the heavy chain. Since each monomer of an immunoglobulin has two heavy and two light chains, an immunoglobulin can bind two antigenic sites.

Of all the immunoglobulin classes, IgG is present in the highest concentration in the plasma and is responsible for most specific antibody reactions in the adult. It is the principal antibody secreted in the secondary response and is the antibody passed from the maternal blood to the fetus that is responsible for protection of the fetus and newborn. Two of the four subclasses of IgG are able to activate complement. Also, macrophages and neutrophils have receptors on their cell surfaces that can bind to IgG.

The antibody IgM is formed first. It is the first class of immunoglobulins to be formed in the fetus and the first in primary infections. It is a large molecule, a pentamer, composed of five monomer units, that is very efficient in agglutinating particles such as viruses. Present in mucosal secretions, breast milk, and saliva, IgA helps prevent antigens from gaining access to the systemic circulation. It is the second most abundant immunoglobulin in the serum (10% to 15%). A fourth immunoglobulin, IgE, is present in allergic reactions such as asthma and hay fever and in parasitic infections, and is also known as reaginic antibody. It is present in minute amounts in the plasma, but in the tissues is bound to the surface of mast cells. Not much is known about IgD. It is present in small amounts in the circulation and is involved in the regulation of immunoglobulin synthesis.

Primary and Secondary Responses

The responses of the immune system are different the first time an antigen is encountered from those of second or subsequent times. The first or primary response takes a longer time to develop and is not as specific nor as sustained as the responses to secondary encounters. Whereas in a primary response IgM is formed first and IgG later, in the secondary response IgG titers are much higher than those generated in the primary response, and they are sustained for a longer period of time (Figure 2.7). That is why vaccinations to a particular microorganism are given several times, to generate clones of lymphocytes that can respond more quickly to the presence of an antigen.

Complement

The complement system is a series of about 20 plasma proteins that acts as a bridge between the specific antibody response and the non-

Figure 2.7 Primary and secondary immune responses. Secondary immune responses are distinguished from primary ones by the decrease in the latent period, greater specific and more sustained response.

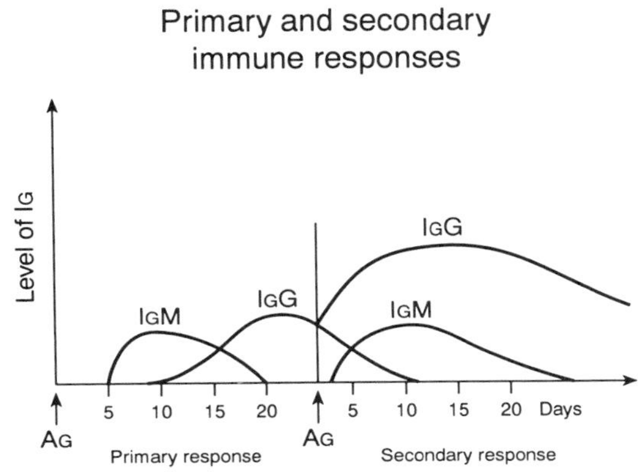

Primary and secondary immune responses

Source: Reprinted with permission from: Gallucci, B. 1987. The immune system and cancer. *Oncology Nursing Forum* 14(6 Suppl): 3–12.

specific inflammatory response. Complement acts to magnify and expand the specific antibody response. The complement proteins circulate as proenzymes or inactive enzymes. When the complement cascade is triggered, often by an antibody-antigen complex, the proteins become active in a series of enzymatic reactions that resemble the blood clotting cascade. The end product of both the classical and the alternative complement pathways is the membrane attack complex. This complex inserts a doughnut-shaped channel into the membrane, which allows lysis of the cell on which the antibody-antigen complex was attached.

When the inactive complement proteins are activated, small polypeptides are released. These small ''split products'' are nonspecific activators of inflammation and act as chemotactic agents, attracting white blood cells to the area; opsonins, enhancing phagocytosis of the antigen; and anaphylactoid agents, inducing the release of histamine, and increasing capillary permeability, which causes edema. These functions are vital to the clearance of microorganisms from the host. Individuals who have a congenital deficiency of one of the complement proteins are at higher-than-normal risk of chronic infections or autoimmune diseases.

T-Cell Responses

The T cell is responsible for cell-mediated immunity, i.e., immunity carried out by cells. This type of immunity protects the body against intracellular organisms such as viruses and parasites, and malignant cells. T cells are also responsible for immunoregulation through secretion of lymphokines. These responses can be broadly divided into two types, the cytotoxic response and the T-helper response.

T-Helper Cell Responses

The T-helper (CD4) cell is the primary cell responsible for initiation of a specific immune response. Moving a T cell from its resting phase requires the binding of the T-cell receptor with a processed antigen, which is in turn bound to a MHC complex; it also requires the presence of various cytokines such as IL–1. Interleukin–1 produced by accessory cells such as macrophages, causes, along with antigen-MHC stimulation, a change in the plasma membrane and then an activation of IL–2 and the IL–2 receptor genes. This production and secretion of IL–2 and its binding to the IL–2 cell-membrane receptor drives the T cell through to the S phase of the cell cycle. The end result is a differentiated T cell that can produce lymphokines which mediate T-cell immunity, and activate cytotoxic T cells, whose function is to directly lyse cells. The T-helper cell is a major producer of lymphokines.

The T-helper response generates a delayed hypersensitivity reaction, the prototype of which is the positive **PPD** reaction. The results of the PPD test are read after 36 to 72 hours, a delayed response that contrasts with

Figure 2.8   Activation of T cells. After a macrophage internalizes and processes antigen, it presents antigen fragments on its surface in conjunction with class II proteins to the helper T cell. Cytokines secreted by the macrophage help the T cell to mature. The activated T cell then secretes additional lymphokines that attract other immune cells to the area, activate cytotoxic T cells, and cause the growth of more T helper cells.

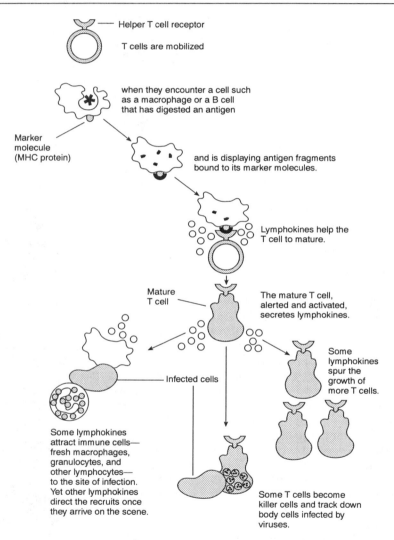

Source: Schindler, L. 1992. *Understanding the Immune System.* NIH pub. no. 90–3229. Bethesda, MD: U.S. Department of Health and Human Services, June 1992, p. 13.)

the B-cell or immediate hypersensitivity response. A typical immediate hypersensitivity response is a penicillin reaction. The T-cell responses control intracellular pathogens such as *Mycobacteria*, fungi, and viruses, and eliminate altered and malignant cells. Graft rejection and graft-versus-host disease are also T-cell responses.

Cytotoxic T-Cell Responses

The cytotoxic T-cell response requires direct physical contact between the cytotoxic T cell (CD8 lymphocyte) and the target cell (Figure 2.8). Generally, the CD8 cells are MHC class I restricted, meaning that the target cells must have MHC class I antigens expressed on their surfaces. Since almost every cell in the body expresses MHC class I antigens, almost every cell can be killed by cytotoxic T cells.

Before directed cell killing begins, specific T-helper cells are stimulated by the antigen. This expanded pool of T-helper cells then produces IL–2. It is in response to both this IL–2 and the antigen presented with the MHC class I molecule that the resting cytotoxic T cell is stimulated to proliferate and differentiate. The killing of the target cell is the result of a series of steps, starting with the joining or conjugation of the cytotoxic T cell and the target cell. Conjugation is dependent on the binding of the T-cell receptor–CD3 complex with the antigen-MHC class I complex on the target cell. A series of membrane changes occur in the cytotoxic T cell generating a signal in the protoplasm. Orientation of the Golgi complexes and granules in the cytotoxic T cell toward the target cell occurs next, then the contents of the granules are released in the space between the cytotoxic T cell and the target cell. The cytotoxic T cell migrates away and is ready to start the cycle again; shortly after, the target cell lyses. Any one cytotoxic T cell can kill multiple target cells and yet not be harmed itself. The target cell is lysed when pores or channels form in the target cell membrane in a manner reminiscent of complement lysis. However, the proteins required for each type of reaction are different molecules.

TUMOR IMMUNOLOGY

The first experimental system used to study tumor biology was the transplantation of tumors between animals. When this work was started in the late-1800s, inbred strains of animals were unknown, thus, what the scientists were really studying was allogeneic transplantation and responses to antigens. Around the same time, Dr. Coley (see Chapter 1) observed tumor regression in a few patients who had serious infections. He devised a vaccine that would simulate a serious infection and tested it in 1200 patients; 270 of these had complete regression of tumor. Now we know that responses to infections, tumors, and transplantation are all related and that insights into the mechanisms of one are relevant to the other two. The other side of understanding immune responses to infections and transplantation is understanding tolerance to self molecules, an area of study that has helped in discovering the way tumors can evade recognition and destruction by the immune system.

Immune Surveillance and Tumor Antigens

In the 1950s, knowledge of the body's reaction to tumors was synthesized by Mac-Farlane Burnett into a theory of a process termed **immune surveillance**. Expressed in somewhat popular terms, the theory states that (1) all individuals form tumor cells; (2) not everyone develops a malignancy; and (3) it is the immune system that prevents the development of tumors. As stated, the theory can not be directly tested because it is almost impossible to prove the negative, an absence of tumors. However, worded differently, this theory implies that tumors have antigens that under appropriate circumstances can be identified by the immune system. In animal models, the tumor antigens are called tumor transplantation antigens, reflecting the design of the experiments to test these ideas. One way to study tumor rejection and tumor-associated transplantation antigens is to inject nonviable tumor cells (obtained from another animal of the same inbred line) into an animal as a vaccine. When the animal is later challenged with live tumor cells, it is able to reject the tumor. A control animal without prior exposure to the tumor cell vaccine is unable to reject the live tumor cells and develops a malignancy.

Because transplantation experiments with live tumor cells are not feasible in humans, tumor antigens are termed **tumor-associated antigens** or **oncofetal antigens**. Very few antigens in humans are associated exclusively with malignancy. Most antigens are also present in other pathologic states or in the fetus. Two tumor-associated antigens that are useful clinically are alpha fetoprotein (AFP) and carcinoembryonic antigen (CEA). Carcinoembryonic antigen is expressed in gastrointestinal and breast cancers, AFP in hepatocellular and testicular cancers. Alpha fetoprotein has been used in a few screening programs for the detection of hepatocellular tumors, but these two antigens are more frequently used as indicators of disease progression. Following surgery for the cancers mentioned above, the plasma concentration of the oncofetal antigen usually drops dramatically. If disease recurs, the levels rise once again. A rise in CEA levels might be the first indicator of relapse. However, CEA levels rise in only 60% to 94% of patients, so a negative CEA report does not guarantee an absence of metastases.

Although tumor antigens have been discovered, not all experimentally induced tumors produce antigens recognized by the immune system and some evoke only a "weak" immune response. This is also true of tumors that arise spontaneously, in animals as well as in humans. On the surface of any tumor cell, however, there are many surface marker molecules, such as differentiation antigens, tissue-specific antigens, and receptors, some of which may be exploited for identifying, classifying, and treating the malignancy. Tumor-infiltrating lymphocytes can recognize some tumor-associated antigens.

In the clinic, tumor antigens are detected by monoclonal antibodies to these antigens. As noted above, these monoclonal antibodies can be used in screening and determining tumor progression. They can also be linked to special stains and used in the diagnosis of the tumor type and subtype. For instance, the CD10 antigen, also known as the common acute lymphoblastic leukemia antigen (CALLA), appears in the leukemic cells of approximately 70% of children diagnosed with acute lymphocytic leukemia. This antigen is also seen in Burkitt's and follicular lymphomas. Tumor antigens can also be used to determine the T- or B-cell lineage and the differentiation state of leukemias. Cells positive for CALLA are of the B-cell lineage. Monoclonal antibodies to surface antigens are used to determine the tissue of origin in undifferentiated or poorly differentiated tumors. Monoclonal antibodies can help distinguish tumors of epithelial and connective tissue origins. In clinical trials, monoclonal antibodies are now being linked with radioactive compounds, traditional chemotherapeutic agents, or toxins to determine their utility either in imaging or as therapy. (See Chapter 7.)

Oncogenes, Tumor-Suppressor Genes, and Tumor Antigens

Cancer is a disease of cell growth and division; underlying this abnormal cellular state are genetic changes. The genetic changes that arise in carcinogenesis include point mutation (the change of one nucleotide base in the gene); gene amplification, alterations in the gene control mechanisms; chromosomal deletions and insertions; and chromosomal abnormalities. As the tumor progresses, more and more genetic changes accumulate. One of the main functions of the gene is to code for proteins. Therefore, if carcinogenesis is initiated with a genetic change and that change results in an altered protein, then that protein could be recognized, allowing diagnosis, and become a target for chemotherapy or biological agents.

The genes that have been associated with carcinogenesis are called **oncogenes**. Oncogenes were first recognized in experimental virology, where it was observed that viral genes could transform cells in culture. When these genes were placed into cell cultures, they caused the **phenotype** of the cell to change and take on the appearance of a tumor cell. Since the cells were in a culture, the process was called **transformation** rather than carcinogenesis. It was then discovered that viral oncogenes had a normal cell equivalent, called **proto-oncogenes**. If these genes were first recognized for their normal function, perhaps then they would be called growth, division, and repair genes instead of oncogenes. These genes are responsible for controlling the highly regulated processes of the cell cycle, that is, the sequencing and coordination of the cell through the G_0, G_1, S, G_2, and mitosis phases. The initiating event in cell growth and division is termed a signal. The signal, which might be a growth factor, hormone, cytokine, or antigens, initiates a complex series of actions at the surface membrane and in the cytoplasm and nucleus. Proto-oncogenes are involved in coding for the proteins that act as growth factors, growth factor receptors, and signaling complexes at the membrane; second messengers in the cytoplasm; and regulators of gene expression.

The existence of tumor-suppressor genes or recessive oncogenes was first hypothesized from epidemiologic data. Knudson developed a mathematical model to explain the difference in age of onset of unilateral and bilateral retinoblastoma. He suggested that individuals with familial disease with increased risk for bilateral disease were born with one defective gene of the pair of maternal and paternal genes that control retinoblastoma. (Most genes in the body, except those on the X and Y chromosomes in males, occur as pairs.) The mutation of one allele of the pair of genes occurs earlier in life in patients with familial disease than in those with unilateral disease. Unilateral disease occurs later in life than bilateral disease and requires that mutations oc-cur in both the maternal and paternal genes; since the presence of at least one functioning gene inhibits the growth of the tumor. Great progress has been made in identifying the tumor-suppressor genes in retinoblastoma, Wilms' tumor, von Recklinghausen's neurofibromatosis, familial adenomatous polyposis, and colorectal carcinomas. These genes have a variety of actions, including suppression of cellular transcription factors, DNA replication, and gene transcription.

Clearly, regulation of normal growth and division is complex and under tight control. This complexity in itself may lead to multiple metabolic errors. There are, however, normal cellular mechanisms that limit or correct for these errors. Oncogene products, growth factors, and growth factor receptors are all linked in this complex regulatory system. In malignant diseases, some of the oncogenes are structurally different from their proto-oncogene counterparts. Other oncogenes are expressed in higher amounts in cancer cells than in normal cells, and tumor-suppressor genes may be entirely lacking in the tumor cells. In the future, the protein products of oncogenes might be targets of immunotherapies such as antibodies directed to growth factor receptor produced by an oncogene; the manufacture of suppressor gene products may lead to the development of new biological agents. (See Chapter 16.)

Immune Responses to Tumors

There is some evidence that almost every immune response that has been identified, including cellular and antibody-mediated immunity, is also generated as a response to tumor cells. Probably the most protective responses to tumors are cellular responses, which are similar to those generated against viruses. The important cells in these reactions are cytotoxic T cells, macrophages, NK cells, and antibody-dependent cytotoxic cells. Since the biology of the tumor changes with tumor progression, it may be that the relative importance of one type of immune response differs at the various tumor stages.

Some lines of evidence for an immune response to tumors come from the study of histopathology. To establish a diagnosis of cancer in humans, biopsied tissue is sent to the pathology laboratory, where it is stained and examined. Some tumors have marked infiltrates, often called a mononuclear infiltrate (lymphocytes and macrophages), which suggests that the tumor has stimulated an immune response in the individual. In some instances (medullary carcinoma of the breast, for example) the presence of a mononuclear infiltrate means a more favorable prognosis for the patient. Other clinical signs that have suggested an immune response to tumors is the waxing and waning of tumors. In such cancers as melanomas, the lesions are visible. Some of the lesions will disappear from one area and other tumor deposits will appear simultaneously at distant sites. It has been suggested that the reason for tumor fluctuations is that the immune responses were able to eliminate the tumor from one small area but not to control the progression of the disease in other areas. Spontaneous regression of a diagnosed malignancy is an extremely rare event, but there have been reports of regression in carcinoma of the kidney, neuroblastoma, choriocarcinoma, and melanoma. Again, immune mechanisms appeared to offer the best explanation for the regression. Although clinical evidence suggests the existence of immune responses to tumors, it does not constitute definitive proof. Animal experiments provide further evidence for immune responsiveness to tumors; the development of a cancer-preventing vaccine would be a definitive proof of the theory of immune surveillance.

Cell-Mediated Cytotoxicity

Cytotoxic T cells can recognize and destroy malignant cells by the same mechanisms they use to recognize and destroy cells infected with viruses. The cytotoxic T-cell receptor attaches to the tumor antigen, which is complexed with the class I MHC antigens. The direct contact and binding results in the release of enzymes and lysis of the tumor cell within a few minutes. As with many other specific cytotoxic T-cell reactions, T-helper cell activation is necessary. The T-helper cells are also activated by the presentation of the tumor antigens linked to MHC on macrophages, and activation of T-helper cells can also result in nonspecific cytotoxicity. These cells release lymphokines, which activate macrophages in the area of the tumor. The activated macrophages release lytic enzymes, proteases, and reactive oxygen intermediates which destroy the tumor cells. In another type of cytotoxicity, antibody-dependent cytotoxicity, antibodies bound to a cytotoxic cell, either an NK cell or a macrophage, cross-link the cytotoxic and tumor cells. This binding creates changes in the cell membrane of the macrophage, causing release of lytic granules and death of the tumor cell. Natural killer cells are also responsible for the killing of tumor cells but, unlike the cytotoxic T cells, NK cells do not need prior exposure to generate a cytotoxic response to the tumor cell.

Antitumor Antibodies

In animal experiments, the injection of tumor cells has resulted in the production of antitumor antibodies. The binding of these antibodies to macrophages can lead to tumor cell lysis as described above in antibody-dependent cytotoxicity. Antitumor antibodies could also act as an opsonin. The binding of antibodies to the surface of tumor cells allows phagocytosis by macrophages to occur more readily. Binding of antibodies may also result in the activation of the complement system and the destruction of the tumor cell. Paradoxically, in some animal models it has been shown that the production of antibodies to tumors interfered with cell-mediated antitumor immune responses. Many of the studies in humans of antitumor antibodies have been conducted in patients with melanoma. Very few of these patients, about 6%, generate antitumor antibodies.

Cytokines

Cytokines are low-molecular-weight regulatory proteins produced by various cells. If these proteins are produced by lymphocytes, they are called lymphokines; if by monocytes, they are referred to as **monokines**. Several cytokines are known to have an antitumor effect; they may act alone or in concert with other cytokines. Interferons, tumor necrosis factors, and interleukin–2 are some of the more well-known cytokines with cytotoxic or antiproliferative effects. For instance, interferon gamma activates NK cells, thereby increasing NK cytotoxicity. The interferons are antiproliferative agents and can increase the expression of MHC antigens, which are necessary for T-cell activation. Tumor necrosis factors are secreted by macrophages, NK cells, and T-helper cells. They can directly lyse tumor cells and act in a synergistic fashion with interferon. The cloning of the genes for cytokines and their commercial production has led to an explosion of knowledge about these powerful cell regulators and to their exploitation for therapeutic purposes.

Tumor Escape Mechanisms

Obviously, when a patient is diagnosed with a malignancy, whatever antitumor immune mechanisms were present were not effective. Several different mechanisms are known by which tumors apparently evade the immune system. Antigenic modulation, one of the escape mechanisms, is readily observed in animal models. For instance, an animal that is immunized to a tumor may produce antibodies to the tumor antigen. The antibodies form complexes with the tumor antigen and are taken into the cell by endocytosis or shed to the environment. As long as the antibodies are present, the antigen is lost from the tumor surface and cannot be recognized by a cytotoxic T cell—killing is prevented. Alternatively, shedding of tumor antigens or tumor antigen-antibody complexes may block the activity of the cytotoxic cells.

In humans, as the tumor progresses, it may be that the tumor cells that are most easily recognized by the immune system are killed. Those tumor cells that are left may not express the tumor cell antigen and are able to proliferate without stimulating an immune response. Tumor cells may be able to "sneak through" the immune surveillance network. According to this theory, so few cells and tumor antigens are present early in the growth of a tumor, that the immune system is not stimulated. Later in the natural history of the tumor, there is a sufficient amount of tumor antigen present to stimulate the immune system, but by then the tumor is too large to be controlled by the immune response.

Cell-adhesion molecules are expressed on most somatic cells in the body. These molecules are necessary for the adherence of cytotoxic cells to a target cell before lysis can ensue. During the natural history of tumors, there are multiple genetic changes that are reflected in the phenotype of the cell. One of the changes that occurs in tumor cells is the loss of these cell-adhesion molecules. With the loss of these molecules, cytotoxic cells cannot bind as tightly to the malignant cells and thus the tumor can escape immune surveillance.

Class I MHC molecules on the target cell and the presence of antigen are necessary for cytotoxic T-cell killing. Transformation of cells to a malignant phenotype occurs along with the loss or a decrease in the expression of class I MHC molecules. Theoretically, the loss of these molecules may allow the tumor cell to escape recognition by the cytotoxic cell.

Besides these mechanisms, tumor cells may produce factors that inhibit immune responsiveness. For instance, tumor cells may secrete prostaglandins, which inhibit inflammation and block synthesis of chemotactic factors. This would limit the number of lymphocytes and monocytes in the area of the tumor.

AUTOIMMUNE DISEASES

Autoimmune diseases are another group of diseases in which biological therapies hold great promise. When the immune system reacts against self antigens, the ensuing state is called **autoimmunity.** Approximately 6% of the population suffer a chronic debilitating autoimmune disease. Autoimmune diseases are classified as (1) organ-specific diseases such as Addison's disease, Graves' disease, myasthenia gravis, and poststreptococcal glomerulonephritis or (2) systemic diseases such as ankylosing spondylitis, multiple sclerosis, rheumatoid arthritis, and systemic lupus erythematosus. The current therapies for autoimmune diseases are mainly those of nonspecific immunosuppression, including pharmacological agents such as steroids and cyclosporine, plasmapheresis, lymph node irradiation, and thymectomy. It has been suggested that more specific biological therapies will become available for these diseases in the future that will have fewer side effects than present therapies and will be directed at the immunological abnormalities.

Autoimmunity is the loss of self tolerance. Normally, lymphocytes that recognize self antigens are eliminated, usually in the fetus, in a process called clonal deletion. Most adults have **clonal anergy,** that is, lymphocytes that can react against self molecules are present in the circulation but do not react. This state of self tolerance must be maintained through regulation of immune responses. As discussed earlier, T-helper cells, T-suppressor cells, the interactions of the MHC antigens and T-cell receptors, and the cytokines are all responsible for regulatory reactions.

All these reactions are currently being studied to determine their role in autoimmune diseases. A great deal of research is now being done to determine the roles of MHC antigens and T-cell receptors in autoimmune diseases. It appears that many autoimmune diseases are associated with MHC class II genes and may result from the inappropriate expression of MHC antigens on cells in the target tissue. The relative risk of developing an autoimmune disease is high for individuals who possess certain MHC alleles. Individuals with the HLA-B27 allele, for instance, have a 90% risk of developing ankylosing spondylitis, and those with the HLA-DR3/DQW8 allele have a 100% risk of developing insulin-dependent diabetes. The exact mechanisms of the pathogenesis of these diseases are being explored in animal models, along with specific therapies directed at the T-helper cell receptors and specific T-cell clones. Autoimmune reactions may involve the B-cell system with the production of autoantibodies, the T-cell system with the inappropriate activation of cytotoxic T cells or T-helper cells, or both T-cell and B-cell immune responses.

Current experimental approaches to autoimmune diseases in animal models include the administration of monoclonal antibodies (Kuby, 1992; Wolsy, 1988). In mice with an autoimmune lupus-like syndrome, treatment with monoclonal antibodies to the CD4 molecule (T-helper cell) and to the IL–2 receptor has led to recovery and relief of symptoms. The administration of anti-CD4 antibodies prevented the lymphocytic infiltration of the pancreas and the relief of diabetic symptoms in another experimental animal model (Waldmann, 1988). Monoclonal antibodies to MHC molecules prevented the development of experimentally induced multiple sclerosis. Many strategies other than monoclonal antibody therapies are also being studied for their ability to modify the inflammatory and immune responses responsible for autoimmune diseases, rejections of transplants, and hypersensitivity states.

SUMMARY

The immune system serves as the body's defense system through the functions of protection from pathogenic organisms, surveillance, and homeostasis. Immune responses are divided into two types—innate and adaptive immunity. Innate or nonspecific defenses involve such mechanisms as intact skin and mucous membranes, the acidic environment of the stomach, the cleansing effect of tears, saliva, exfoliation of the skin, and the inflammatory response. These defenses form the body's first line of defense against pathogens. White blood cells, neutrophils, basophils, and eosinophils are important primarily in nonspecific defenses.

If innate immunity fails, adaptive immunity is enlisted. Specific immune responses recognize foreign antigens while tolerating self molecules. The hallmarks of adaptive immunity are memory and specificity. A additional property of specific immune responses is their ability to react in a more specific and sustained fashion upon the second and subsequent encounters with the antigen. Lymphocytes and macrophages are primarily involved in specific immune reactions. Lymphocytes can be classified as B cells responsible for the production of antibodies (immunoglobulins); T cells are important in cytotoxic and regulatory reactions.

The immunoglobulin receptor on the B cell and the T-cell receptor are responsible for the specific recognition of the antigen. The major histocompatibility genes control interactions among cells of the immune system. These genes code for molecules (MHC antigens) on cell surfaces that are recognized by T lymphocytes which require the antigen to be complexed to self MHC antigens for recognition. Cytokines are powerful mediators released during inflammatory and immune reactions. Although separate, there is significant interaction between innate and adaptive immunity and both are typically required to effect a sufficient response to eliminate pathogens.

The theory of immune surveillance implies that the immune system is capable of recognizing and destroying tumors. When a tumor is diagnosed in a patient, theoretically that tumor has evaded or sneaked through the immune surveillance system. Under appropriate conditions the immune system can recognize tumor associated antigens. T-cell responses to tumor cells resembles immune responses to viruses. B-cell responses to tumors also occur. Both activated macrophages and natural killer cells can lyse tumor cells, natural killer cells without prior exposure.

Rapid advances in technology such as genetic engineering and recombinant DNA technology, coupled with a more complete understanding of the immune response and the molecular basis of oncogenesis have led to the utilization of biological proteins in the treatment of cancer. Numerous cytokines; interferons, interleukins, hematopoietic growth factors, tumor necrosis factor and monoclonal antibodies, are now in clinical investigation or have received regulatory approval. As research continues to progress, new avenues of treatment will become available.

Oncogenes when functioning normally regulate cellular growth, division and differentiation. Suppressor genes or recessive oncogenes inhibit the development of the malignant phenotype in a cell. In the future, protein products of oncogenes or suppressor gene products may be used as biological therapy.

Autoimmune states (glomerulonephritis, systemic lupus, arthritis) are currently being investigated as to the underlying immunologic abnormalities. In the future, biologicals may also be manufactured that will control these illnesses.

References

Boon, T. 1993. Teaching the immune system to fight cancer. *Scientific American* 268 (3): 82–89.

Brostoff, J., Scadding, G., Male, D., et al. (eds.). 1991. *Clinical Immunology*. Philadelphia: J.B. Lippincott.

Burnet, F.M. 1976. *Immunology, aging, and cancer: Medical aspects of mutation and selection*. San Francisco: W.H. Freeman.

Claman, H. 1992. The biology of the immune response. *Journal of the American Medical Association* 268(20): 2790–2796.

Dale, M., and Foreman, J. 1989. *Textbook of Immunopharmacology*. Chicago: Year Book Medical Publishers.

Gallucci, B. 1987. The immune system and cancer. *Oncology Nursing Forum* 14(Suppl 6): 3–12.

Grady, C. 1988. Host defense mechanisms: An overview. *Seminars in Oncology Nursing* 4(2): 86–94.

Griffin, J. (ed.). 1986. *Hematology and Immunology: Concepts for Nursing*. Norwalk, CT: Appleton-Century Crofts.

Heberman, R. (ed.). 1993. Miniseries on the Interleukins. *Cancer Investigations* Volume 11.

Hubbard, S., Greene, P., and Knobf, M. (eds). 1993. *Current Issues in Cancer Nursing Practice*. Philadelphia: J.B. Lippincott Co.

Jaffe, H., and Sherwin, S. 1991. Immunomodulators. In Stiles, D., and Terr, A. (eds.). *Basic and Clinical Immunology*. Norwalk, CT: Appleton and Lange, pp. 780–785.

Jaret, P. 1986. Our immune system: the wars within. *National Geographic* 169(6): 702–735.

Knudson, A. 1977. Genetic predisposition to cancer. In Haitt, H., Watson, J., and Winsten, J. (eds.). *Origin of Human Cancer*. Cold Spring Harbor Conferences on Cell Proliferation Volume 4. Cold Spring Harbor, NY: Cold Spring Harbor Laboratory, pp. 45–52.

Kuby, J. (ed.). 1992. *Immunology*. New York: W.H. Freeman and Company.

Kuby, J. 1992. Chp 17 Autoimmunity. In Kuby, J. (ed.). *Immunology*. New York: W.H. Freeman and Company, pp. 383–403.

Kunkel, S., and Remick, D. (eds). 1992. *Cytokines in Health and Disease*. New York: Marcel Dekker.

Life, Death and The Immune System. 1993. *Scientific American* 269(3): 52–144.

Mudge-Grout, C. 1992. *Immunologic Disorders*. St. Louis: Mosby Year Book.

Oppenheim, J., and Shevach, E. (eds). 1990. *Immunophysiology: The Role of Cells and Cytokines in Immunity and Inflammation*. New York: Oxford University Press.

Rieger, P., Harle, M., and Rumsey, K. 1992. The Immune System. In Rumsey, K., and Rieger, P. (eds). *Biological Response Modifiers: A Self-Instructional Manual for Health Professionals*. Chicago, IL: Precept Press, Inc., pp. 3–34.

Roitt, I. (ed). 1991. *Essential Immunology* 7th ed. Boston: Blackwell Scientific Publications.

Roitt, I., Brostoff, J., and Male, D. (eds). 1993. *Immunology* 3rd ed. St. Louis: C.V. Mosby.

Schindler, L. 1992. *The Immune System: How it Works*. U.S. Department of Health and Human Services. Bethesda, MD: National Institutes of Health (NIH publication #92–3229).

Stites, D., and Terr, A. (eds). 1991. *Basic and Clinical Immunology* 7th ed. Norwalk, CT: Appleton and Lange.

Thomson, A. (ed). 1991. *The Cytokine Handbook*. San Diego: Academic Press, Inc.

Virella, G. (ed). 1993. *Introduction to Medical Immunology*, 3rd ed. New York: Marcel Dekker.

Waldmann, T. 1986. The structure, function and expression of interleukin-2 receptors on normal and malignant lymphocytes. *Science* 232: 727–732.

Wolsy, D. 1988. Treatment of autoimmune disease with monoclonal antibodies. *Progress in Allergy* 45: 106–120.

Workman, M., and Ellerhorst-Ryan, J. (eds). *Nursing Care of the Immunocompromised Patient*. Philadelphia, PA: W.B. Sanders.

CHAPTER 3 | Dosing and Scheduling Biological Response Modifiers

Paula Trahan Rieger, RN, MSN, OCN

Biological approaches to cancer treatment have progressed rapidly over the last decade and many biological response modifiers (BRMs) have now been approved for clinical use. However, the optimal dose, route of administration, and schedule are still not known for the majority of BRMs and will most likely differ for each disease treated. Many questions have been raised as to what constitutes optimal dosing and how it should be achieved in clinical trials. Indeed, an array of terms is used to describe the optimal dose for BRMs: optimal biological dose (OBD), optimal immunomodulatory dose, biologically optimal dose, biologically active dose, optimal biological response modifier dose, and maximum tolerated dose (MTD). The aim of this chapter is to define optimal biological dosing and to discuss issues surrounding BRM dosing and the combination of these agents with other types of therapy. A description of the basic concepts of pharmacokinetics and pharmaco-dynamics as they relate to dosing provides a foundation for understanding concerns related to dosing. Methods of evaluating biological effects and analysis of end points (therapeutic outcomes) in the treatment of cancer will serve as clinical examples to highlight these points. The interferons and granulocyte-macrophage colony-stimulating factor (GM-CSF) will be used as primary clinical examples.

DRUG DEVELOPMENT

The process of developing a new drug is both time consuming and costly. In general, the development of BRMs parallels that of chemotherapeutic agents. Both endeavors begin with the discovery of a new agent. For chemotherapeutic agents, the next step is extraction or synthetic formulation. For biological agents, this step involves the discovery of the gene or determination of the DNA sequence that codes for the biological protein. With hybridomas, for example, this phase includes selection of the hybridoma producing the desired monoclonal antibody. Biological activities are documented and animal studies to evaluate toxicity and mechanisms of action follow. If, at that point, an agent appears to have clinical usefulness, the company developing the drug files an investigational new drug application (**INDA**). The cost of a single INDA can run into millions of dollars. Having been declared an investigational new drug, the new agent then enters clinical trials for evaluation in humans. The purpose of phase I trials is to determine the MTD and recommend a schedule of administration. The MTD is the dose at which, within the design of that trial, side effects become unacceptable to the physician and the patient. In phase II trials, therapeutic activity with respect to a given disease is tested. When an agent reaches phase III trials, its usefulness is compared to the standard therapy for that particular disease. At this point, if the agent appears promising, a new drug application (NDA) is made to the Food and Drug Administration (FDA). Dosage, route, schedule, toxicity, and indications for the agent are then specified (Oldham, 1991).

Problems inherent in this system are many. The time it takes to move a drug through the approval process is often as long as eight to ten years, and the costs can run as high as $80–100 million. Only companies with substantial resources are able to persevere through the lengthy and expensive approval process (Oldham, 1991). In addition, the current system is often not sufficiently flexible to optimize the development of BRMs. The majority of advances in biotherapy have been made through empirical discoveries rather than based on rational principles. (Creekmore et al., 1991).

OPTIMAL BIOLOGICAL DOSING

Animal models have demonstrated that there may be a wide disparity between the MTD and the OBD for biological agents. The **OBD** may be defined as the minimum dose at which biological activity is maximally stimulated (Creekmore et al., 1991). Parameters deemed important for treating a particular disease with BRMs must be determined so that the optimal desired response may be assessed. Within the current framework of drug development, several crucial issues unique to BRMs are not addressed: BRM diversity and selectivity, the **cytokine cascade**, the existence of physiological mechanisms/receptors for BRMs because they are natural products, and the measurement of biological effects within the context of clinical trials (Talmadge, 1992; Creekmore et al., 1991).

Diversity and Selectivity

Biological response modifiers are both diverse and selective. Owing to their **pleiotropic** nature, many have more than one mechanism of action (Balkwill and Burke, 1989; Sporn and Roberts, 1988). Determination of which biologic effect yields the antitumor effect when a BRM is given for a particular disease is often unknown. For example, the most important antitumor action of interferon-alpha (IFN-α) may be due to either immunomodulatory effects or antiproliferative effects. The approach to dosing would be very different depending on which effect is to be maximally stimulated (Creekmore et al., 1991; Mihich, 1987). The relationship of dosing to antitumor activity is not the same for biological agents as it is for chemotherapeutic agents.

Moreover, BRMs are much more selective than are chemotherapeutic agents. Most function as receptor-mediated molecules; that is, select cells bear receptors for a given agent. Monoclonal antibodies are an excellent example of a group of agents with high selectivity.

The Cytokine Cascade

The biology of the immune system is complex. This system contains a multitude of cells that communicate with each other through secretion of a variety of cytokines or biological proteins that act as messengers. (See Chapter 2.) The term *cytokine cascade* is used to describe the network of interactions which occur through mutual cytokine induction, through transmodulation of cell surface receptors and by **synergistic, additive,** or **antagonistic** interactions that affect the function of a target cell (Balkwill and Burke, 1989; Kelso, 1989). The assessment of a cytokine's action often occurs *in vitro* or in animal models. It is difficult to determine whether such activities will also be seen when the agent is given *in vivo*. The ultimate response of a cell may be determined by the number of different messages it receives concurrently at its surface (Sporn and Roberts, 1988).

Toxicity of Natural Products

The toxicity of BRMs may need to be viewed differently from that of chemotherapy. Because BRMs are naturally found in the body, we would expect them to have a less acute and/or milder cumulative toxic effect. To a certain extent this is true, for when administration of biological agents is stopped, side effects generally resolve very quickly. This characteristic may be related to the fact that both receptors and physiological mechanisms for these natural body proteins are already in place (Oldham, 1991).

Measurement of Biological Effects in Clinical Trials

The issue of evaluating biological effects within the context of clinical trials is gaining increasing attention. How does administration of a BRM affect the normal cytokine cascade? What is the predominant antitumor effect? What is the rationale for using a given BRM in treating a particular disease given the underlying pathophysiology? Because a degree of sophistication has now been reached in the use of biotherapy, these questions need to be addressed.

Table 3.1 Factors affecting drug absorption

Factor	Definition
Bioavailability	The percentage of drug that is absorbed. Dosage forms of a drug from different manufacturers may differ in their bioavailability.
Solubility	The ability of a medication to dissolve and form a solution.
Concentration	The relative content of a component (strength or potency). The more concentrated a drug, the more rapidly it will be absorbed.
Circulation	The amount of blood flow available to carrry the drug to the site of action.
Route	Method by which medication can be introduced into the body. Possible routes are: oral, via mucous membranes, via inhalation, and parenteral. Places the drug near the absorbing surface for absorption into the vascular system.

The concepts of pharmacokinetics, pharmacodynamics, and measurement of response can be used to understand BRM dosing issues and to evaluate the aforementioned issues in more detail.

PHARMACOKINETICS AND DOSE DETERMINATION

Pharmacokinetics may be defined simply as what the body does to the drug (Benet *et al.*, 1990). In essence, the end effect of a drug depends on its ultimate concentration at the site of action. The pharmacokinetic phase comprises an agent's absorption, distribution to the site of action, biotransformation, and excretion. This entire phase may be affected by such individual differences as body weight, age, disease state, immune factors, psychological factors, environmental factors, and timing of the dose (chronobiology). A brief review of this phase will serve as a foundation for understanding related dosing issues.

Administration of a drug to a patient may occur through a variety of possible routes, the most common being intramuscular (IM), subcutaneous (SC), intravenous (IV), and oral (PO). The drug must then be absorbed so that it can make its way into the systemic circulation. **Absorption** is the rate at which the drug leaves the site of administration and the extent to which this occurs. This process involves the passage of the drug across the surface of cell membranes. Once the drug enters the blood, it can circulate either independently or while bound to plasma proteins. Factors affecting absorption include bioavailability, solubility, concentration, circulation, and route (Table 3.1).

Once absorption occurs, the drug must then make its way to the site of action. This process is termed **distribution.** For most biological agents, the site of action is receptors on target cells. Factors affecting the distribution process are blood flow, drug properties such as solubility, and binding ability. Drugs generally bind to plasma proteins or physiological receptors after which an equilibrium is reached between the concentration of drug in the blood and in plasma and target receptors or in certain tissue reservoirs such as fat cells. **Plasma concentration** is the amount of both free and bound drug in the plasma. The maximal effect of a drug usually occurs when the peak level of concentration is reached.

Biotransformation, or metabolism, refers to the enzymatic alteration of the drug. Generally occurring in the liver, it can be affected by factors such as genetics, pre-existing liver disease, or the concomitant administration of other drugs.

Lastly, drugs are excreted through the liver and kidneys in either altered (as metabolites) or natural form. The **clearance** of a drug is a measure of the speed at which the drug leaves the system. The rate of clearance will impact the frequency of administration. For example, a drug with a low clearance rate requires less frequent administration than a drug with a high clearance rate (Kuhn, 1991; Benet *et al.*, 1990).

The ability to relate these concepts to the clinical evaluation of biological agents is important. For example, in phase I trials, pharmacologic studies relate the concentration of drug in the circulation to the concentration needed at the site of action to obtain the desired biological effect. These studies represent a way to quantify the relationship between dose and the effect of a drug.

The results of a pharmacologic study can be plotted on a pharmacology curve (Figure 3.1). In this case, the **area under the curve (AUC)** defines the exposure of the target cell to the drug and is a function of the concentration of the drug and time. Half-life is defined as the time it takes for the concentration of drug in the blood to decrease by 50% (Benet *et al.*, 1990).

The pharmacokinetic profiles of IFN-α and GM-CSF serve to illustrate these concepts. Figure 3.2 depicts administration of IFN by the intramuscular route. The pharmacology curve for IM administration of IFN shows a slow and gradual absorption from the muscle into the bloodstream, with a gradual decline over the course of one to two days. Escalation of the IFN dose shows higher levels of the drug initially, with a slower clearance time. Peak serum concentrations are generally achieved four to six hours after injection, with maximum observed serum concentrations increasing with dose (Gutterman *et al.*, 1982).

The pharmacology curves of colony-stimulating factors are similar to those seen with IFN. For GM-CSF administered intravenously, the serum concentration is very high initially but falls rapidly over several hours (Figure 3.3A). When GM-CSF is given subcutaneously, a more gradual absorption is seen, with the peak in the serum concentration occurring after approximately two to four hours depending on the dose (Figure 3.3B, C, D) (Morstyn *et al.*, 1989; Cebon *et al.*, 1988).

Pharmacologic studies in phase I trials are clinically important because the results are used to determine the appropriate route, dose, and schedule for administration of a drug. The concentration of drug needed at the site of

Figure 3.1 Linear medication curve shows the biological half-life of a medication. A dose of 500 mg of the drug, which has a half-life of 3 hours, is given at point X. At 3 hours, 250 mg are excreted; at 6 hours, an additional 125 mg are excreted; at 9 hours, an additional 62.5 mg are excreted. This continues for approximately 5 half-lives.

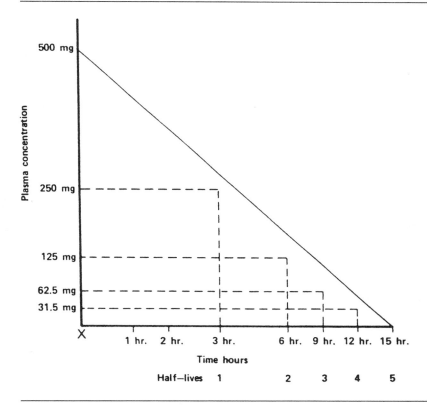

Source: Reprinted with permission from publisher F.A. Davis. Kuhn, M. (1991). The phase of drug action. In Kuhn, M. (ed.) 2nd ed. *Pharmacotherapeutics: A Nursing Approach.* Fig. 4.6, pp. 79.

action can be obtained by the dose that yields this concentration in the blood. This information can also be correlated clinically with side effects. Peak concentrations of drug often relate to the peak occurrence of side effects. Again, IFN serves as an excellent model. Fever and chills are generally seen two to four hours after injection, which correlates with the beginning of a peak concentration in the blood. When drugs are given by the intra-venous route, side effects in general are seen much more quickly.

The primary pharmacokinetic factors affecting the concentration of drug in the blood, therefore the patient's response, include the rate and amount of drug absorbed, the distribution of the drug to the site of action, biotransformation of the drug, and excretion or elimination of the drug from the body. These are key principles in determining the

Figure 3.2   The mean serum concentrations of IFN as measured by the bioassay with MDBK (bovine kidney) cells as target cells. The numbers of patients measured at 3, 9, 36, 72, 108, and 198 million unites are 16, 16, 16, 16, 14, and 5, respectively.

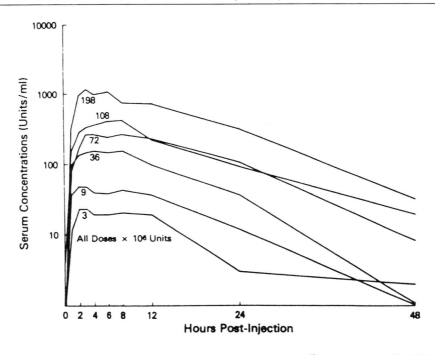

Source: Reproduced with permission from Gutterman, J., *et al.* Recombinant leukocyte A interferon: Pharmacokinetics, single-dose tolerance, and biologic effects in cancer patients. *Annals of Internal Medicine* 1982, 96: 549–555. Figure 2, p. 551.

proper dose and schedule for administration of a drug.

PHARMACODYNAMICS AND DOSE DETERMINATION

Pharmacodynamics defines what the drug does to the body. It deals with the biochemical and physiological effects and mechanisms of action of the drug (Ross, 1990). Most BRMs are receptor-mediated molecules. After interaction with cell surface receptors, these molecules stimulate certain functions, induce secondary messengers, or suppress select immune functions. The interferons can be used as a model to illustrate this point. They have several biological actions: antiviral effects, immunomodulatory and antiproliferative activity, oncogene regulation, and metabolic and phenotypic alterations of cell surface proteins. The interferons are receptor mediated, and once bound, cause the induction of secondary messengers inside the cell (Balkwill, 1989).

If the biological actions of IFN were to be assessed, what response parameters would be measured? Useful parameters include the activation of natural killer cells; β_2-microglobulin production which relates to the induction of major histocompatibility complex antigens, and neopterin production which relates to the

Figure 3.3   Pharmacokinetics of human GM-CSF in humans: (A) 0.3 µg/kg administered intravenously(IV), (B) 1 µg/kg administered subcutaneously (SC), (C) 3 µg/kg SC, and (D) 10 µg/kg SC. Serum levels are expressed as means of triplicate determination ± SD. GM-CSF was injected at time 0.

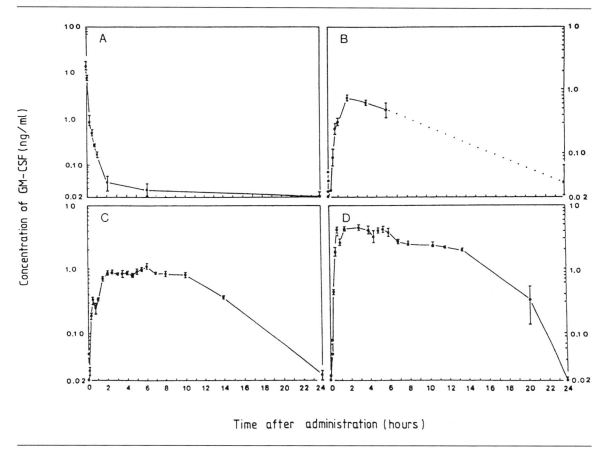

Time after administration (hours)

Source: Reprinted with permission from Cebon, J., *et al*, 1988. Pharmocokinetics of human granulocyte-macrophage colony-stimulating factor using a sensitive immunoassay. *Blood* 72(4): 1340–1347. Figure 6, p. 1344.

activation of macrophages. (Aulitzky *et al.*, 1989; Huber and Herold, 1989; Borden *et al.*, 1987).

Aulitzky *et al.* (1989) evaluated the effects of IFN-gamma on biological responses in 16 patients with renal cell cancer and observed a bell-shaped response curve. As the concentration of drug increased, responses also increased to a certain point. Past a certain dose, however, responses began to decrease or plateau. An evaluation of β_2-microglobulin in-

duction at IFN-gamma doses of 10, 100, and 500 µg once weekly is depicted in Figure 3.4. At the lowest dose, there was minimal induction of β_2-microglobulin levels. A significant increase in levels was seen at the 100-µg dose, but levels were not greatly increased at the 500-µg dose even though toxic effects were significantly more severe. This illustrates how the MTD may differ from the biologically optimal dose. The MTD (500 µg) was not the dose at which maximal biological activity was ob-

Figure 3.4   Kinetics of β_2-microglobulin serum levels after the first application of different dose levels of IFN-gamma. Median values and range of all determinations performed in 16 patients with renal cell carcinoma are demonstrated.

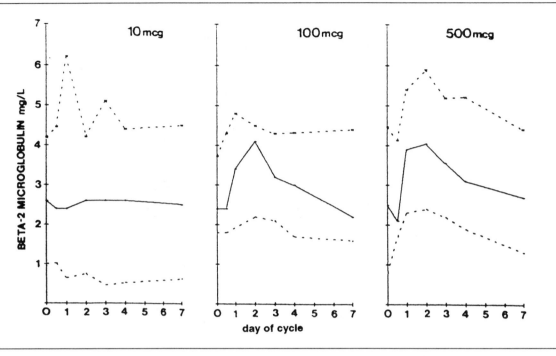

Source: Reprinted with permission from Aulitzky, W., *et al,* 1989. Successful treatment of metastatic renal cell carcinoma with a biologically active dose of recombinant interferon-gamma. *Journal of Clinical Oncology* 7(12): 1875–1884. Figure 1, p. 1878.

tained (100 µg) as determined by the aforementioned parameters. Neopterin levels showed a similar pattern (Figure 3.5). In the next phase of the study, Aulitzky *et al.* treated patients at the biologically optimal dose of 100 µg IFN-gamma and found some that did respond to this dose. This is an example of how clinical trials might be designed that begin to evaluate the issue of biologically optimal dosing in conjunction with determination of MTD.

A key to determining the OBD is identifying which biological effects contribute to the antitumor effect. With most BRMs, it is difficult to say which biological property is responsible for the primary antitumor effect in a given disease. With IFNs, OBD may differ for different types of tumors. For example, hairy cell leukemia responds to very low doses of IFN-α. For the treatment of renal cell cancer, moderate doses of IFN-α are needed, whereas for treatment of Kaposi's sarcoma, much higher doses of IFN-α are required to produce clinical responses.

The evaluation of GM-CSF serves as an additional clinical example. Hematopoietic growth factors are substances involved in the maturation and differentiation of hematopoietic cells. They are also able to enhance the function of these cells (Metcalf, 1990). For example, GM-CSF can enhance the function of neutrophils and macrophages. Key functions of neutrophils in the body include the ability to move to an area of inflammation or

Figure 3.5 Kinetics of neopterin serum levels after the first application of different dose levels of IFN-gamma. Median values and range of all determinations performed in 16 patients with renal cell carcinoma are demonstrated.

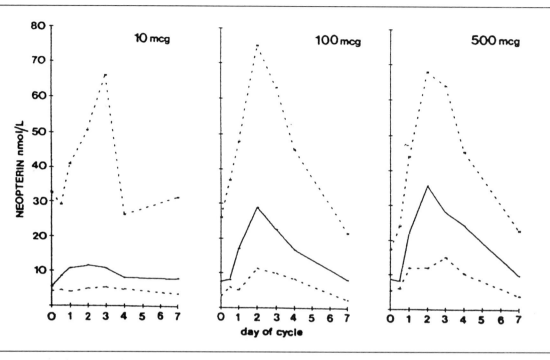

Source: Reprinted with permission from Aulitzky, W. et al, 1989. Successful treatment of metastic renal cell carcinoma with a biologically active dose of recombinant interferon-gamma. *Journal of Clinical Oncology 7(12): 1875–1884.* Figure 1, p. 1878.

infection and to phagocytize foreign bodies (Wiernik, 1989).

A simple way to evaluate the biological effects of hematopoietic growth factors is examination of peripheral blood cell counts. For example, early phase I trials with GM-CSF demonstrated increasing numbers of white blood cells as the dose was increased, with a rapid decline in counts once therapy was discontinued (Figure 3.6.) (Vadhan-Raj *et al.*, 1988). Lower doses, at which there are minimal toxic effects, may be adequate to stimulate the desired number of white blood cells. A case study reported by Kurzrock *et al.* (1991) provides an example of how a lower dose may provide the desired therapeutic goal. A patient with chronic lymphocytic

leukemia being treated for neutropenia was started on GM-CSF at 150 µg/m² daily. At this dose, levels of eosinophils increased, but no changes were observed in the number of neutrophils. Escalation of the dose to 300 µg/m² daily resulted in very high levels of eosinophils with only minimal elevation of neutrophil levels. At this point, the patient experienced an episode of eosinophilic pneumonia and required treatment in the intensive care setting. Following recovery, therapy was reinitiated at a lower dose of 75 µg/m² daily. The eosinophil count began to fall, and the neutrophil count began to rise. A reduction of the dose to 10 µg/m² daily resulted in excellent stimulation of neutrophils with no stimulation of eosinophils (Figure 3.7).

Figure 3.6 White blood cell counts and absolute granulocyte counts (neutrophils and bands) in patients with solid tumors treated with recombinant human (rh) GM-CSF. The rhGM-CSF was administered by IV bolus injection on day 1, followed by continuous intravenous infusion (solid bar) from days 2 to day 14. After a 2-week rest period, a second 2-week cycle by intravenous continuous infusion was repeated. Each of the five patients traced here received rhGM-CSF at a dose of 30 (◇–◇), 60 (▲–▲), 120 (O–O), 120 (●–●), or 250 (■–■) μg/m² of body surface area.

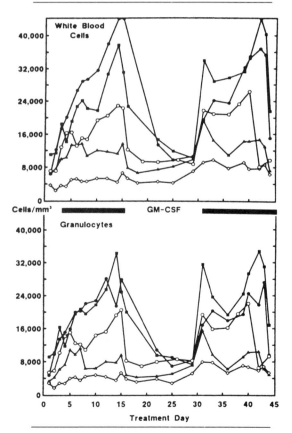

Source: Reprinted with permission from Vadhan-Raj, S. *et al,* 1988. Stimulation of hematopoiesis in patients with bone marrow failure and in patients with malignancy by recombinant human granulocyte-macrophage colony-stimulating factor. *Blood* 72(1): 134–141. Figure 1, p. 136.

Although this case study demonstrates the experience of only one patient, it does provide an interesting example of how a smaller dose may produce the desired biological effect. Future trials with larger sample populations will be required to document this effect.

As discussed previously, the endogenous normal cellular cytokine cascade appears to be delicately balanced. The therapeutic use of a BRM may occasionally produce unintended biological effects. A controversial point surrounding the use of GM-CSF was that neutrophils appeared to not function properly. Work by Peters *et al.* (1988) evaluated the function of neutrophils by measuring their margination, phagocytosis, peroxide production, and migration in patients receiving GM-CSF. Evaluation of these functions demonstrated that margination, phagocytosis, and peroxide production levels were similar both before and after therapy, whereas neutrophil migration was decreased. Neutrophils tended to stay in the bloodstream because of the concentration gradient that resulted from GM-CSF administration. It is uncertain whether decreased neutrophil migration has a negative clinical effect.

Clinical studies evaluating levamisole provide another relevant example of OBD. Although levamisole was approved in 1990 for use in standard adjuvant therapy for patients with Dukes' stage C colon cancer, little is known about its optimal dose and schedule or the mechanism by which it exerts its antitumor effects (Janik *et al.*, 1993). A recent phase I study by Janik *et al.* evaluated levamisole alone and in combination with IFN-gamma in treating patients with advanced cancers. Patients were placed on one of two arms: those with advanced disease in whom standard therapy had failed and those with either renal cancer or melanoma who received adjuvant therapy. The main objective of the trial was to determine the MTD and immunomodulatory activity of levamisole alone and in combination with IFN-gamma. Immunologic monitoring involved measurement of neopterin levels, flow cytometric **immuno-**

Figure 3.7   The course of the peripheral blood absolute neutrophil and eosinophil counts of a patient with chronic lymphocytic leukemia during treatment with varying doses of subcutaneously administered GM-CSF is depicted. The daily dose of GM-CSF is shown in the shaded area, with the empty spaces representing times when GM-CSF was withheld. (A dose of 100 $\mu g/m^2$ is approximately equivalent to 2–5 $\mu g/kg$.) There were no significant changes in monocyte, lymphocyte, platelet, and reticulocyte counts.

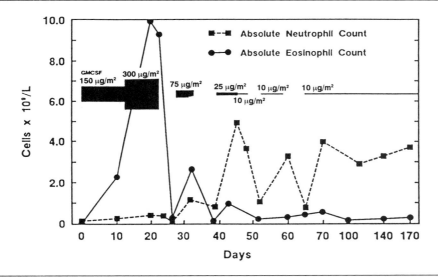

Source: Reprinted with permission from Kurzrock, R., *et al.* 1991. Differential dose-related haematologic effects of GM-CSF in pancytopenia: Evidence supporting the advantage of low- or high-dose administration in selected patients. *British Journal of Haematology* 78: 352–358. Figure 1, p. 353.

phenotyping, and natural killer cell assays. In both groups, it appeared that a threshold dose of 5.0 mg/kg of levamisole was needed to induce levels of both neopterin and soluble interleukin–2 receptor (sIL–2R). Expression of monocyte surface markers associated with activation increased in response to treatment with levamisole alone at this dose level, but multiple doses were needed to induce this effect.

These data suggest that monocytes were activated *in vivo*. Increased levels of sIL–2R suggest that T cells were activated by levamisole with subsequent secretion of IFN-gamma. Monocytes may then have been stimulated by IFN-gamma to make neopterin.

Natural killer cell activity was not reproducibly elevated above baseline, regardless of levamisole dose.

In this study, therefore, the MTD of levamisole alone and in combination with interferon-gamma was 5.0 mg/kg, which was also the optimal immunomodulatory dose. The reported dose of levamisole when used as adjuvant therapy in other cancers (Quirt *et al.*, 1991; Moertel *et al.*, 1990) is below the MTD, and also below the OBD according to calculations by Janik *et al.* These data argue for additional trials evaluating higher doses of levamisole with alternative schedules. These trials should include both immunologic and clinical end points.

A recent article by Mäas *et al.* (1993) reviews the issue of high-dose versus low-dose interleukin-2 (IL–2). In many trials, IL–2 has been used like a chemotherapeutic agent (i.e., at the MTD). Therapy at these doses appears to best stimulate nonspecific antitumor activity (lymphokine-activated killer cell, or LAK activity). Therapy with low doses of IL–2, however, preferentially stimulates a specific antitumor immune response. Many studies have evaluated the immunological effects of IL–2 administration both in animal models and in patients with cancer. High-dose IL–2 causes an increase in the number of lymphocytes in the peripheral blood and induces LAK activity. In addition, cytokines such as interferon-gamma, IL–1, IL–6, and tumor necrosis factor are released. If LAK cell cytotoxicity is the predominant antitumor mechanism, then IL–2 therapy should be effective against a wide range of different tumors. To date, however, IL–2 therapy has been found to be effective primarily in patients with melanoma and renal cell cancer; tumors known to be very immunogenic. These facts may suggest the involvement of a specific antitumor reaction. Over the last few years, data have been accumulated indicating that tumor-specific T cells are essential for the therapeutic effect of IL–2 alone or in combination with LAK cells. Mäas *et al.* argue for the use of low IL–2 doses which give optimal stimulation of a specific immune reaction, particularly the intratumoral application of low doses of IL–2 which does not induce toxic effects.

SCHEDULING

Dose is not the only important factor in achieving maximal biological effects; scheduling may also have an impact. A study by Vadhan-Raj *et al.* (1992) evaluated the scheduling of GM-CSF after chemotherapy in patients with sarcoma to determine a schedule that would best abrogate myelosuppression. In the initial schedule, chemotherapy with CyADIC (cyclophosphamide, doxorubicin and dacarbazine) was given on days 1 through 5

and GM-CSF was administered on days 8 through 21 by continuous intravenous infusion following the second cycle of chemotherapy (Figure 3.8). Although the rate of neutrophil recovery was enhanced, severe neutropenia was not eliminated. A modified schedule was then initiated to allow earlier administration of GM-CSF. The CyADIC treatment was compressed from 5 to 3 days, and GM-CSF was infused immediately following the completion of the second cycle of chemotherapy. On the modified schedule, GM-CSF significantly reduced both the degree and the duration of neutropenia and incidence of mucositis, and it allowed for higher doses of chemotherapy in 17 patients. These findings suggest that the timing of administration of growth factors and chemotherapy has a great impact on the degree of myeloprotection. This clinical study illustrates the point that optimal dose may not be the only factor important in obtaining the desired biological effect.

BIOTHERAPY IN COMBINATION THERAPY

As more success is achieved with the use of BRMs in the treatment of cancer, the next logical step in assessing these agents is evaluation of their combination with other biological agents or with other therapies (chemotherapy or radiotherapy) to improve their therapeutic indices. Issues such as the rationale for selecting a certain combination and the dose and schedule to be used remain important. This section will review reasons for using combination therapy and will specifically analyze the rationale for combining biotherapy with chemotherapy, while highlighting several clinical examples. Issues related to the toxicity of these combinations will also be discussed.

Goals of Combination Therapy

The ultimate goal of cancer therapy is patient survival. The first principle in reaching this goal is that the patient must first achieve a

Figure 3.8 Schema of the initial therapeutic schedule of CyADIC and GM-CSF (A) and the modified therapeutic schedule (B).

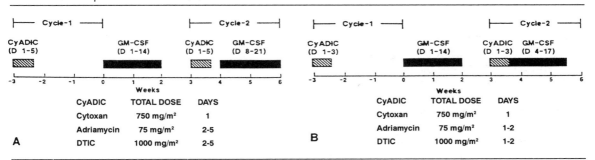

Source: Reprinted with permission from Vadhan-Raj, S., et al. 1992. Abrogating chemotherapy-induced myelosupression by recombinant granulocyte-macrophage colony-stimulating factor in patients with sarcoma: Protection at the progenitor cell level. *Journal of Clinical Oncology* 10(8): 1266–1277. Figure 1, p. 1268.

complete response. When the patient has maintained this response over a defined time frame (usually five years), he or she can then be considered cured. The question then arises as to how available therapies can be better utilized to achieve cure.

One approach is the use of combination therapies with the intent of increasing response rates. Two agents would ideally provide better results than one alone. Generally, when agents are combined, it is because they have demonstrated synergistic, not just additive, effects. A useful illustration of the difference between synergistic and additive effects is as follows: with additive effects, 1 + 1 = 2, whereas with synergy, 1 + 1 = 4.

To design an effective combination regimen, several issues including dosing and scheduling issues and the rationale for combining agents must be addressed. An ideal combination would also have less severe toxicity than either agent alone. A discussion of the combination of biotherapy with other biological agents, chemotherapy, or radiotherapy follows to illustrate how these principles are being investigated.

Although certain BRMs used singly have been observed to induce responses, only a small percentage of patients receiving the single agents have achieved long-standing remission or cure. The major opportunity for suc-

cess may rest on rational combinations of BRMs. Due to their redundant and pleiotropic nature, combinations of cytokines may be synergistic or antagonistic; amplification or limitation of a response may also occur through the cytokine cascade when one cytokine induces the synthesis of another (Kelso, 1989). Determination of effective combinations through *in vitro* work or animal models should serve as the foundation for designing effective combinations.

Combinations of Biological Response Modifiers

A variety of combinations of BRMs have now been tested clinically. A brief overview of combinations is given here, with more thorough overviews provided in certain chapters. Combinations of different IFNs, IFN and IL–2, IFN or IL–2 with monoclonal antibodies, and tumor necrosis factor with IFN or IL–2 are representative of the major combinations undergoing evaluation (Mulé and Rosenberg, 1991; Gilewski and Golomb, 1990; Mulé and Rosenberg, 1989).

Numerous clinical trials have evaluated the combination of IFN and IL–2 in patients with advanced malignancies. The rationale for combining IL–2 and IFN is based on their differing mechanisms of action: IL–2 appears to act primarily as an immunomodulator, whereas IFN has antiproliferative effects. However, IFN may also serve to augment the expression of histocompatibility antigens on tumor cells, making them more susceptible to IL–2-sensitized lymphocytes (Figlin, 1992). Even though potent synergism is seen *in vitro* with this combination, its mechanism is as yet undetermined. To date, most responses to this combination are seen in patients with renal cell cancer or melanoma. Only prospective randomized trials will be able to determine the true value of this combination.

A newer area of exploration involves combinations of monoclonal antibodies and other BRMs. The proposed rationale for using monoclonal antibodies and IL–2 lies with the antibody's reaction with target cells and mediation of tumor destruction through binding complement or via effector cells by **antibody-dependent cell mediated cytotoxicity.** In short, IL–2 would be used to stimulate LAK effector cells (Mulé and Rosenberg, 1991). With IFNs, up-regulation of tumor-associated antigens or major histocompatibility antigens on tumor cells may serve to improve targeting of antibodies to tumor cells. Clinical trials evaluating these combinations are in early stages.

Investigation of the many possible combinations of biological agents is just beginning. It is unlikely that all possible combinations of the 20-plus known cytokines will be tested (Kelso, 1989). It is crucial, therefore, that *in vitro* and animal model data be used to guide the rational combination of these agents. When clinical successes are seen, prospective randomized trials must then be used to delineate the full benefit.

Biological Response Modifiers and Chemotherapy

Rationale

The combination of biotherapy with chemotherapy is currently an area of active investigation. The interaction of cytokines and cyto-

Figure 3.9   Interaction of cytokines and cytotoxic drugs.

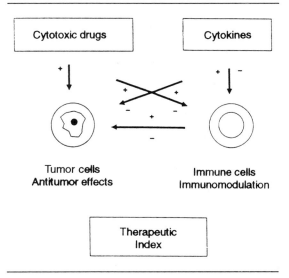

Source: Reprinted with permission from Kreuser, E., *et al.* 1992. Interactions between cytokines and cytotoxic drugs: Putative molecular mechanisms in experimental hematology and oncology. *Seminars in Oncology* 19(2) (Suppl 4): 1–7. Figure 1, p. 3.

toxic drugs may occur on several levels (Figure 3.9) (Kreuser, 1992). The rationale for using combinations of biotherapy and chemotherapy includes differing mechanisms of actions (in essence a two-pronged approach to attacking the tumor), modulation of the pharmacokinetics or action of the chemotherapeutic agent on key enzymes, alteration of drug-resistance mechanisms, and alteration of cell cycle kinetics. Further rationale includes modifications in the permeability of the vascular system that allow increased accumulation of chemotherapeutic drugs at the tumor site, nonoverlap of toxicities, reduction of the tumor burden, use of one modality as maintenance therapy, and use of one modality to improve patient tolerance of cytotoxic agents (Krueser, 1992; Pazdur, 1992; Parmiani and Rivoltini, 1991).

It is useful to explore in more depth the concept of differing mechanisms of action. Chemotherapy targets rapidly dividing cells and through various mechanisms causes cell

Table 3.2 Cytotoxic drug-cytokine interactions: levels of mechanisms

Tumor Cells	Host Cells
Cellular Modulation	Immunomodulation
Enzymes	Natural killer cells
Topoisomerase	Monocytes
Thymidylate synthase	Macrophages
Thymidine kinase	Cytotoxic T lymphocytes
Pyrimidine phosphorylase	
DNA	Pharmacologic modulation
Gene Expression	Liver cells
Receptors	
Adhesion receptors	
Growth factor receptors	
Cytokine receptors	
Cell cycle phase	
G_0/G_1 arrest	
G_0/G_1 recruitment	
Effects on tumor-cell vasculature	

Source: Reprinted with permission from Kreuser, E., *et al.* 1992. Interactions between cytokines and cytotoxic drugs: Putative molecular mechanisms in experimental hematology and oncology. *Seminars in Oncology* 19(2) Suppl 4: 1–7. Table 3, p.3.

death. Biological response modifiers, which are sometimes termed *biomodulators,* modulate biological responses through various actions including: (1) augmenting the patient's antitumor response (e.g., stimulation of effector cells or increased production of cytokines); (2) decreasing suppressor mechanisms; (3) increasing the patient's immunological defenses; (4) increasing the patient's ability to tolerate damage by cytotoxic modalities; (5) changing membrane characteristics of the tumor cell to make it more susceptible to killing by chemotherapeutic agents; (6) preventing or reversing transformation; (7) or decreasing the ability of tumor cells to metastasize (Kreuser, 1992; Mitchell, 1988).

The term *biomodulation* may also be used in another context. When agents are combined, one agent can cause the biochemical modulation of another. A definition of this type of modulation would be the enhancement of the antitumor activity of an effector agent by a second agent (Schmoll *et al.*,1992). With biochemical modulation, the modulator manipulates the metabolic pathway of a cytotoxic drug to increase the efficacy or selective

protection of normal tissue or both. Cytokines can also serve as biochemical modulators, with multiple levels of interaction between chemotherapy and cytokines possible. Targets of modulation include specific enzymes of drug metabolism, receptors for adhesion or growth, cell cycle phases, gene expression, and the immune system (Table 3.2) (Kreuser, 1992).

Dosing

Issues of dosing already have been reviewed. Although the hope is that combining agents will decrease the amount of each that is needed, this may not be the case. Again, the desired biological effect must be identified so that the proper dose can be administered.

Scheduling

To avoid one agent negating the effects of the other or to obtain maximum benefit, scheduling issues are of the utmost importance when combining chemotherapy with biotherapy. *In vitro* work can be used as a guide to determine whether biotherapy should be given before, during, or after chemotherapy. A primary

Table 3.3 Immunosuppressive activity of chemotherapeutic agents

Class of Agent	Demonstrated	Relatively Little
Alkylating Agents	Cyclophosphamide Nitrosoureas	Busulfan, Dimethyl busulfan, Dacarbazine
Antibiotics	Daunorubicin	Bleomycin, Doxorubicin Mithramycin
Folic Acid Antagonists	Methotrexate	
Purine analogues	6-Mercaptopurine Azathioprine	
Pyrimidine analogs	5-FU, Cytarabine	
Vinca alkaloids	Vincristine Vinblastine	

Source: Reprinted with permission from Gilewski, T., and Golomb, H. 1990. Design of combination biotherapy studies: Future goals and challenges. *Seminars in Oncology* 17(1) (Suppl 1): 3–10. Table 1, p. 4.

question that must be answered in determining sequence is whether the chemotherapy agent being used is immunosuppressive. Typically, chemotherapy is given before biotherapy. Proposed reasons for using this sequence include: reducing the tumor burden, allowing for recovery from the immunosuppressive effects of chemotherapy, eliminating suppressor influences (such as CD8+ cells), and altering tumor cell membranes, which may lead to exposure of antigens, thereby increasing the susceptibility of tumor cells to lysis by immune cells. Table 3.3 illustrates the relative immunosuppressive activity of various chemotherapeutic agents (Gilewski and Golomb, 1990). It is interesting to note that not all chemotherapy agents are immunosuppressive, and the immunosuppressive effects in those that are are dependent on dose.

Clinical Examples

Interferon-alpha again serves as a clinical example to illustrate the principles of combination therapy. Many *in vitro* studies using both

Table 3.4 Cytotoxic drugs with activity modulated by IFNs

Cisplatin	Cyclophosphamide
Doxorubicin	Fluorouracil
Melphalan	Methotrexate
Mitomycin	Mechlorethamine
Vinblastine	Vincristine
Dactinomycin	ACNU
Carmustine	Bleomycin
Cytarabine	Difluoromethylornithine
Neocarzinostatin	(DFMO)
Prednisone	Peplomycin
	Thioguanine

Source: Reprinted with permission from Wadler, S., and Schwartz, E. 1992. Principles in the biomodulation of cytotoxic drugs by interferons. *Seminars in Oncology* 19(2) (Suppl 3): 45–48. Table 2, p. 47.

tumor cell lines and animal tumor models have analyzed the activity of IFN-α in combination with other cytotoxic agents. Preclinical data have identified a variety of chemotherapeutic agents that are positively modulated by IFN (Table 3.4), including at least one from every class of chemotherapeutic drugs: alkylating agents, mitotic spindle inhibitors, anthracyclines, heavy metals, antibiotics, antimetabolites, and steroids. (Wadler and Schwartz, 1992). This broad spectrum of activity suggests at least two possible mechanisms. Either IFN-α possesses a single fundamental action that affects nearly every aspect of cell growth and replication, or it acts at multiple levels, with different actions predominating in different cell types. In all likelihood, the predominant mechanism of action depends on the cytotoxic drug employed (Wadler and Schwartz, 1992).

One of the most exciting areas to emerge in the study of combination therapy has been the evaluation of the combination of IFN-α with 5-fluorouracil (5-FU). *In vitro* studies demonstrated that synergy was both dose and schedule dependent and was seen only when IFN-α was given before or concurrently with 5-FU (Sznol and Longo, 1993). Proposed explanations for this synergy include the ability of IFN-α to increase plasma levels of active metabolites of 5-FU, decrease resistance to

5-FU by inhibiting overexpression of thymidylate synthase, alter the cell cycle to enhance antiproliferative effects, activate the patient's immunological defense mechanisms, and induce direct but separate antiproliferative effects (Kreuser, 1992; Schuller *et al.*, 1992; Wadler and Schwartz, 1992; Wadler *et al.*, 1992; Meadows *et al.*, 1991). Initial studies by Wadler *et al.* (1989) showed a 76% rate of response to this combination in patients with colon cancer, although most responses were only partial remissions. Further clinical evaluation of this combination by Wadler and other investigators (Kemeny and Younes, 1993; Pazdur, 1992; Pazdur *et al.*, 1992; Wadler and Wiernick, 1990) demonstrated efficacy in a lower percentage of patients. (See Chapter 4.) Although the combination of 5-FU and IFN-α may represent an improvement in the treatment of colon cancer, there are many questions to be answered and problems to be resolved before optimal benefit from this combination can be achieved.

The combination of IL–2 and chemotherapy has also been evaluated. The use of low-dose cyclophosphamide to eliminate suppressor influences prior to administration of IL–2 was evaluated by Mitchell in 1992. A 26% rate of response to this combination was reported in patients with melanoma. The median survival period of responders in the study was 18 months, as compared to the historical overall survival period of 12 months in melanoma patients with recurrent disease. Although these data did not conclusively prove that the combination regimen resulted in greater longevity, there was a strong suggestion to that effect. However, one clear discovery of the study was that patients do not need to achieve a complete remission to have an increased lifespan with a good quality of life. Although the overall response rate of 26% was not better than traditional response rates to chemotherapy with dacarbazine, nitrosoureas, vindesine/vinblastine, and cisplatin alone, the suggestion of improved survival and relative lack of toxicity certainly warrants further exploration.

A large number of experiments have evaluated the combination of chemotherapy and IL–2 in animal models. In most cases, these combinations are effective only if the host immune system is intact and if the tumor is sensitive to IL–2 (i.e., immunogenic). Possible explanations of the beneficial effect of adding chemotherapy to treatment with IL–2 include modulation of the immune system as noted in the example above, alteration of the tumor-cell membrane to increase immunogenicity, and debulking of the tumor. To date, many different combinations of chemotherapy with IL–2 or IL–2 and IFN-α have been tested in the clinical setting. Results have been negative or inconclusive at best in most phase I and phase II trials. To determine if biological therapy definitely enhances the effects of chemotherapy, randomized phase III trials are necessary (Legha and Buzaid, 1993; Sznol and Longo, 1993).

Biotherapy may also be used as maintenance therapy after chemotherapy. Mandelli *et al.* (1990) evaluated the use of IFN-α as maintenance therapy in patients with multiple myeloma and found improved duration of response that translated into overall improved survival in the group that received IFN. This statistically significant advantage was seen only in patients who had achieved an objective response to induction chemotherapy. The rationale for the use of IFN-α as maintenance therapy includes its ability to reduce the capacity for self renewal in myeloma cells, its modulation of oncogene expression, and its antiproliferative activity (Cooper, 1991).

The introduction of hematopoietic growth factors to combination regimens was an attempt to use biological agents to significantly reduce the toxicity associated with chemotherapy. In general, the effectiveness of chemotherapy in treating most tumors is limited by two major problems: drug resistance and the toxic effects of the drug in normal tissues. Even though hematopoietic growth factors represent a major breakthrough in treating the problem of chemotherapy-induced myelosuppression, several problems remain. Although these agents are highly effective in amelioriation of myelosuppression, increased doses of chemotherapy may lead to other organ toxicities upon which hematopoietic growth factors have no protective effect or in which myelosuppression may not be the dose-limiting toxic effect of a chemotherapeutic agent. Also, whether more dose-intensive chemotherapy will lead to improved response and prolonged overall survival has not yet been determined. Large scale studies are needed to prove that dose-intensive therapies with hematopoietic growth factor support can be administered with acceptable toxicity and costs (Canelos and Demetri, 1993; Demetri and Griffin, 1990).

Future Issues in Combinations of Biotherapy and Chemotherapy

Although exciting results are beginning to emerge from the use of combination chemotherapy and biotherapy, many issues remain that must be addressed. Often, agents are combined solely because each has shown clinical activity in treating a given disease. A clinical trial, however, should be based on a firm preclinical rationale rather than an empirical approach. Elucidation of the mechanisms of action of BRMs and chemotherapeutic agents, as well as an understanding of mechanisms of synergism are musts in applying a rational approach to combination therapy. Refinement of dose, schedule, and route of administration will then be facilitated. The use of animal models has focused mostly on evaluating schedules, sequencing, and doses rather than on understanding the mechanisms of synergism (Parmiani and Rivoltini, 1991), and until more predictive preclinical models are available, the design of combination trials must rely partly on reasonable evaluation of preclinical data and partly on empiricism (Sznol and Longo, 1993). If heightened responses are seen, evaluation of remission rates and durability of response must be assessed through large-scale randomized trials. Future directions include targeting therapy by using monoclonal antibodies with biotherapy, chemotherapy, or radiotherapy attached and

the introduction of new hematopoietic growth factors or combinations of growth factors that can further abrogate chemotherapy-induced suppression of bone marrow. Exciting possibilities remain for the combination of very different modalities that will ultimately lead to improved patient responses, cure rates, and survival rates.

Biotherapy and Radiotherapy

Evaluation of combinations of radiotherapy and biotherapy remains at an early stage (Hallahan *et al.*, 1993). A handful of clinical trials have investigated the concomitant use of IFN-α and radiotherapy or tumor necrosis factor and radiotherapy (Devine *et al.*, 1991). One mechanism of radiation cytotoxicity is oxidative damage to DNA by ionizing radiation. *In vitro* work suggests that tumor necrosis factor cytotoxicity results from the generation of superoxide radicals or other reactive oxygen species. Work by Hallahan *et al.*, (1990) demonstrated that interaction between tumor necrosis factor and radiation is observed only when tumor necrosis factor is added several hours before irradiation. Experiments in animal models have also demonstrated that IFN-α may act as a radiosensitizer, but the mechanism of this enhanced response is unknown. A future area of study involves the use of monoclonal antibodies conjugated to radioisotopes to selectively deliver radiation to the tumor site. This form of therapy, known as radioimmunotherapy, remains in the early stages of development.

Toxicity

Toxicity remains an important issue when considering combination therapy. In theory, the use of combinations of biotherapy and chemotherapy would capitalize on the fact that these agents have essentially nonoverlapping toxic effects. Toxicities are often additive with BRMs, unless lower doses are utilized. The most common side effects of biological agents—constitutional symptoms, fatigue, anorexia, changes in mental status, reversible changes in lab values, and allergic reactions—differ significantly from those of chemotherapy (bone marrow suppression with resultant anemia, thrombocytopenia and neutropenia, nausea and vomiting, mucositis, and alopecia). Nurses caring for patients receiving combination therapies should be aware of the expected toxic effects of individual agents, and should also assess for unexpected adverse reactions. Such unexpected adverse effects seen with combinations of IFN-α and 5-FU include increased incidence and severity of mucositis, diarrhea, neurotoxicity (dependent on patient age and degree of liver involvement), and prolonged granulocytopenia (Kemeny and Younes, 1992; Pazdur, 1992). With combinations of IFN-α and IL–2 major treatment-limiting toxic effects were neurologic (e.g., confusion) gastrointestinal (e.g., nausea and vomiting), and fatigue (Figlin, 1992; Rosenberg *et al.*, 1989).

OUTCOMES OF THERAPY

The final area to consider with respect to dosing in biotherapy is determination of the outcome of therapy. An essential component of determining the appropriate dose of a drug is determining how long therapy should be administered. This decision ultimately hinges on measurement of a clinical response. As we gain sophistication in the use of biological agents and as successes are seen in various disorders, questions of when to stop therapy will arise. In some diseases, achieving a complete response is the desired goal, whereas in other situations, it may be argued that stabilizing disease with improved quality of life is an appropriate goal (Mitchell, 1992). Typically, the time period required to achieve responses with BRMs is longer than that required with chemotherapy; hence, caution must be exercised to avoid halting therapy prematurely.

For many diseases, technology has changed the way response to therapy is evaluated. Patients with chronic myelogenous leukemia provide an interesting illustration

of technology's role in changing the definition of response and ultimately of cure in certain diseases. Traditionally, hematologic remission (normalization of peripheral blood counts) was used as the bench mark for evaluating response. Cytogenetic analysis now provides a more precise determination of when therapy should be discontinued. The use of **cytogenetics**, the study of cytology in relation to **genetics**, to measure response in patients with this disease facilitated a more accurate determination of complete response.

Cytogenetics specifically looks at the behavior of **chromosomes** during **mitosis** and **meiosis** (Heim and Mitelman, 1987). Bone marrow smears of the majority of patients with chronic myelogenous leukemia exhibit the **Philadelphia chromosome**, a shortened chromosome number 22, as a marker for this disease. The classic Philadelphia (Ph[1]) chromosome results from a **translocation** between chromosomes 9 and 22, which results in the production of a new protein (Kurzrock, 1988). Interferon-alpha, which is used to treat patients with chronic myelogenous leukemia, has demonstrated the ability to suppress the Philadelphia chromosome in some patients (Talpaz *et al.*, 1991). The degree of disappearance of the Philadelphia chromosome from the bone marrow is now used to determine response. Technology has progressed even further with the introduction of molecular analysis. This technique, which involves the use of molecular probes that can identify the altered gene produced in the translocation, can be used to monitor therapies even more precisely. Molecular analysis provides for the evaluation of both dividing and nondividing cells and detects minute amounts of the Philadelphia chromosome in patients (Yoffe, 1987). For example, a patient who shows a complete disappearance of the Philadelphia chromosome by cytogenetic analysis may still exhibit a small amount of disease with this new technique.

Although cure is generally the desired goal, with many BRMs only partial or minor responses are seen. In a small percentage of these patients, however, disease may remain stable or quiescent for long periods of time. If stabilization of disease and improved quality of life were valued as a desired therapeutic goal, then less sophisticated means of determining response could be used to evaluate response. Measurement of quality of life, an active focus in oncology research (Till, 1992), can also be used to evaluate the outcome of therapy in conjunction with more traditional diagnostic tests.

SUMMARY

The issue of attaining the optimal biological dose (OBD) is complex, and at this point there are more questions than answers. Determination of the OBD often appears insurmountable because of the complexity of biological proteins. Indeed, an OBD must be determined not only for each agent but also for each disease that agent may be used for.

Parameters crucial to immune function must be identified and measured so that pertinent mechanisms of response for a given disease can be identified (Osband and Ross, 1990). With IFN-α pinpointing whether the antiproliferative effect or the immunomodulatory effect is most dominant will determine optimum dose. Doses are generally much higher when antiproliferative effects are desired. Basic knowledge about the pathophysiology of the disease, tumor antigenicity, the pleiotropic mechanisms of host defenses, the mode of action of a BRM, and the dynamic status of these defenses must be improved so that therapy may be more selectively applied. Furthermore, "each sick patient is immunologically deficient in his or her own way" (Osband and Ross, 1990), and if factors predictive of response were identified, they could be used to target therapy to individual patients most likely to respond.

An ideal phase I biotherapy study would thus include determining an agent's bioavailability, pharmacokinetic properties, biological response, and toxicity all in the context of escalating doses and with a dose-response

curve to be assessed for each property (Oldham, 1991; Osband and Ross, 1990). Creekmore et al. (1991) have suggested the development of a two tiered phase I trial: phase Ia to determine MTD and phase Ib to determine the optimal dose for achieving the desired biological effect(s). As previously discussed, the desired biological response and MTD of a biological agent may occur at different doses.

In the development of BRMs, patient selection, dose escalation, measurement of biological effect, determination of optimal dose and route of administration will need to be assessed differently than for chemotherapeutic agents. The question of the amount of tumor burden as it relates to patient selection remains an issue. Because certain kinds of BRMs may work only in a specific patient population, more selectivity in patient eligibility may be required. Such selectivity is now required to a certain extent for studies involving monoclonal antibodies, and it may need to be instituted for other BRMs as well. Determining the underlying pathophysiology of a disease will allow for the more rational selection of a BRM or combination of agents in treating a given disease. Dose escalation studies are traditionally conducted with successive groups of patients receiving higher doses. For BRMs, however, dose escalation may need to occur for each patient. With natural body proteins, toxic effects are not expected to be as severe as with chemotherapy drugs. For studies with a given patient, we should be able to increase doses without the fear of excess toxicity. The dose and route of administration should be determined by pharmacokinetics, as well as by biological effects. The desired antitumor effect to be stimulated should also be considered. One may argue, for example, that a serum concentration may not even be necessary to have a biological effect (Kelso, 1989); perhaps it is more important that secondary messengers be set in motion by the biological agent. These same principles apply for the rational design of combination therapies. Although exciting results are beginning to emerge from clinical studies, a great deal remains to be learned about designing effective combinations. Determination of underlying mechanisms of action will provide the cornerstone for designing these combinations.

Determination of when to stop therapy can be viewed from two sides. To cure a patient, obtaining a complete remission must be the ultimate goal. Biotherapy is often regarded as less than desirable because few complete remissions (CRs) are obtained with biological agents. However, could stable disease be viewed as a desirable end point? In cases where the course of disease is slowed or quiescent, is this not a potentially valuable goal? With diseases in which biological therapy has shown efficacy, technology is beginning to provide the capability to more precisely measure responses. With these advances, the selection of end points for determining the clinical usefulness of BRMs may need to be re-evaluated.

The ultimate role of biotherapy in the treatment of cancer remains uncertain. Determination of the appropriate dose and schedule in treating a given disease and determination of rational combination therapies lie at the core of this challenge.

References

Aulitzky, W., Gastl, G., Aulitzky W., *et al.* 1989. Successful treatment of metastatic renal cell carcinoma with a biologically active dose of recombinant interferon-gamma. *Journal of Clinical Oncology* 7(12): 1875–1884.

Balkwill, F. 1989. Interferons. In Balkwill, F. (ed). *Cytokines in Cancer Therapy*. Oxford: Oxford University Press, pp. 8–53.

Balkwill, F., and Burke, R. 1989. The cytokine network. *Immunology Today* 10(9): 299–304.

Benet, L., Mitchell, J., and Sheiner L. 1990. Pharmacokinetics: The dynamics of drug absorption, distribution, and elimination. In Gilman, A., Rall, T., Nies, A., and Taylor, P. (eds). *The Pharmacological Basis of Therapeutics* 8th ed. New York: Pergamon Press, pp. 3–32.

Borden, E., Paulnock, D., Spear, G., *et al.* 1987. Biological response modification in man: Measurement of interferon-induced proteins. In Baron, S., Dianzani, F., Stanton, G., and Fleischmann, W. (eds). *The Interferon System: A Current Review to 1987*. Austin, Texas: University of Texas Press, pp 423–429.

Canellos, G., and Demetri, G. 1993. Myelosuppression and "conventional" chemotherapy: What price, what benefit? *Journal of Clinical Oncology* 11(1): 1–2.

Cebon, J., Dempsey, P., Fox, R., *et al.* 1988. Pharmacokinetics of human granulocyte-macrophage colony-stimulating factor using a sensitive immunoassay. *Blood* 72(4): 1340–1347.

Cooper, R. 1991. A review of the clinical studies of alpha-interferon in the management of multiple myeloma. *Seminars in Oncology* 18(5) (Suppl 7): 18–29.

Creekmore, S., Longo, D., and Urba, W. 1991. Principles of the clinical evaluation of biologic agents. In DeVita, V., Hellman, S., and Rosenberg, S. (eds). *Biologic Therapy of Cancer*. Philadelphia: J.B. Lippincott Co., pp. 67–86.

Demetri, G., and Griffin, J. 1990. Hematopoietic growth factors and high-dose chemotherapy: Will grams succeed where milligrams fail? *Journal of Clinical Oncology* 8(5): 761–764.

Devine, S., Vokes, E., and Weichselbaum, R. 1991. Chemotherapeutic and biologic radiation enhancement. *Current Opinion in Oncology* 3: 1087–1095.

Figlin, R., Bellegrun, A., Moldawer, N., *et al.* 1992. Concomitant administration of recombinant human interleukin-2 and recombinant interferon alfa-2a: An active outpatient regimen in metastatic renal cell carcinoma. *Journal of Clinical Oncology* 10(3): 414–421.

Gilewski, T., and Golomb, H. 1990. Design of combination biotherapy studies: Future goals and challenges. *Seminars in Oncology* 17(1) (Suppl 1): 3–10.

Gutterman, J., Fine, S., Quesada, J., *et al.* 1982. Recombinant leukocyte A interferon: Pharmacokinetics, single-dose tolerance, and biologic effects in cancer patients. *Annals of Internal Medicine* 96: 549–555.

Hallahan, D., Haimovitz-Friedman, A., Kute, D., *et al.*, 1993. The role of cytokines in radiation oncology. In DeVita, V., Hellman, S., and Rosenberg, S. (eds). *Important Advances in Oncology*. Philadelphia: J.B. Lippincott Co., pp. 71–81.

Hallahan, D., Beckett, M., Kuff, D., *et al.* 1990. The interaction between recombinant human tumor necrosis factor and radiation in 13 human tumor cell lines. *International Journal of Radiation Oncology Biology Physics* 19: 69–74.

Heim, S., and Mitelman, F. 1987. *Cancer Cytogenetics*. New York: Alan R. Liss, Inc.

Huber, C., and Herold, M. 1989. The importance of patient monitoring in clinical cytokine trials: Use of serum markers to define biologically active doses. *Cancer Surveys* 8(4): 809–815.

Janik, J., Kopp, W., Smith II, J., *et al.* 1993. Dose-related immunologic effects of levamisole in patients with cancer. *Journal of Clinical Oncology* 11(1): 125–135.

Kelso, A. 1989. Cytokines: Structure, function and synthesis. *Current Opinion in Immunology* 2: 215–225.

Kemeny, N., and Younes, A. 1992. Alfa-2a interferon and 5-fluorouracil for advanced colorectal carcinoma: The

Memorial Sloan-Kettering Experience. *Seminars in Oncology* 19(2) (Suppl 3): 171–175.

Kreuser, E., Wadler, S., and Thiel, E. 1992. Interactions between cytokines and cytotoxic drugs: Putative molecular mechanisms in experimental hematology and oncology. *Seminars in Oncology* 19(2) (Suppl 4): 1–7.

Kuhn, M. 1991. The phases of drug action. In Kuhn, M. (ed). *Pharmacotherapeutics: A Nursing Process Approach.* 2nd ed. Philadelphia: F.A. Davis Co., pp. 69–87.

Kurzrock, R., Gutterman, J., and Talpaz, M. 1988. The molecular genetics of Philadelphia chromosome-positive leukemias. *New England Journal of Medicine* 319: 990–998.

Kurzrock, R., Talpaz, M., Gomez, J. *et al.* 1991. Differential dose-related haematologic effects of GM-CSF in pancytopenia: Evidence supporting the advantage of low-over high-dose administration in selected patients. *British Journal of Haematology* 78: 352–358.

Legha, S., and Buzaid, A. 1993. Role of recombinant interleukin-2 in combination with interferon-alfa and chemotherapy in the treatment of advanced melanoma. *Seminars in Oncology* 20(6) (Suppl 9): 27–32.

Mäas, R., Dullens, H., and Otter, W. 1993. Interleukin–2 in cancer treatment: Disappointing or (still) promising? A review. *Cancer Immunology and Immunotherapy* 36: 141–148.

Mandelli, F., Avvisati, G., Madori, S., *et al.* 1990. Maintenance treatment with recombinant interferon alfa–2B in patients with multiple myeloma responding to conventional induction chemotherapy. *New England Journal of Medicine* 322(20): 1430–1434.

Meadows, L., Walther, P., and Ozer, H. 1991. Alpha-interferon and 5-fluorouracil: Possible mechanisms of antitumor action. *Seminars in Oncology* 18(5) (Suppl 7): 71–76.

Metcalf, D. 1990. The colony-stimulating factors: Discovery, development and clinical applications. *Cancer* 5(10): 2185–2195.

Mihich, E. 1987. Modulation of antitumor immune responses. *Cancer Detection and Prevention* (Suppl 1): 399–407.

Mitchell, M. 1992. Chemotherapy in combination with biomodulation: A 5-year experience with cyclophosphamide and interleukin–2. *Seminars in Oncology* 19(2)(Suppl 4): 80–87.

Mitchell, M. 1988. Combining chemotherapy with biological response modifiers in treatment of cancer. *Journal of the National Cancer Institute* 80: 1445–1450.

Moertel, C., Fleming, T., MacDonald, J., *et al.* 1990. Levamisole and fluorouracil for adjuvant therapy of resected colon carcinoma. *New England Journal of Medicine* 322: 352–358.

Morstyn, G., Lieschke, G., Sheridan, W., *et al.* 1989. Pharmacology of the colony-stimulating factors. *Trends in Pharmacological Sciences* 10: 154–159.

Mulé, J., and Rosenberg, S. 1991. Combination cytokine therapy: Experimental and clinical trials. In DeVita, V.,

Hellman, S., and Rosenberg, S. (eds). *Biologic Therapy of Cancer.* Philadelphia: J.B. Lippincott Co., pp. 393–416.

Mulé, J., and Rosenberg, S. 1989. Immunotherapy with lymphokine combinations. In DeVita, V., Hellman, S., and Rosenberg, S. (eds). *Important Advances in Oncology.* Philadelphia: J.B. Lippincott Co., pp. 99–126.

Oldham, R. 1991. Developmental therapeutics and the design of clinical trials. In Oldham, R. (ed). *Principles of Cancer Biotherapy* 2nd ed. New York: Marcel Dekker, pp. 49–63.

Osband, M., and Ross, S. 1990. Problems in the investigational study and clinical use of cancer immunotherapy. *Immunology Today* 11: 193–195.

Parmiani, G., and Rivoltini, L. 1991. Biologic agents as modifiers of chemotherapeutic effects. *Current Opinion in Oncology* 3: 1078–1086.

Pazdur, R. 1992. Combination of fluorouracil and interferon: Mechanisms of interaction and clinical studies. In Holdstein, A., and Garaci, E. (eds). *Combination Therapies.* New York: Plenum Publishing Corp., pp.73–78.

Pazdur, R., Moore, D., and Bready, B. 1992. Modulation of fluorouracil with recombinant alfa interferon: M.D. Anderson clinical trial. *Seminars in Oncology* 19(2) (Suppl 3): 176–179.

Peters, W., Stuart, A., Affronti, M., *et al.* 1988. Neutrophil migration is defective during recombinant human granulocyte-macrophage colony-stimulating factor infusion after autologous bone marrow transplantation in humans. *Blood* 72: 1310–1315.

Quirt, J., Shelley, W., Pater, J., *et al.* 1991. Improved survival in patients with poor-prognosis malignant melanoma treated with adjuvant levamisole: a phase III study by the National Cancer Institute of Canada clinical trials group. *Journal of Clinical Oncology* 9: 729–735.

Rosenberg, S., Lotze, M., Yang, J., *et al.* 1989. Combination therapy with interleukin–2 and alpha-interferon for the treatment of patients with advanced cancer. *Journal of Clinical Oncology* 7(12): 1863–1874.

Ross, E. 1990. Pharmacodynamics: Mechanisms of drug action and the relationship between drug concentration and effect. In Gilman, A., Rall, T., Nies, A., and Taylor, P. (eds). *The Pharmacological Basis of Therapeutics* 8th ed. New York: Pergamon Press, Inc., pp. 33–48.

Schmoll, H., Hiddemann, W., Rustum, Y., *et al.* 1992. Introduction: The emerging role for biomodulation of antineoplastic agents. *Seminars in Oncology* 19(2) (Suppl 3): 1–3.

Schuller, J., Czejka, M., Schernthaner, G., *et al.* 1992. Influence of interferon alfa–2b with or without folinic acid on pharmacokinetics of fluorouracil. *Seminars in Oncology* 19(2) (Suppl 3): 93–97.

Seeber, S. 1992. Combining cytokines and cytotoxic drugs in the treatment of cancer: Summary and outlook. *Seminars in Oncology* 19(2) (Suppl 4): 102–103.

Sporn, M. and Roberts, A. 1988. Peptide growth factors are multifunctional. *Nature* 332: 217–219.

Sznol, M. and Longo, D. 1993. Chemotherapy drug interactions with biological agents. *Seminars in Oncology* 20(1): 80–93.

Talmadge, J. 1992. Development of immunotherapeutic strategies for the treatment of malignant neoplasms. *Biotherapy* 4(3): 215–236.

Talpaz, M., Kantarjian H., Kurzrock R., *et al.* 1991. Interferon-alpha produces sustained cytogenetic responses in chronic myelogenous leukemia. *Annals of Internal Medicine* 114: 532–538.

Vadhan-Raj, S., Broxmeyer, H., Hittelman, W., *et al.* 1992. Abrogating chemotherapy-induced myelosuppression by recombinant granulocyte-macrophage colony-stimulating factor in patients with sarcoma: Protection at the progenitor cell level. *Journal of Clinical Oncology* 10(8):1266–1277.

Vadhan-Raj, S., Buescher, S., LeMaistre, A., *et al.* 1988. Stimulation of hematopoiesis in patients with bone marrow failure and in patients with malignancy by recombinant human granulocyte-macrophage colony-stimulating factor. *Blood* 72(1): 134–141.

Wadler, S., and Schwartz, E. 1992. Principles in the biomodulation of cytotoxic drugs by interferons. *Seminars in Oncology* 19(2) (Suppl 3): 45–48.

Wadler, S., and Schwartz, E. 1990. Antineoplastic activity of the combination of interferon and cytotoxic agents against experimental and human malignancies: a review. *Cancer Research* 50: 3473–3486.

Wadler, S., Schwartz, E., Goldman, M., *et al.* 1989. Fluorouracil and recombinant alfa–2a-interferon: an active regimen against advanced colorectal carcinoma. *Journal of Clinical Oncology* 7(12): 1769–1775.

Wadler, S., and Wiernik, P. 1990. Clinical update on the role of fluorouracil and recombinant interferon alfa–2a in the treatment of colorectal carcinoma. *Seminars in Oncology* 17: 16–21.

Wiernik, P. 1989. Neutrophil function in infection. *Mediguide to Infectious diseases* 9(1): 1–8.

Yoffe, G., Blick, M., Kantarjian, H., *et al.* 1987. Molecular analysis of interferon-induced suppression of Philadelphia chromosome in patients with chronic myeloid leukemia. *Blood* 69(3): 961–963.

PART 2

Major Categories of Biological Agents

CHAPTER 4 | The Interferons

Nancy P. Moldawer, RN, MSN

Robert A. Figlin, MD, FACP

It has been known since the early 1930s that cells infected with viruses are capable of protecting other cells from viral infection. In 1957, Isaacs and Lindenmann discovered the protein that partially explained this phenomenon and named it interferon (IFN) (Isaacs and Lindenmann, 1957). Within a few years, the antiproliferative and immunomodulatory cellular effects of this molecule had been identified. It is now known that there are three major species of IFN: alpha (a), beta (b), and gamma (g). In the early 1970s, Cantell and co-workers developed techniques for purifying IFN-a from donated human blood (Cantell *et al.*, 1975). Although this method proved to be costly and time consuming and resulted in an impure product, it instigated the testing of this molecule as an antitumor agent. At the same time, the birth of the biotechnology industry and, more specifically, recombinant DNA technology, allowed the production of highly purified IFN mole-

cules; in 1981, human clinical trials with recombinant IFN-a began.

In 1986, just a few years after its introduction as an anticancer agent, IFN-a was approved by the Food and Drug Administration (FDA) for its significant role in the treatment of hairy cell leukemia. Shortly thereafter, in 1989, IFN-a received its second FDA approval for the treatment of AIDS-related Kaposi's sarcoma. In the United States, IFN has been approved by the FDA for the treatment of six different diseases (Table 4.1). Two of these are viral diseases: condyloma acuminatum (genital warts) and non-A, non-B/C hepatitis, and hepatitis B. A third, chronic granulomatous disease, is an inherited immune disease characterized by severe, recurrent infections of the skin, lymph nodes, liver, lungs, and bone. Because treatment with IFN-g led to a 70% reduction of serious infections in patients with this disease (Gallin *et al.*, 1991), this agent was approved in 1990.

Table 4.1 Indication for interferon therapy approved by the FDA

Disease	Agent
Hairy cell leukemia	IFN-α
Kaposi's sarcoma in AIDS	IFN-α
Non-A, non-B/C hepatitis	IFN-α
Hepatitis B	IFN-α
Condyloma acuminatum	IFN-α
Multiple sclerosis	IFN-β
Chronic granulomatous disease	IFN-γ

In 1993, IFN-β was approved for the treatment of multiple sclerosis. Moreover, IFNs are now licensed in more than 40 countries for at least a dozen therapeutic indications of viral or neoplastic origin.

Today, the IFNs are referred to as the prototype biological agent and have undergone the most intensive molecular, preclinical, and investigational scrutiny. Interferon therapy has an established role in the treatment of several advanced malignancies. Numerous phase II and phase III trials have demonstrated its efficacy, and additional studies have shown its ability to induce responses in refractory neoplasms, to modify chromosomal disorders in chronic myelogenous leukemia, and more recently, to modulate the activity of cytotoxic, biological, and differentiating agents.

This chapter will focus on the role of IFN treatment in the 1990s and highlight possible future applications of this molecule in cancer treatment.

BIOLOGICAL ACTIVITY

The IFN family comprises a very complex set of proteins and glycoproteins. Because of this heterogeneity, it is not surprising that several attempts have been made to classify these agents.

Three major species of human IFN are recognized and designated IFN-α, IFN-β, and IFN-γ (Stewart *et al.*, 1980). IFN-α is produced by leukocytes (B cells, T cells, null cells, and macrophages) after exposure to B cell antigens, viruses, foreign cells, or tumor cells. In-terferon-β is produced by fibroblasts after exposure to viruses or foreign nucleic acids. Interferon-γ often called "immune interferon," is produced by T lymphocytes after stimulation with T-cell mitogens, specific antigens, or interleukin–2 (Fleischmann *et al.*, 1984). (See Table 4.2.)

The genes known to encode for IFN-α have been assigned to chromosome 9; 16 distinct protein sequences for IFN-α have been described (Sehgal, 1982). Only a single protein species apiece has been identified for both IFN-β and -γ (Borden, 1984).

Antiviral Effects

The IFNs have very high antiviral specific activity and are protective against both DNA and RNA viruses (Samuel, 1988). When a cell is infected with a virus, it synthesizes and releases interferon into the extracellular space. The IFN then binds to receptors on other cells and is internalized. The IFN-induced cells then produce several enzymes that can regulate the process of viral protein synthesis. The two best studied of these enzymes are 2′-5′-oligoadenylate synthetase and a protein kinase. Indirectly, the IFNs may mediate antiviral effects by stimulating cytotoxic T lymphocytes to lyse virally infected cells.

Intercellular Protein Changes

The effect of IFN at the cellular level is initiated by the IFN molecule binding to a cell-surface membrane receptor (Pestka, 1983). Competitive binding studies indicate that IFN-α and -β interact with one cell surface receptor, whereas IFN-γ interacts with a different receptor (Williams, 1983). After binding to the cell-surface membrane, human IFN is rapidly internalized and degraded (Feinstein *et al.*, 1985). The anticancer activity of IFN probably results from a number of different mechanisms, including induction of intracellular proteins, enhancement of immune effector cells, and changes in cellular surface structures. Two enzymes appear to play major

Table 4.2   Interferon types in clinical use

Type	Subtype	Manufacturer
Alpha (α)	Recombinant alpha-A (IFN alpha-2a) Roferon®-A	Hoffmann-La Roche
	Recombinant alpha-2 (IFN alpha-2b) Intron®-A	Schering-Plough
	Lymphoblastoid (IFN alpha-N1) Wellferon®	Burroughs Wellcome
Beta (β)	Recombinant beta ser-17 (IFN beta-1b) Betaseron®	Chiron Corporation–Manufacturer Birlex Laboratories–Distributor
Gamma (γ)	Recombinant gamma (IFN gamma) Actimmune®	Genentech

roles in IFN activity. Exposure of cells in culture to IFN results in an increase in production of the enzyme 2′-5′-oligoadenylate synthetase (Ball, 1982; Bale, 1979). This enzyme, which can affect RNA transcription and translation, may ultimately inhibit protein and DNA synthesis in both normal and neoplastic cells (Revel *et al.*, 1980). The second class of enzymes activated by IFN is the protein kinases. Protein kinase activation inhibits peptide chain initiation. The exact relationship of these observations to IFN's anti-cancer activity remains undetermined.

ANTIPROLIFERATIVE EFFECTS

Interferon-α has antiproliferative effects on some malignant tumor cells. *In vitro* inhibition of hematologic tumors by IFN-α has been observed in Burkitt's lymphoma, lymphocytic lymphoma, acute myelogenous leukemia, chronic myelogenous leukemia, chronic lymphocytic leukemia, and multiple myeloma (Denz *et al.*, 1985; Salmon *et al.*, 1983; Borden *et al.*, 1982; Chadha and Srivastava, 1981; Balkwill and Oliver, 1977). Other studies have suggested that IFN-α has a greater inhibitory effect on cells of hematopoietic origin than either IFN-β or -γ. What's more, non-dividing tumor cells (Cell cycle phases G_0 and G_1)

appear to have increased sensitivity to the antiproliferative activity of human IFN (Creasey *et al.*, 1980; Horoszewicz *et al.*, 1979). That there is a direct antiproliferative effect is supported by studies of transplanted human tumors in immunodeficient nude mice in which the immunomodulatory effects of IFN are minimal. A dose-dependent inhibition of growth is observed in these models, but it lasts only for the duration of IFN exposure (Balkwill *et al.*, 1982; Yoshitake *et al.*, 1976).

Immunomodulatory Activity

The anticancer effects of IFN have been attributed to several of its immunomodulatory activities, but the most relevant appears to be its effects on natural killer (NK) cells and macrophages. *In vitro* work shows that IFN increases the killing potential of NK cells by recruiting pre-NK cells and enhancing the cytotoxic activity of activated NK cells. In clinical trials, both the dose and route of IFN administration have been shown to affect NK cell activity significantly. Lower dosages of IFN seem to result in greater NK cell activity. IFN-γ appears to enhance the activity of macrophages more than IFN-α or -β.

Another mechanism whereby IFN may exert its antitumor activity is by its effects on

Table 4.3 Clinical activity of interferon in hematologic malignancies

| | Treatment | | In Combination with | | |
| | | | | | |
Indications	Single Agent	Adjuvant	Biological Response Modifier	Chemotherapy	Other
Hairy cell leukemia	✓				
Chronic myelogenous leukemia	✓			*	BMT*
Non-Hodgkins lymphoma					
Low grade	✓	or as maintenance*		✓	
Intermediate grade/high grade	*			*	
T-cell lymphoma	✓				Phototherapy*
Multiple myeloma	✓	maintenance, adjuvant after BMT*		*	

  * = considered experimental
  ✓ = studies support indications
BMT = Bone Marrow Transplant

oncogene expression. It is now believed that the neoplastic transformation of normal cells to malignant cells is regulated by the expression of cellular oncogenes. In small clinical trials, treatment with IFN has been shown to be associated with significant decreases in oncogene expression.

CLINICAL EXPERIENCE— INTERFERON-ALPHA

Hematologic Malignancies and Lymphomas

Table 4.3 summarizes the uses of IFNs in hematologic malignancies and lymphomas.

Hairy Cell Leukemia

Hairy cell leukemia (HCL) is a rare, chronic lymphoproliferative disorder that typically affects middle-aged men. It has characteristic clinical features that include splenomegaly, pancytopenia, and the presence of distinctive irregular projections on lymphoid cells in the bone marrow, peripheral blood, and reticuloendothelial system.

Since 1958, when the disease was initially described (Bouroncle et al., 1958), splenectomy has been the treatment of choice. This treatment has effectively reversed severely depressed blood counts, and these remissions can last up to several years. However, because this approach does not address the bone marrow involvement of this disease, the majority of patients experience relapse. In 1984, IFN was introduced as a treatment for HCL by Quesada et al., (1984). In their initial study, seven patients with progressive disease were treated with daily intramuscular doses of 3 million international units (MIU) of partially purified IFN-α. Peripheral blood counts normalized in all patients. The authors' report of three complete remissions and four partial remissions was based on bone marrow examination (defined as hairy cells absent from bone marrow). During the 1980s, multiple clinical trials utilized IFN in comparable dosing regimens consisting of 3 to 6 MIU administered intramuscularly or subcutaneously; the results were similar to those of the first trial (Berman et al., 1990; Lauria et al., 1988; Ratain et al., 1988; Skotnicki et al., 1988; Golomb et al., 1987; Foon et al., 1986; Quesada et al., 1986; Hagberg et al., 1985; Jacobs et al., 1985).

In general, treatment of HCL with IFN leads to a high overall response rate (80%) with normalization of peripheral blood counts, but few complete bone marrow remissions (<5%). Interferon treatment for HCL generally lasts about 12 months, and at these doses patients experience only minor toxic effects. The high frequency of beneficial responses led to approval by the FDA of IFN-α for treatment of HCL in 1986.

The treatment of HCL with IFN-α has recently been challenged by the development of newer drugs. Pentostatin, or 2'-deoxycoformycin (DCF), exerts its biological activity by inhibiting the enzyme adenosine deaminase, and was reported by Spiers et al. in 1984 to have clinical activity in HCL. Subsequent trials of this drug have demonstrated that it yields a higher percentage of complete remissions than IFN-α with excellent durability of response. Trials have been conducted to compare its effectiveness with that of IFN-α. This drug has also been demonstrated to be non-cross-resistant with IFN and to be effective in HCL patients who are unresponsive to IFN. Two recently published studies have evaluated a regimen of alternating cycles of pentostatin and IFN (Habermann et al., 1990; Martin et al., 1990). Because of evidence that IFN-α and DCF are clinically non cross-resistant and that patients who do not respond to IFN-α may respond to DCF, Martin et al. studied their combination (1990). The rate of improvement in peripheral blood counts was comparable to that for single-agent DCF (Johnston et al., 1988) and more rapid than responses to IFN alone (Foon et al., 1986, Golomb et al., 1986; Quesada et al., 1984). In contrast to other reports, no patient who received the combination achieved a pathologic complete remission. This may have been due in part to the study's frequent sampling of bone marrow, allowing detection of minimal residual disease. Pentostatin (Nipent®) is now approved by the FDA for the treatment of IFN-α-refractory HCL (Physician's Desk Reference, 1994).

Cladribine, or 2-CdA, is a second drug evaluated in the treatment of HCL. This drug is a chlorinated purine nucleoside resistant to degradation by adenosine deaminase. Once administered, a resultant accumulation of 2-CdA nucleotides occurs in cells with high levels of deoxycytidine kinase to 5'-nucleotidase activity (e.g., lymphocytes and monocytes). Within the cell, 2-CdA is metabolized into a triphosphate derivative that ultimately causes cell death. Initial investigations with 2-CdA in 12 patients with HCL found a marked response (eleven CRs and one PR) with a single 7-day course. Subsequent studies confirm the efficacy of this agent in the treatment of HCL (Estey et al., 1992; Tallman et al., 1992). In 1993, the FDA approved cladribine (Leustatin®) for the treatment of HCL (Physician's Desk Reference, 1994).

Thus, there are several proven effective and durable therapies for HCL, although none are considered curative. Several questions remain unanswered in the efforts to identify a curative treatment for HCL. Splenectomy, the mainstay of therapy for HCL, has been replaced by treatment with IFN, DCF, and cladribine. The Southwest Oncology Group–Intergroup study (SWOG No. 8694) is currently randomizing patients to receive DCF or IFN-α. These studies will determine the relative efficacy and toxicity of these two agents as well as their effects on survival and quality of life. The advantages of pentostatin or cladribine therapy over IFN (Golomb et al., 1992) are the shorter duration of therapy than required with IFN-α therapy and an improved rate of complete response. Phase III trials are underway in patients with newly diagnosed HCL who are randomly assigned to undergo splenectomy or receive IFN-α therapy.

Myeloproliferative Disorders

Chronic Myelogenous Leukemia Chronic myelogenous leukemia (CML) is a disorder characterized by a cytogenic abnormality, namely, reciprocal translocation between chromosomes 9 and 22.

The disease occurs in three phases: a chronic phase that is characterized by an increased number of granulocytes with normal cellular maturation; an accelerated phase, although vaguely defined, characterized by increased peripheral blasts and basophils; and an acute phase, known as the blastic phase, with impaired maturation and characterized by more than 30% blasts in the marrow or peripheral blood . Blastic transformation precedes the onset of acute leukemia and is uniformly fatal (Kantarjian et al., 1993).

The traditional treatment approach in patients in the chronic phase has been with single-agent hydroxyurea or busulfan. These agents have extended median survival to 30 to 40 months, but neither of these agents suppresses the positive Philadelphia (Ph[1]) chromosome, nor prevents the progression to blast crisis. Aggressive combination chemotherapy has had only a modest effect on the survival rate of patients with CML (Kantarjian et al., 1985; Koeffler and Golde, 1981). Transplantation with allogeneic bone marrow has produced encouraging results, but only in the small fraction of patients for whom human leukocyte antigen (HLA)-identical bone marrow can be found (McGlave et al., 1984; Speck et al., 1984).

Use of recombinant IFN-α in the treatment of CML was first reported by Talpaz et al. (1986). In this study, recombinant IFN-α was given to 17 patients at 5 MIU/m² of body surface area intramuscularly each day. This regimen was effective in inducing hematologic remissions in 14 patients with early, benign phase, Ph[1] CML. Eight patients with hematologic remission had accompanying cytogenetic improvement. When this trial, which was conducted at the University of Texas M. D. Anderson Cancer Center, Houston, Texas, was expanded, hematologic complete remission (normalization of blood counts) was achieved in 71% of CML patients (Talpaz et al., 1987).

Several U.S. and European trials have confirmed these initial findings and more than 350 patients with CML have been entered in one of several IFN-α trials. The Ph[1] chromosome has been suppressed to varying degrees in 35%–40% of these individuals.

Interferon dosages required to produce these responses are moderate and cause mild to moderately severe side effects in treated patients. Treatment duration is prolonged with a median time to response of 12 months. Studies of combinations of IFN with concomitant chemotherapeutic agents such as hydroxyurea or cytarabine are ongoing; preliminary results suggest that these combinations yield cytogenetic response rates higher than those produced by IFN alone, although this remains to be confirmed (Kantarjian et al., 1992; Talpaz et al., 1992). Although many issues remain to be defined, a number of general statements can be made regarding IFN-α therapy in CML. Unlike conventional chemotherapy, IFN produces frequent (35%–45%) and sustained suppression of the Ph[1] chromosome. These data are encouraging, but whether these results translate into an extended chronic phase, delayed emergence of blastic transformation, or prolonged survival is still under investigation.

The Italian Cooperative Study Group recently reported the results of a randomized trial in which IFN-α–2a was compared to hydroxyurea (conventional therapy) in over 300 nonblastic, Ph[1] patients with CML (Italian Cooperative Study Group on Chronic Myeloid Leukemia, 1994). During the initial 14 months of therapy, patients in both treatment arms demonstrated identical hematologic responses. Since that time, patients in the IFN group have shown less transformation to blast crisis, a greater number of cytogenetic responses, and prolonged remission duration and survival: 87% of the IFN patients are alive after five years, whereas 40% of the chemotherapy group are alive.

Essential Thrombocythemia and Polycythemia Vera Because the condition of thrombocytopenia appears to be relieved in patients with CML treated with IFN, investigators have treated patients with other myeloproliferative disorders, such as essential thrombocythemia with IFN on the assumption that IFN might have the same cytoreductive properties in this disorder. Essential thrombocythemia is a myeloproliferative disorder characterized by an increase in the number of circulating platelets. Most of the clinical morbidity associated with this disease comprises bleeding and thrombosis. As recently summarized (Schiffer, 1991; Silver, 1990; Giles *et al.*, 1988), in doses lower than those required to produce the cytogenetic effects seen in CML, IFN effectively reduces platelet counts in patients with essential thrombocythemia. Similarly, IFN has been investigated in the treatment of polycythemia vera, a condition characterized by deranged growth of various components of the myeloid system, especially excessive production of red blood cells. Patients treated with IFN had reductions both in the number of phlebotomies required and in platelet counts. Dose regimens of 3 to 5 MIU/m² three times weekly are well tolerated. Patients with these disorders survive for long periods with their disease, but it is unlikely that they will be able to tolerate IFN for a prolonged period. However, IFN therapy may offer some benefit to certain patients during certain phases of their disease.

B-Cell Malignancies

Multiple Myeloma Although multiple myeloma, a disease characterized by uncontrolled proliferation of malignant plasma cells, responds initially to a variety of chemotherapeutic agents, once it becomes refractory to first-line therapies, further responses and prolonged survival are difficult to achieve. Early clinical trials demonstrated that single-agent IFN therapy can affect the level of abnormal serum proteins and can modify the course of the disease in some patients. As a result, several strategies for the use of IFN have been employed in the treatment of multiple myeloma. As a single agent, recombinant IFN-α demonstrates response rates of 10%–20% in previously treated patients with

multiple myelomas and 50% in previously untreated patients (Oken *et al.*, 1990; Quesada *et al.*, 1986; Costanzi *et al.*, 1985). Although occasional long-term remissions have been seen, IFN-α does not have a meaningful impact on the overall management of myeloma patients when used as a single agent. However, recent prospective randomized studies using IFN-α–2b to maintain chemotherapy-induced remissions have been encouraging. To study the efficacy of IFN as maintenance therapy, patients in whom the disease has not progressed after 12 months of initial chemotherapy were randomized to receive either IFN for two years or no treatment. Data from this study demonstrated that response duration and median survival were significantly longer in the group that received IFN maintenance therapy: the treated group had an advantage over the control group of 12 to 13 months (Mandelli *et al.*, 1990). The Southwest Oncology Group (SWOG) is currently performing a similar trial of IFN as maintenance therapy to confirm these results (SWOG 8624). The Cancer and Acute Leukemia Group B has conducted a randomized study comparing melphalan and prednisone with melphalan, prednisone and IFN-α in the initial treatment of patients with multiple myeloma (Cooper *et al.*, 1990). In contrast with the maintenance IFN protocol, the simultaneous administration of IFN with chemotherapy showed no benefit to myeloma patients.

The Eastern Cooperative Oncology Group (ECOG) is evaluating a regimen that combines IFN with chemotherapy in alternating cycles. The chemotherapy regimen consists of two initial induction cycles of the combination of vincristine, carmustine, melphalan, cyclophosphamide and prednisone (VBMCP) followed by alternating cycles of IFN-α and VBMCP; treatment continues for two years. Preliminary analyses show the response duration and median survival to be one year longer than previously observed in patients with multiple myeloma, suggesting that VBMCP alternating with IFN is an effective new regimen for the treatment of this disease (Oken *et al.*, 1990b). This study is based on the prior phase II work of investigators Oken *et al.* (1988), who administered alternating cycles of VBMCP with IFN-α and achieved a 41% incidence of complete and near complete responses with this regimen.

Non-Hodgkin's Lymphoma
Based on consistently demonstrated activity in phase I trials, especially in the indolent (low-grade) lymphomas, several phase II studies were undertaken to define more precisely the rate and duration of response to IFN in patients with lymphomas. In a phase II trial, Foon *et al.*, (1984) reported initial response rates ranging from 14%–54%. Dosages used in this study were very high and were associated with significant morbidity. Higher response rates appeared to correlate with the histologic subtype of lymphoma categorized as low-grade malignancy under the "working formulation" classification system. The response rate was 54% in tumors so classified. Other investigators have demonstrated IFN's effectiveness in the low-grade lymphomas when even lower, less toxic dosages are administered (O'Connell *et al.*, 1986; Wagstaff *et al.*, 1986). An important observation in these early studies was that patients previously treated with chemotherapy and/or radiation therapy were still able to achieve a very good response to IFN-α. A question that remains, however, is whether IFN can be used effectively as initial therapy in patients with low-grade lymphomas. IFN-α as a single agent has shown less efficacy in the intermediate-and high-grade lymphomas (Foon *et al.*, 1984)

Several studies have been undertaken specifically to answer the questions of whether IFN can contribute to the conventional chemotherapy treatment of non-Hodgkin's lymphoma and when IFN should be administered in relation to chemotherapy. Although standard chemotherapy can produce excellent remissions in 75% to 90% of patients, maintaining the remission in this group of patients is the major clinical challenge. IFN has been combined with chemotherapy regimens in an attempt to improve the duration of response and survival. Trials involving chemotherapy and IFN have come forth from animal studies of lymphoma, which demonstrated the effectiveness of IFN either alone or in combination with cytotoxic therapy (Mowskowitz *et al.*, 1982; Slater *et al.*, 1981; Gresser *et al.*, 1978; Chirigos and Pearson, 1973). Additional data supporting the effectiveness of IFN-α in combination with a chemotherapy regimen come from the demonstrated *in vivo* synergy between IFN and two cytotoxic agents, doxorubicin and cyclophosphamide, in xenograft models.

Hawkins *et al.* (1985) reported one of the earliest studies of the combination of IFN-α with chemotherapy. In this phase I study, which included patients with lymphoma, IFN was introduced in mid-cycle of the 21-day COPA regimen (cyclophosphamide, doxorubicin, vincristine, and prednisone). Delays in treatment and anemia were reported in patients receiving the highest dose level of IFN, but no other unexpected toxic effects occurred. Thus, these investigators demonstrated that a chemotherapy and IFN combination was feasible. Several of the cooperative groups in the United States are conducting prospective randomized trials to evaluate patients with non-Hodgkin's lymphoma. ECOG has completed accession to a trial comparing moderately aggressive chemotherapy, in the form of COPA, with COPA plus recombinant IFN-α in untreated patients with clinically aggressive low-grade ("B" symptoms [fever, night sweats, weight loss] only) and intermediate-grade non-Hodgkin's lymphoma. Smalley *et al.* (1992) report that these two regimens produced comparable objective responses, but the regimen containing IFN was more effective in prolonging the time to treatment failure and the duration of complete response. The IFN regimen also was more effective in prolonging survival. Previous studies have reported an association between prognostic factors such as the absence of bulky disease, low degree of extranodal involvement, and absence of B symptoms with both the level of response to cytotoxic therapy and the duration of response. In this study, IFN proved to be an additional factor of importance, being associated with prolonged relapse-free and overall survival. Other studies have examined the combination of standard therapy chlorambucil and IFN in the treatment of indolent lymphomas. Clark *et al.* (1984; 1989) administered a combination of IFN (6 MIU intramuscularly, days 1–5 and 8) and chlorambucil in 13 previously treated lymphoma patients. Responses were noted in five patients, four of whom had low-grade lymphomas. The toxic effects reported in this study were tolerable. A phase III trial (Peterson *et al.*, 1993) was initiated to evaluate the benefits of adding IFN to the standard therapy, single-agent cyclophosphamide. Preliminary analysis of induction therapy with this regimen in 531 patients has demonstrated that the addition of IFN-α to cyclophosphamide for induction appears to result only in increased toxicity. The effect IFN-α will have on long-term follow-up remains to be determined.

Cutaneous T-cell Lymphoma Cutaneous T-cell lymphomas (mycosis fungoides and the Sézary Syndrome) are non-Hodgkin's lymphomas characterized by a malignant proliferation of mature helper T lymphocytes; these lymphomas present with skin infiltration and an indolent clinical course. Effective therapies include topical mechlorethamine, psoralen plus ultraviolet light, total skin electron-beam irradiation, and systemic chemotherapy. Although high response rates and complete remissions have been reported, the remissions are difficult to maintain, and prolonged survival is rarely reported. The limited efficacy of conventional cytotoxic drugs in the treatment of mycosis fungoides has led to the use of biological therapy in the treatment of this disorder. Several phase II clinical trials of IFN have been performed (Covelli *et al.*, 1987; Olsen *et al.*, 1987; Bunn *et al.*, 1984). The response rate is variable: about 79% of previ-

ously untreated patients responded, whereas the response rates in pretreated patients ranged between 45% and 70%. The average duration of response has been about nine months in previously treated patients. Bunn *et al.* evaluated recombinant IFN-α 2a in patients with cutaneous T-cell lymphoma, administering a dose of 50 MIU/m^2 three times weekly in previously treated patients. Nine of 20 patients responded (two completely and seven partially). Responses in both cutaneous and extracutaneous sites were reported (Bunn *et al.*, 1989; Olsen *et al.*, 1989). These results were confirmed by other investigators who treated patients with skin involvement only with either 3 MIU daily or escalating doses from 3 to 36 MIU for 10 weeks. Three patients responded completely and 10 partially. From these results the authors concluded that there is a dose-response relationship (Bunn *et al.*, 1989). In a phase I dose-escalation trial, the dose of IFN-α was increased from 6 to 30 MIU intramuscularly three times weekly in combination with psoralen plus ultraviolet light irradiation (PUVA). A complete response was obtained in 12 patients (80%), with an overall objective response rate of 93%. The median duration of response is 17 months. The maximal tolerated dose of IFN-α–2a given in combination with PUVA is reported to be 12 MIU/m^2 (Springer *et al.*, 1991).

In the treatment of mycoses fungoides and Sézary syndrome, IFN-α can induce significant responses in both previously treated and untreated patients, but future trials are looking at combining IFN-α with other treatment modalities to determine exactly what impact IFN has in this disease.

Solid Tumors

Table 4.4 summarizes the uses of IFNs in solid tumors. In solid tumors, the objective response rates from treatment with single-agent IFN have not been as high as those for the hematologic malignancies and lymphomas. Despite this, IFN has significant activity in

Table 4.4 Clinical activity of interferon in solid tumors

			In Combination with		
Indications	Single Agent	Adjuvant	Biological Response Modifier	Chemotherapy	Other
Kaposi's sarcoma (AIDS)	✓				AZT ✓
Renal cell CA	✓	*	IL-2 ✓		Cellular Therapy*
Melanoma	✓	*	IL-2 *	*	
Colorectal CA				*	
Carcinoid tumors	✓				Octreatide*
Ovarian CA	✓ IP				
Squamous cell CA					
Skin					13-*cis*-retinoic acid*
Cervix					13-*cis*-retinoic acid ± RT*

* = considered experimental	RT = Radiation Therapy	CA = Cancer
✓ = studies support indication	AZT = Azidothymidine	IL-2 = Interleukin-2
IP = Intraperitoneal		

solid tumors, often when combined with cytotoxic chemotherapy or biological or differentiating agents.

AIDS-Related Kaposi's Sarcoma

Kaposi's sarcoma, once a rare malignancy of the skin, is now occurring in epidemic proportions in association with the acquired immunodeficiency syndrome (AIDS). Although chemotherapy has induced responses in individuals with Kaposi's sarcoma (Mitsuyasu and Groopman, 1984; Hymes et al., 1981) its use in AIDS is of little long-term benefit because of poor bone marrow tolerance and the risk of further immunosuppression in already severely immunocompromised individuals (Mitsuyasu, 1989).

Prior to the recognition of human immunodeficiency virus 1 (HIV–1) as the causative agent of AIDS, several studies were conducted, in groups of homosexual men with Kaposi's sarcoma at various stages of the disease, that were based on evidence that IFN had a therapeutic effect in viral diseases. Krown and colleagues (1983) reported the earliest phase I trial of recombinant IFN-α in AIDS-related Kaposi's sarcoma. Five of 12 patients had major objective responses to IFN (three complete and two partial). These data have been confirmed in larger groups of patients treated with IFN-α–2a (Krown et al., 1986a and 1986b; Real et al., 1986; Krown et al., 1984) and IFN-α–2b (Volberding and Mitsuyasu, 1985; Groopman et al., 1984; Mitsuyasu et al., 1984). Objective response rates approaching 30% were reported when IFN was administered in high doses (> 20 MIU/m^2) (Abrams and Volberding, 1987). It appears that higher dosages (10–36 MIU daily) and very high doses (> 36 MIU daily) have been associated with better response rates than lower doses (Goldstein and Laszlo, 1986).

Several characteristics have been found to be associated with higher response rates that affect the outcome of therapy in patients with AIDS-related Kaposi's syndrome (Mitsuyasu et al., 1986; Vadhan-Raj et al., 1986). They include early stage disease, absence of opportunistic infections, absence of circulating IFN before treatment, and relative preservation of lymphocyte and T-helper subsets (Gelmann et al., 1985; Rios et al., 1985; Krigel et al., 1983). Although no clear-cut immunologic improvement has been observed in AIDS patients treated with IFN-α, opportunistic infections were less frequently diagnosed and survival was improved in a subset of treated patients (Mitsuyasu, 1988). There is recent evidence that IFN-α has an inhibitory effect on HIV, both *in vivo* and *in vitro*, which has suggested that IFN-α has another important mechanism of action in patients with HIV infection.

The combination of azidothymidine (AZT) and IFN-α has been observed to have a synergistic antiretroviral effect both *in vivo* and *in vitro* (Hartshorn et al., 1987). Several pilot studies based on these findings have been conducted with this combination. Tumor response rates between 33% and 63%, as well as *in vivo* antiviral effects, have been reported (Krown et al., 1989; Fischl et al., 1988; Mullen et al., 1988). In studies in which doses of IFN-α–2a ranged from 4.5 to 18 MIU, given in combination with AZT at either 100 mg or 200 mg every 4 hours, tumors regressed at every dose level, with higher doses producing more responses (Hartshorn et al., 1987). Tumor remissions were seen with much lower doses of IFN in the combination regimen than were required with IFN alone. Responses occurred even in patients with prior opportunistic infections and other poor prognostic features. Myelotoxicity and hepatotoxicity were the dose-limiting side effects of this combination.

Interferon-α is an important investigational agent in patients with HIV infection without Kaposi's sarcoma. Its well-documented efficacy against AIDS-related Kaposi's sarcoma led to its being approved by the FDA as a therapy for that condition. There is a strong relationship between CD4+ cell count and response rate, those patients with a higher CD4+ cell count tend to respond better with improvement in their lesions.

Gastrointestinal Malignancies

Although IFN-α has shown therapeutic activity in several hematologic malignancies, its performance as a single agent in adenocarcinomas and other solid tumors has been disappointing. Colon carcinoma is a solid tumor with a low rate of response to all agents, including IFN, but 5-fluorouracil (5-FU) may induce a relatively brief partial response in 15% to 20% of patients. Preclinical studies and early pharmacokinetic studies suggest that the coadministration of IFN and 5-FU elevates serum levels of the chemotherapeutic agent from 1.5-fold to 64-fold (Grem et al., 1990; Lindley et al., 1990). Recombinant IFN-α–2a has been shown to enhance the cytotoxic effect of 5-FU *in vitro*; in a pilot clinical trial by Wadler et al., the combination induced a partial response in 63% of the patients (Wadler and Wiernik, 1990; Wadler et al., 1984). To confirm these findings, a phase II clinical trial (Wadler et al., 1991) was conducted by ECOG in 1989. The treatment regimen consisted of 5-FU (750 mg/m^2/day for five days) as a continuous infusion followed by weekly outpatient bolus therapy and IFN (9 MIU) subcutaneously three times per week beginning day 1. The objective response rate was 42%, including one clinical complete response and 14 partial responses. Doses were modified for gastrointestinal, hematologic, and neurologic toxic effects and for fatigue.

Phase II clinical trials of recombinant IFN-α and 5-FU in advanced colorectal carcinoma showed that the combination had a greater therapeutic effect than would be expected for 5-FU alone (Wadler et al., 1991; Huberman et al., 1990; Kemeny et al., 1990; Pazdur et al., 1990; Wadler and Wiernik, 1990). To better understand the efficacy and safety of the combination, an international multicenter randomized trial in 234 patients was conducted and reported by York et al. (1993). Patients with advanced colorectal carcinoma were randomized to receive 5-FU alone at a dose of 750 mg/m²/day by a five day continuous infusion followed by a weekly dose or the same 5-FU schedule with IFN-α–2a at a dose of 9 MIU three times a week. The complete and partial remission rates were 20% in the group that received only 5-FU and 25% in those patients who received the combination. Although mild nausea, vomiting, diarrhea, and stomatitis were common side effects in both groups, fever and fatigue were more common in the patients who received IFN. In this randomized study, the combination of 5-FU and IFN-α–2a had activity similar to that of 5-FU alone with no prolongation of remission duration or survival.

In another phase III trial, 496 patients with advanced colorectal cancer were randomized to receive either 5-FU plus IFN-α–2a or 5-FU plus leucovorin (Kocha, 1993). The overall response rates were 21% in the IFN group and 18% in the leucovorin group, indicating that these two regimens yield more or less equal periods of response and survival. Severe diarrhea, nausea and vomiting, and stomatitis were more common in the leucovorin arm, whereas fatigue, somnolence, and fever were more frequent in the IFN arm. The combination of 5-FU and IFN, therefore, appears comparable to either high-dose 5-FU or the combination of 5-FU and leucovorin, but none of the three has clear-cut superiority.

Renal Cell Carcinoma

Renal cell carcinoma is the most common malignancy of the kidney. Only half of the patients who present with local disease are cured by surgery, and those with metastatic disease have a median survival of approximately 10 months. Neither chemotherapy nor radiation therapy has a significant role in the treatment of metastatic renal cell carcinoma.

For a long time, patients with metastatic renal cell carcinoma have been treated on a variety of investigational protocols. The majority of these protocols have involved the use of biological response modifiers. In 1983, the University of California, Los Angeles (Dekernion et al., 1983) and the University of Texas M.D. Anderson group (Quesada et al., 1983) reported independently on the regression of metastatic renal cell carcinoma with partially purified human leukocyte IFN. Objective responses (complete and partial) occurred in 16.5% and 26% of patients, respectively. Numerous phase II trials have confirmed a reproducible objective response rate of 15% to 20%. Responses are independent of the type of IFN-α used and correlate positively with prior nephrectomy, good performance status, a long disease-free interval, and lung as the predominant site of metastasis. The median duration of response averages 6 to 10 months, with few durable complete remissions. Minasian and colleagues (Minasian et al., 1988) from the Memorial Sloan-Kettering Cancer Center reported a large single-institution experience with IFN-α in 159 patients with metastatic renal cell cancer. The overall response rate was 10% (two complete and 14 partial responses). The median response duration was 12.2 months, and the median survival was 11.4 months. Only 3% of patients were alive at five years. Although the response rate of 10% is lower than those reported elsewhere, it is within the range for the overall clinical experience with IFN-α. This report demonstrated the need for continued investigation for more effective therapies for advanced renal cell carcinoma and supports the investigation of combinations of new agents with IFN-α–2a.

In an attempt to improve the therapeutic index of IFN therapy in patients with renal cell carcinoma, there has been great interest in the combination of interleukin–2 (IL–2) and IFN-α. In experimental murine models, the combination of IL–2 and IFN-α has greater antitumor effects than either agent alone (Cameron et al., 1988). Many phase I trials combined different administration schedules (intravenous bolus versus continuous infusion) and doses of both IL–2 and IFN. These studies reported that this combination of cytokines had antitumor activity. Figlin and his colleagues at UCLA (1992) conducted a phase

II trial in which IFN-α was combined with a low-dose continuous infusion of IL–2 in an attempt to lower the toxicity of this IL–2-based regimen. Thirty patients with metastatic renal cell carcinoma were treated with IFN-α–2a at a dose of 6 MIU/m²/day on days 1 and 4 of each treatment week, with an IL–2 dose of 2 million IU/m²/day for four days. Patients received four weeks of treatment followed by a two-week rest. Except for the first four days of treatment, all therapy was administered on a out-patient basis. The objective response rate for this group of patients was 30% (nine partial responses). Two partial responders were found to have pathologic complete remissions after surgery, and a third patient with a pathologic complete remission had a surgical complete remission after a nephrectomy. Median survival for this group of responding patients to date is 34 months. These results have been confirmed by Vogelzang et al. (1993) who administered both cytokines as subcutaneous injections using similar dosages and schedules.

In a randomized trial, IFN-α–2a has been administered as adjuvant therapy to patients at risk of relapsing from their kidney cancer (Porzolt, 1992). Results have demonstrated no differences in survival duration or time to treatment failure in patients who did not receive IFN compared to those patients who did.

Metastatic Melanoma

The treatment of disseminated melanoma continues to be a frustrating problem for the cancer specialist. The median survival period of untreated patients is 5 to 6 months, and fewer than 20% of patients survive 1 year (Heimdal et al., 1989). Despite the large number of systemic single-agent or multidrug chemotherapeutic regimens available, the overall objective rates of response have been documented as ranging from 15% to 40% (McClay and Mastrangelo, 1988). Very few complete responses have been documented, and the majority of responses are short-lived. The need for new drugs and drug combinations for this group of patients is clear. Clinical studies in which disseminated melanoma was treated with either IFN-α–2a or –2b as a single agent have demonstrated response rates between 10% and 20% (Sertoli et al., 1989; Creagan et al., 1988; Creagan et al., 1986a; Creagan et al., 1986b; Dorval et al., 1986; Legha, 1986; Creagan et al., 1984; Hawkins et al., 1984; Kirkwood and Ernstoff, 1984; Robinson et al. 1984; Ernstoff et al., 1983).

In attempts to improve response rates, IFN-α has been combined with chemotherapeutic regimens with some promising initial results. In a phase II trial by Margolin et al., (1992) at the City of Hope Hospital, Duarte, California, 42 patients with melanoma were treated with cisplatin and a low dose of subcutaneous IFN-α. Three patients achieved complete response, and seven had partial responses. The overall objective response rate was 24%. In a different trial (Falkson et al., 1991), 64 patients were randomized to receive either dacarbazine (DTIC), the standard medical treatment for melanoma, or DTIC plus IFN. Objective responses were documented in six patients on DTIC alone and in 16 patients on DTIC plus IFN. Median time to relapse and median survival were significantly longer in the patients who received the combination.

In another phase II study (Pyrhonen et al., 1992), IFN-α was combined with one of the more effective four-drug combination chemotherapy regimens for metastatic melanoma. The four-drug chemotherapy regimen comprised DTIC, vincristine, bleomycin, and lomustine (CCNU). Of 45 evaluable patients, the objective response rate was 62%; six patients (13%) achieved a complete response and 22 (49%) a partial response. These results demonstrate that treatment results in metastatic melanoma may be improved with an out-patient chemotherapy regimen and low doses of leukocyte IFN.

In efforts to prolong survival for early stage melanoma patients, a randomized controlled trial of high-dose IFN-α–2b was undertaken in high-risk, surgically resected melanoma patients (Kirkwood *et al.*, 1993). Results from this trial are pending.

Ovarian Cancer

Two studies have been conducted that demonstrate the role of intraperitoneal recombinant IFN-α (Willemse *et al.*, 1990; Berek *et al.*, 1985) in patients with persistent epithelial ovarian cancer. Berek *et al.*, 1985 reported complete responses in four of the 11 patients whose disease was re-evaluated by surgery, which suggests that IFN may prove useful in the treatment of ovarian cancer. Responses were noted after 4 to 6 cycles of 50 MIU of recombinant IFN-α–2a, and the toxicity of the treatment was acceptable.

Carcinoid Tumors

Carcinoid tumors of the intestinal tract are thought to arise from cells in the base of the intestinal crypts. Chemotherapy with single agents or combination regimens may yield response rates ranging from 20% to 40%. Human leukocyte IFN has demonstrated significant effects on hormone levels and tumor growth in patients with malignant carcinoid tumors (Oberg *et al.*, 1986). A randomized controlled study comparing streptozocin plus 5-FU (the standard therapy) to IFN in 20 patients with malignant carcinoid tumors demonstrated that human leukocyte IFN produced significantly better antitumor responses and a higher degree of subjective improvement than the standard therapy (Oberg *et al.*, 1989). This type of therapy appears to have promise in the treatment of malignant carcinoid tumors.

Squamous Carcinomas of the Skin or Cervix

Several preclinical and clinical studies provide a rationale for evaluating the combination 13-*cis*-retinoic acid and IFN-α. Preclinical data indicate that the two drugs have different mechanisms of action (Lotan *et al.*, 1990;

Pitha, 1990; Grossberg *et al.*, 1989; Evans, 1988; Langer and Pestka, 1988; Pestka *et al.*, 1987; Sporn *et al.*, 1986) and show enhanced activity when they are used in combination in a variety of human hematologic and solid tumor cell lines (Frey *et al.*, 1991; Higuchi *et al.*, 1991; Peck and Bollag, 1991; Marth *et al.*, 1989; Gallagher *et al.*, 1987; Hemmi and Breitman, 1987; Marth *et al.*, 1986). Data on the use of each agent singly suggest that each, when used systemically at high doses, produces response rates of 40% to 50% (less than 15% complete responses) in locally advanced skin cancer. The two drugs also have non-overlapping and reversible toxic effects; 13-*cis*-retinoic acid causes primarily mucocutaneous side effects (Bollag, 1983; Lippman *et al.*, 1987) whereas IFN-α causes a flu-like syndrome and fatigue (Goldstein and Laszlo, 1988; Quesada *et al.*, 1986).

In the first phase II trial of systemic therapy in metastatic squamous cell carcinoma of the skin, Lippman *et al.* at the University of Texas M. D. Anderson Cancer Center reported on the combination of 13-*cis*-retinoic acid and IFN-α–2a (Lippman *et al.*, 1992a). This carcinoma is extremely common, and although 90% of patients are cured by local therapy, the remaining 10%, which represent tens of thousand of cases, often suffer severe disfigurement with cosmetic deformities as a result of their treatment. The purpose of the trial by Lippmann was to evaluate whether a high rate of complete responses could be achieved by using a combination of these two agents in patients in whom local therapy had failed or who had regional and/or distant metastases. Ultimately, seven patients had complete responses and 12 had partial responses.

The combination of 13-*cis*-retinoic acid and IFN-α–2a has also recently been reported by Lippmann *et al.* (1992b) to be effective in the treatment of squamous cell carcinoma of the cervix. Twenty-six patients with locally advanced bulky disease received daily oral 13-*cis*-retinoic acid (1 mg/kg) and subcutaneous recombinant human IFN-α–2a (6 MIU). Fifty percent (13 patients) achieved major responses (one complete, 12 partial). Side effects were mild. Studies of the long-term response rates, response durations, and survival duration are still ongoing, and further study is needed before defining this regimen's role in squamous cell carcinoma of the cervix. Lippman *et al*. (1993) have designed follow-up trial of a combination of concomitant 13-*cis*-retinoic acid, IFN and radiotherapy for treating locally advanced cancer of the cervix. The preliminary results of this study included an overall response rate of 81% (56% complete). The dose-limiting toxic effect of the regimen is radiation proctitis. These data indicate that 13-*cis*-retinoic acid and IFN-α–2a can be integrated with radiotherapy in an attempt to improve survival rates in locally advanced cervical cancer.

Non-Oncologic Indications for Interferon-α Therapy

Hepatitis

Several multicenter clinical trials have demonstrated that IFN has significant activity in the treatment of chronic hepatitis B (Coppens *et al*., 1990; Perillo *et al*., 1990; Fattovich *et al*., 1989; Saracco *et al*., 1989). Approximately 30% to 50% of patients with chronic hepatitis infection respond to IFN-α therapy. Remissions of chronic hepatitis B following IFN therapy are reported to be of long duration and are often associated with loss of viral hepatitis B surface antigen (Korenman *et al*., 1991). Several studies have indicated that treatment of chronic hepatitis B with a sufficient dose of IFN-α for at least six months slows progression of disease and can result in long-term remission. Current strategies to increase response rates include combining IFN-α with other antiviral or immunomodulatory agents.

IFN-α recently was approved by the FDA for chronic active non-A, non-B/C hepatitis, for which there previously had been no consistently effective treatment. In two controlled studies, serum alanine aminotransferase levels were normalized and liver function was improved in approximately 48% of the patients who received IFN-α. Unfortunately, a significant number of patients experienced relapse six months after treatment ended, indicating that prolonged treatment may be required for the beneficial effects to continue (DiBisceglie *et al*., 1989; Davis *et al*., 1989).

Toxicity Profile

The toxicity profile of IFN-α is dependent on the dose, the route of administration and the treatment schedule. The occurrence of side effects in patients receiving IFN can be predictable, and these side effects have often been categorized according to their frequency (Table 4.5). The majority of the side effects associated with IFN are constitutional. They include fatigue, fever, chills, myalgias, headache, and anorexia, and are often referred to as a flu-like syndrome. These flu-like symptoms are reported almost universally following the initial injections: the appearance of subsequent **tachyphylaxis** depends on the type of IFN used, the dose, the route, and the schedule of administration. These symptoms are generally controlled with acetaminophen prior to IFN administration; the acetaminophen is usually required only with the initial injections. Administration of the IFN during the evening or at bedtime has been successful in minimizing the effects of peak toxicity, which usually occurs 2 to 3 hours after administration. The fatigue associated with IFN therapy is often chronic and may require a dose reduction.

The hematologic effects of IFN therapy include leukopenia, anemia, and thrombocytopenia. The white blood cell counts are usually lowered by 40% to 60%, but they usually rebound rapidly to normal after discontinuation of therapy. Infectious sequelae do not increase in IFN-induced leukopenia, and granulocytopenia is rarely dose-limiting. Anemia is generally seen with chronic therapy but is rarely severe. Mild thrombocytopenia has been reported in 5% to 50% of patients but generally is not clinically significant. Patients

Table 4.5 Toxicity profile of interferon

	Frequent	Less Frequent
Acute	Fever	Nausea
	Chills	Vomiting
	Malaise	Diarrhea
	Headache	
	Anorexia	
Chronic	Fatigue	Mild neutropenia
	Weight loss	Elevated liver enzymes
	Alopecia (mild)	Thrombocytopenia
		Central nervous system
		Depression
		Confusion
		Mental slowing
		Mild proteinuria

previously treated with chemotherapy and/or radiation may be more susceptible to the hematologic side effects of IFN.

The most frequent neurologic side effects of IFN are alteration in mental status such as slowed thinking, difficulty concentrating, and problems with memory. With higher doses, more significant toxicity such as somnolence, lethargy, and confusion may occur. Anorexia is commonly reported, and weight loss may occur with prolonged treatment. The occurrence of nausea, vomiting, or diarrhea is related to dose, but these effects tend to be mild and self-limiting. The most common renal toxic effect is mild proteinuria, but nephrotic syndrome and acute renal insufficiency have been reported. Transaminase elevation, usually mild, has occurred more often in the presence of pretreatment hepatic abnormalities and is dose related. Patients given IFN at high doses may experience hypotension, tachycardia, skin rashes, and peripheral neuropathies. Patients receiving IFN require frequent laboratory monitoring and regularly scheduled visits with their physician. However, almost all of the signs and symptoms of IFN use appear to be rapidly and fully reversible following discontinuation of therapy.

Some patients treated with IFN-α develop neutralizing antibodies to the IFN preparation. The incidence of development of these antibodies depends on which IFN-α preparation is used and which assay system is employed (Antonelli *et al.*, 1991; Figlin *et al.*, 1988). The relationship between the presence of neutralizing antibodies and the clinical efficacy of IFN-α is under investigation. Itri *et al.* (1987) reviewed the incidence of antibodies in 617 patients treated with IFN-α–2a and found no deleterious effect on response rate, time to or duration of response, or survival duration among patients who developed neutralizing antibodies to IFN-α–2a.

CLINICAL EXPERIENCE— INTERFERON-β

Interferon-β is produced primarily by fibroblasts and epithelial cells. Its biological effects are similar to those of IFN-α and may be summarized as antiviral, immunomodulatory, and antiproliferative. The use of IFN-β in the treatment of cancer remains investigational.

Multiple Sclerosis

Multiple sclerosis (MS) is a common neurologic disease that causes severe disabilities to those afflicted. Extensive research has failed to identify the cause of MS, but an immunologic basis is strongly suggested. The utility of IFN-α in MS has been evaluated because of its immunoregulatory properties. Trials of IFN-α or -β have reported reduced clinical exacerbations and disease activity in patients who received one of these agents. A multicenter, randomized, double-blind, placebo-controlled trial of interferon beta-1b (IFN-β) in 372 patients with relapsing-remitting multiple sclerosis showed significant reductions in exacerbation rates, severity of exacerbations, and accumulation of magnetic resonance imaging (MRI) abnormalities in patients on the treatment arm. In general, therapy was well tolerated. The proposed mechanism of action for interferon in this population is unknown, however, the immunoregulatory properties of

IFN-β and its ability to inhibit IFN-γ synthesis may be important. (IFN-β Multiple Sclerosis Study Group, 1993). In June 1993, the Food and Drug Administration approved IFN-β for clinical use in MS.

CLINICAL EXPERIENCE— INTERFERON-γ

Interferon-γ shares many properties with IFN-α and -β, but has many differences as well. It shows greater antiproliferative activity than the other IFNs, but is more likely to result in myelosuppression. Hypotension is also a more common toxic effect of IFN-γ (at higher doses) than of the other two IFNs. Interferon-γ appears to be a more potent immune stimulator of monocytes and class II HLA activity than IFN-α or -β. Interferon-γ is an approved immunomodulatory agent for the treatment of chronic granulomatous disease and has modest activity at biologically active doses in renal cell carcinoma (Aulitzky et al., 1989).

REGULATORY APPROVALS

Interferon-γ was first approved by the FDA in 1986 for its significant role in the treatment of hairy cell leukemia. Since then, the IFNs have been approved for a total of six diseases. In other countries, there are a minimum of 12 therapeutic indications of viral or neoplastic origin. For a summation of regulatory approvals in the United States for the IFNs, see Table 4.1.

SUMMARY

Interferon-α was the first pure human protein found to be effective in the treatment of cancer. Just over 10 years ago, when this molecule was introduced into the clinical arena, it was hailed as a wonder drug and "magic bullet" by the media. For patients, the medical community, and the drug industry, that announcement was the beginning of an arduous period of watching and waiting for clinical results to come forth. Today IFN has clearly demonstrated its usefulness in inducing regressions in both hematologic malignancies and solid tumors. Some of its antitumor effects have been dramatic, others only partial or relatively brief in duration. The IFNs have been shown to have only limited potential as single-agents; the most important issue now is how to best integrate IFN with existing treatment modalities to improve clinical outcomes in certain malignancies. Several studies are underway and have reported encouraging results.

The most important future direction for research on IFNs and, possibly their greatest value will be in prolonging the disease-free interval and, ultimately, survival. This may be accomplished by administration of adjuvant IFN to patients at high risk for recurrent disease after surgery. Prospectively randomized clinical trials of IFN-α must be performed to test this technique. The rationale that IFN may be most effective when tumor burden is low will lead to continued studies of IFN as maintenance therapy after chemotherapy-induced tumor "debulking" in multiple myeloma and low grade lymphomas.

A different approach is the combination of IFN with differentiating agents such as the retinoids. Such combinations have been associated with the regression of advanced squamous carcinomas of the skin or cervix, suggesting that IFN has an influence on cellular differentiation.

In early clinical trials in patients with AIDS, an unexpected finding was that therapy with IFN-α improved Kaposi's sarcoma, a vascular tumor associated with HIV infection. Because it is known that IFNs also inhibit angiogenesis, combination studies of novel angiogenesis inhibitors in vascular tumors or as metastasis prevention agents are warranted. Over 10 years after its entry into clinical trials, IFN remains an active agent in laboratory and clinical investigations as we attempt to improve the lives of cancer patients.

References

Abrams, D., and Volberding, P. 1987. Alpha interferon of AIDS-associated Kaposi's sarcoma. *Seminars in Oncology* 14(2 suppl 2): 43–47.

Antonelli, G., Currenti, M., Turriziani, O., *et al.* 1991. Neutralizing antibodies to interferon alpha: Relative frequency in patients treated with different interferon preparations. *Journal of Infectious Diseases* 163(4): 882–885.

Aulitzky, W., Gastl, G., Aulitzky, M., *et al.* 1989. Successful treatment of metastatic renal cell carcinoma with a biologically active dose of recombinant interferon gamma. *Journal of Clinical Oncology* 7(12): 1875–1884.

Bale, L. 1979. Induction of 2'–5'-oligoadenylate synthetase activity and a new protein by chick interferon. *Virology* 94 (2): 282–296.

Balkwill, F., Moodie, E., Freedman, V., *et al.* 1982. Human interferon inhibits the growth of established human breast tumors in the nude mouse. *International Journal of Cancer* 30 (3): 231–235.

Balkwill, F., and Oliver, R. 1977. Growth-inhibitory effects of interferon on normal and malignant human haemopoietic cells. *International Journal of Cancer* 20 (4): 500–505.

Ball, L. 1982. 2'–5'-oligoadenylate synthetase. In Boyer, P. (ed). *The Enzymes.* New York: Academic Press, pp. 281–313.

Berek, J., Hacker, N., Lichtenstein, A., *et al.* 1985. Intraperitoneal recombinant alpha interferon for 'salvage' immunotherapy in persistent epithelial ovarian cancer. *Cancer Treatment Reviews* 12(1):23–32.

Berman, E., Heller, G., Kempin, S., *et al.* 1990. Incidence of response and long-term follow-up in patients with hairy cell leukemia treated with recombinant interferon alfa–2a. *Blood* 75(4): 839–845.

Bollag, W. 1983. Vitamin A and retinoids: From nutrition to pharmacotherapy in dermatology and oncology. *Lancet* 1(8329): 860–863.

Borden, E. 1984. Progress toward therapeutic application of interferons, 1979–1983. *Cancer* 54(11): 2770–2776.

Borden, E., Hogan, T., and Voelkel, J. 1982. Comparative antiproliferative activity *in vitro* of natural interferons alpha and beta for diploid and transformed human cells. *Cancer Research* 42: 4948–4953.

Bouroncle, B., Wiseman, B., and Doan, L. 1958. Leukemic reticuloendotheliosis. *Blood* 13 (7): 609–630.

Bunn, P., Ihde, D., and Foon, K. 1989. The role of recombinant interferon alpha–2a in the therapy of cutaneous T-cell lymphomas. *Cancer* 57(8): 1689–1695.

Bunn, P., Foon, F., and Ihde, D. 1984. Recombinant leukocyte A interferon: An active agent in advanced cutaneous T-cell lymphomas. *Annals of Internal Medicine* 101(4): 484–487.

Cameron, R., McIntosh, J., and Rosenberg, S. 1988. Synergistic antitumor effects of combination immunotherapy with recombinant interleukin–2 and recombinant hybrid alpha-interferon in the treatment of established murine hepatic metastases. *Cancer Research* 8(6): 1637–1649.

Cantell, K., Hervonen, S., and Morgensen, K. 1975. *Human leukocyte interferon production, purification and animal experiments.* In Waymouth, C. (ed). *In Vitro.* Baltimore: Baltimore Tissue Culture Association, pp. 35–38.

Chadha, K., and Srivastava, B. 1981. Comparison of the antiproliferative effects of human fibroblast and leukocyte interferons on various leukemic cell lines. *Journal of Clinical Hematology Oncology* 11: 55–60.

Chirigos, M., and Pearson, J. 1973. Cure of murine leukemia with drug and interferon treatment. *Journal of the National Cancer Institute* 51(4): 1367–1368.

Clark, R., Dimitrov, N., and Axelson, J. 1989. A Phase II trial of intermittent leukocyte interferon and high-dose chlorambucil in the treatment of non-Hodgkin's lymphoma resistant to conventional therapy. *American Journal of Clinical Oncology* 12(1): 75–77.

Clark, R., Dimitrov, N., Axelson, J., *et al.* 1984. Leukocyte interferon as a possible biological response modifier in lymphoproliferative disorders resistant to standard therapy. *Journal of Biological Response Modifiers* 3(6): 613–619.

Cooper, M., Dear, K., McIntyre, O., *et al.* 1990. A randomized study comparing melphalan/prednisone with or without alpha 2b interferon in newly diagnosed multiple myeloma. *Blood* 76(10): 345a (abstract).

Coppens, J., Cornu, C., Lews, E., *et al.* 1989. Prospective trial of recombinant leukocyte interferon in chronic hepatitis B: A 10-month follow-up study. *Liver* 9(5): 307–313.

Costanzi, J., Cooper, M., Scarffe, J., *et al.* 1985. Phase II study of recombinant alpha–2 interferon in resistant multiple myeloma. *Journal of Clinical Oncology* 3(5): 654–659.

Covelli, A., Cavalieri, R., Coppola, G., *et al.* 1987. Recombinant leukocyte A interferon (IFN-rA) as initial therapy in mycosis fungoides and Sézary syndrome. *Proceedings of the American Society of Clinical Oncology* 6: 189 (abstract).

Creagan, E., Schaid, D., Ahmann, D., *et al.* 1988. Recombinant interferons in the management of advanced malignant melanoma; updated review of 5 prospective clinical trials and long-term responders. *American Journal of Clinical Oncology* 11(6): 652–659.

Creagan, E., Ahmann, D., Frytak, S., *et al.* 1986a. Recombinant leukocyte a interferon in the treatment of disseminated malignant melanoma. Analysis of complete long-term responding patients. *Cancer* 58(12): 2576–2578.

Creagan, E., Ahmann, D., Frytak, S., *et al.* 1986b. Phase II trials of recombinant leukocyte A interferon in disseminated malignant melanoma. Results in 96 patients. *Cancer Treatment Reports* 70(5): 619–624.

Creagan, E., Ahmann, D., Green, S., *et al.* 1984. Phase II study of recombinant leukocyte A interferon in disseminated malignant melanoma. *Journal of Clinical Oncology* 2(9): 1002–1005.

Creasey A.A., Bartholomew, J., and Merigan, T. 1980. Role of G_0-G_1 arrest in the inhibition of tumor cell growth by interferon. *Proceedings of the National Academy of Sciences USA* 77(3): 1471–1475.

Davis, B., Balart, L., Schiff, E., *et al.* Hepatitis Interventional Therapy Group. 1989. Treatment of chronic hepatitis C with recombinant interferon alpha: A multicenter, randomized, controlled trial. *New England Journal of Medicine* 321(22): 1501–1506.

Dekernion, J., Sarna, G., Figlin, R., *et al.* 1983. Treatment of renal cell carcinoma with human leukocyte (alpha) interferon. *The Journal of Urology* 130: 1063–1066.

Denz, H., Lechleitner, M., Marth, C., *et al.* 1985. Effect of human recombinant alpha–2 and gamma interferon on the growth of human cell lines from solid tumors and hematologic malignancies. *Journal of Interferon Research* 5 (1): 147–157.

Di Bisceglie, A., Martin, P., Kassianides, C., *et al.* 1989. Recombinant interferon alpha therapy for chronic hepatitis C: A randomized, double-blind placebo-controlled trial. *New England Journal of Medicine* 321(22): 1506–1510.

Dorval, T., Palangie, T., Jouve, M., *et al.* 1986. Clinical phase II trial of recombinant DNA interferon (interferon alfa 2b) in patients with metastatic malignant melanoma. *Cancer* 58(2): 215–218.

Ernstoff, M., Reiss, M., Davis, C., *et al.* 1983. Intravenous (IV) recombinant alfa interferon (IFN-alfa–2) in metastatic melanoma. *Proceedings of the American Society of Clinical Oncology* 2: 57 (abstract).

Estey, E., Kurzrock, R., Kantarjian, H., *et al.* 1992. Treatment of hairy cell leukemia with 2-chlorodeoxyadenosine (2-CdA). *Blood* 79: 882–887.

Evans, R. 1988. The steroid and thyroid hormone receptor superfamily. *Science* 240(4854): 889–895.

Falkson, C., Falkson, G., and Falkson, H. 1991. Improved results with the addition of interferon alfa–2b to dacarbazine in the treatment of patients with metastatic malignant melanoma. *Journal of Clinical Oncology* 9(8):1403–1408.

Fattovich, B., Brollo L., Boscaro, S., *et al.* 1989. Long-term effect of low-dose recombinant interferon therapy in patients with chronic hepatitis B. *Journal of Hepatology* 9(3): 331–337.

Feinstein, S., Traub, A., LaZar, A., *et al.* 1985. Studies on cell binding and internalization of human lymphoblastoid interferon. *Journal of Interferon Research* 5(1): 65–67.

Figlin, R., Belldegrun, A., Moldawer, J., *et al.* 1992. Concomitant administration of recombinant human interleukin–2 and recombinant interferon alfa–2A: An active outpatient regimen in metastatic renal cell carcinoma. *Journal of Clinical Oncology* 10(3): 414–421.

Figlin, R., Dekernion, J., Mukamel, E., *et al.* 1988. Recombinant interferon alfa–2a in metastatic renal cell carcinoma: Assessment of antitumor activity and anti-interferon antibody formation. *Journal of Clinical Oncology* 6(10): 1604–1610.

Fischl, M., Reese, J., Dearmas, L., *et al.* 1988. Phase I study of interferon-alpha and AZT in patients with AIDS-related Kaposi's sarcoma. *Fourth International Conference on AIDS* 1:253 (abstract).

Fleischmann, W., Klimpel, G., Tyring, S., *et al.* 1984. Interferon and cancer: Current use and novel approaches. In Sunkara P. (ed). *Novel Approaches to Cancer Chemotherapy*. Orlando: Academic Press, pp. 1–22.

Foon, K., Maluish, A., Abrams, P., *et al.* 1986. Recombinant leukocyte A interferon therapy for advanced hairy cell leukemia. *American Journal of Medicine* 80(3): 351–356.

Foon, K., Sherwin, S., Abrams, P., *et al.* 1984. Treatment of advanced non-Hodgkin's lymphoma with recombinant leukocyte interferon. *New England Journal of Medicine* 311(18): 1148–1152.

Frey, J., Peck, R., and Bollag, W. 1991. Antiproliferative activity of retinoids, interferon-alpha and their combination in five human transformed cell lines. *Cancer Letters* 57(3): 223–227.

Gallagher, R., Lurie, K., Leavitt, R., *et al.* 1987. Effects of interferon and retinoic acid on the growth and differentiation of clonogenic leukemic cells from acute myelogenous leukemia patients treated with recombinant leukocyte-alpha A interferon. *Leukemia Research* 11(7): 609–691.

Gallin, J., Malech, H., Weening, R., and the International Chronic Granulomatous Disease Cooperative Study Group. 1991. A controlled trial of recombinant human interferon gamma to prevent infection in chronic granulomatous disease. *New England Journal of Medicine* 324: 509–516.

Gelmann, E., Preble, O., Steis, R., *et al.* 1985. Human lymphoblastoid interferon treatment of Kaposi's sarcoma in the acquired immunodeficiency syndrome. *American Journal of Medicine* 78(5): 737–741.

Giles, F., Gray, A., Brozovic, M., *et al.* 1988. Alpha-interferon therapy for essential thrombocythaemia. *Lancet* 2(8602): 70–72.

Goldstein, D., and Laszlo, J. 1988. The role of interferon in cancer therapy: A current perspective. *Cancer* 38(1): 259–278.

Goldstein, D., and Laszlo, J. 1986. Interferon therapy in cancer: From imaginon to interferon. *Cancer Research* 46(9): 4315–4329.

Golomb, H., Ratain, M., Mick, R., *et al.* 1992. The treatment of hairy cell leukemia: An update. *Leukemia* 2(1): 24–27.

Golomb, H., Fefer, A., Golde, D., *et al.* 1987. Sequential evaluation of alpha–2b interferon treatment in 128 patients with hairy cell leukemia. *Seminars in Oncology* 14(1): 13–17.

Golomb, H., Jacobs, A., Fefer, A., *et al.* 1986. Alpha–2 interferon therapy of hairy-cell leukemia: A multicenter study of 64 patients. *Journal of Clinical Oncology* 4(6): 900–905.

Grem, J., Allegra, C., McAtee, N., *et al.* 1990. Phase I study of interferon alfa–2a (IFN-A), 5-fluorouracil (5-FU) and high-dose leucovorin (LV) in metastatic gastrointestinal cancer. *Proceedings of the American Society of Clinical Oncology* 9:70 (abstract).

Gresser, I., Maury, C., and Tovey, M. 1978. Efficacy of combined interferon-cyclophosphamide therapy after diagnosis of lymphoma in AKR mice. *European Journal of Cancer* 14(1): 97–99.

Groopman, J., Gottlieb, M., Goodman, J., *et al.* 1984. Recombinant alpha–2 interferon therapy for Kaposi's sarcoma associated with the acquired immunodeficiency syndrome. *Annals of Internal Medicine* 100(5): 671–676.

Grossberg, S., Taylor, J., and Kushnaryov, V. 1989. Interferon receptors and their role in interferon action. *Experientia* 45(6): 508–513.

Habermann, T., Cassileth, P., Bennett, J., *et al.* 1990 A phase II trial for the evaluation of alpha–2A interferon (Roferon A) (Alpha-IFN) followed by 2'-deoxycoformycin (pentostatin) (dCF) in the therapy of hairy cell leukemia (HCL) in previously splenectomized patients. *Blood* 76 (suppl 1): 277a.

Hagberg, H., Alm, G., Bjorkholm, M., *et al.* 1985. Alpha interferon treatment of patients with hairy cell leukemia. *Scandinavian Journal of Hematology* 35(1): 66–70.

Hartshorn, K., Vogt, M., Chou, T., *et al.* 1987. Synergistic inhibition of human immunodeficiency virus *in vitro* by azidothymidine and recombinant alpha A-interferon. *Antimicrobiology Agents in Chemotherapy* 31(2): 168–172.

Hawkins, M., McCure, C., Speyer, J., *et al.* 1984. Recombinant alfa–2 interferon (IFN alpha–2) (SCH 30500) in patients with metastatic malignant melanoma (MMM). An ECOG pilot study. *Proceedings of the American Society of Clinical Oncology* 3: 51 (abstract).

Hawkins, M., O'Connell, M., Schiller, J., *et al.* 1985. Phase I evaluation of recombinant A interferon alpha (rIFN-Alpha) in combination with COPA chemotherapy (I-COPA). *Proceedings of the American Society of Clinical Oncology* 4: 229 (abstract).

Heimdal, K., Hannisdal, E., and Gundersen, S. 1989. Regression analysis of prognostic factors in metastatic melanoma. *European Journal of Clinical Oncology* 25(8): 1219–1223.

Hemmi, H., and Breitman, T. 1987. Combinations of recombinant human interferons and retinoic acid synergistically induced differentiation of the human promyelocytic leukemia cell line HL–60. *Blood* 69(2): 501–507.

Higuchi, T., Hannigan, G., Malkin, D., *et al.* 1991. Enhancement by retinoic acid and dibutyryl cyclic adenosine 3'-5'-monophosphate of the differentiation and gene expression of human neuroblastoma cells induced by interferon. *Cancer Research* 51(15): 3958–3964.

Horoszewicz, J., Leong, S., and Carter, W. 1979. Noncycling tumor cells are sensitive targets for the antiproliferative activity of human interferon. *Science* 206(4422): 1091–1093.

Huberman, M., Bering, H., Tessitore, J., *et al.* 1990. 5-Fluorouracil (5FU) plus recombinant alpha interferon (Roferon A) in advanced colorectal cancer. *Proceedings of the American Society of Clinical Oncology* 9: 116 (abstract).

Hymes, K., Cheung, T., Greene, J., *et al.* 1981. Kaposi's sarcoma in homosexual men: A report of eight cases. *Lancet.* 2(8247): 598–599.

IFNβ Multiple Sclerosis Study Group, 1993. Interferon beta-1b is effective in relapsing-remitting multiple sclerosis. I. Clinical results of a multicenter, randomized, double-blind, placebo-controlled trial. *Neurology* 43: 655–661.

Isaacs, A., and Lindenmann, J. 1957. Virus interference. I. The interferon. *Proceedings from the Royal Society Service* B147: 258–267.

Italian Cooperative Study Group on Chronic Myeloid Leukemia, 1994. Interferon alfa-2a as compared with conventional chemotherapy for the treatment of chronic myeloid leukemia. *New England Journal of Medicine* 330: 820–825.

Itri, L., Campion, M., Dennin, R., *et al.* 1987. Incidence and clinical significance of neutralizing antibodies in patients receiving recombinant interferon alfa–2a by intramuscular injection. *Cancer* 59(3): 668–674.

Jacobs, A., Champlin, R., and Golde, D. 1985. Recombinant alpha–2 interferon for hairy cell leukemia. *Blood* 65(4): 1017–1020.

Johnston, J., Eisenhauer, E., Corbett, W., *et al.* 1988. Efficacy of 2'-deoxycoformycin in hairy cell leukemia: A study of the National Cancer Institute of Canada Clinical Trials Group. *Journal of the National Cancer Institute* 80: 765–769.

Kantarjian, H., Deisseroth, A., Kurzrock, R. *et al.* 1993. Chronic myelogenous leukemia: A concise update. *Blood* 82(3): 691–703.

Kantarjian, H., Keating, M., Estey, E., *et al.* 1992. Treatment of advanced stages of Philadelphia chromosome-positive chronic myelogenous leukemia with alpha interferon and low dose cytosine arabinoside. *Proceedings of the American Society of Clinical Oncology* 11: 260 (abstract).

Kantarjian, H., Vellekoop, L., McCredie, K., *et al.* 1985. Intensive combination chemotherapy (ROAP 10) and splenectomy in the management of chronic myelogenous leukemia. *Journal of Clinical Oncology* 3(2): 192–200.

Kemeny, N., Kelsen, D., Derby, S., *et al.* 1990. Combination 5-fluorouracil and recombinant alpha-interferon in advanced colorectal carcinoma: Activity but significant toxicity. *Proceedings of the American Society of Clinical Oncology* 9: 109 (abstract).

Kirkwood, J., and Ernstoff, M. 1984. Interferons in the treatment of human cancer. *Journal of Clinical Oncology* 2(4): 336–352.

Kirkwood, J., Hunt, M., Smith, T., *et al.* 1993. A randomized controlled trial of high-dose IFN alfa–2b for high-risk melanoma. The ECOG Trial EST–1684. *Proceedings of the American Society of Clinical Oncology* 12: 1331 (abstract).

Kocha, W. 1993. 5-Fluorouracil (5-FU) plus interferon alfa–2a (Roferon-A) versus 5-Fluorouracil plus leucovorin (LV) in metastatic colorectal cancer—results of a multi-center, multinational phase III study. *Proceedings of the American Society of Clinical Oncology* 12: 562 (abstract).

Koeffler, H., and Golde, D. 1981. Chronic myelogenous leukemia: New concepts. *New England Journal of Medicine.* 304(21): 1269–1274.

Korenman, J., Baker, B., Waggoner, J., et al. 1991. Long-term remission of chronic hepatitis B after alpha interferon therapy. *Annals of Internal Medicine* 114(8): 629–634.

Krigel, R., Laubenstein, L., and Muggia, F. 1983. Kaposi's sarcoma: A new staging classification. *Cancer Treatment Report* 67(6): 531–541.

Krown, S., Bundow, D., Gansbacher, B., et al. 1989. Interferon alpha + AZT in AIDS-associated Kaposi's sarcoma: Final results of a phase I trial. *V. International Conference. AIDS WBP 374.* (abstract).

Krown, S., Real, F., Gold, J., et al. 1986a. Therapeutic trials of interferon alfa–2a (IFNα2a) in AIDS-related Kaposi's sarcoma (KS/AIDS). Proceedings, International Conference on AIDS, Paris, France, June 23–25, 1986. *Communication* 88: 35 (abstract).

Krown, S., Gold, J., Real, F., et al. 1986b. Interferon alfa–2a + vinblastine (VLB) in AIDS-associated Kaposi's sarcoma: Therapeutic activity, toxicity, and effects on HTLV-III/LAV viremia. *Journal of Interferon Research* 6: 3 (abstract), Supplement 1.

Krown, S., Real, F., Krim, M., et al. 1984. Recombinant leukocyte A interferon in Kaposi's sarcoma. *Annals of the New York Academy of Sciences* 437: 431–438.

Krown, S., Real, F.,Cunningham-Rundles, S., et al. 1983. Preliminary observations on the effect of recombinant leukocyte A interferon in homosexual men with Kaposi's sarcoma. *New England Journal of Medicine* 308(18): 1071–1076.

Langer, J., and Pestka, S. 1988. Interferon receptors. *Immunology Today* 9(12): 393–400.

Lauria, F., Foa, R., Raspadori, D., et al. 1988. Treatment of hairy cell leukemia with alpha interferon (alpha IFN). *European Journal of Cancer Clinical Oncology.* 24(2): 195–200.

Legha, S. 1986. Interferons in the treatment of malignant melanoma. A review of recent trials. *Cancer* 57(8): 1675–1677.

Lindley, C., Bernard, S., Gavigan, M., et al. 1990. Interferon-alpha increases 5-fluorouracil (5FU) plasma levels 64-fold within one hour: Results of a phase I study. *Journal of Interferon Research* 10: 132 (suppl).

Lippman, S., Kavanagh, J., Paredes-Espinoza, M., et al. 1993. 13-Cis-retinoic acid, interferon-alpha 2a and radiotherapy for locally advanced cancer of the cervix. *Proceedings of the American Society of Clinical Oncology* 12: 816 (abstract).

Lippman, S., Parkinson, D., Itri, L., et al. 1992a. 13-Cis-retinoic acid and interferon alpha–2a: Effective combination therapy for advanced squamous cell carcinoma of the skin. *Journal of the National Cancer Institute* 84(1): 235–241.

Lippman, S., Kavanagh, J., Paredes-Espinoza M., et al. 1992b. 13-Cis-retinoic acid plus interferon alpha–2a: Highly active systemic therapy for squamous cell carcinoma of the cervix. *Journal of the National Cancer Institute* 84(1): 241–245.

Lippman, S., Kessler, J., Meyskens, F. 1987. Retinoids as preventive and therapeutic anticancer agents. *Cancer Treatment Report* 71(4): 391–405 (part I), 493–515 (part II).

Lotan, R., Francis, G., Freeman, C., et al. 1990. Differentiation therapy. *Cancer Research* 50(12): 3453–3464.

Mandelli, F., Giuseppe, A., Amadori, S., et al. 1990. Maintenance treatment with recombinant interferon alpha–2b in patients with multiple myeloma responding to conventional induction chemotherapy. *New England Journal of Medicine* 322(20): 1430–1434.

Margolin, K., Doroshow, J., Akman, S., et al. 1992. Phase II trial of cisplatin and alpha-interferon in advanced malignant melanoma. *Journal of Clinical Oncology* 10(10): 1574–1578.

Marth, C., Kirchebner, P., and Daxenbichler, G. 1989. The role of polyamines in interferon and retinoic acid medidated synergistic antiproliferative action. *Cancer Letters* 44(1): 55–59.

Marth, C., Daxenbichler, G., and Dapunt, O. 1986. Synergistic antiproliferative effect of human recombinant interferons and retinoic acid in cultured breast cancer cells. *Journal of the National Cancer Institute* 77(5): 1197–1202.

Martin, A., Nerenstone, S., Urba, W., et al. 1990. Treatment of hairy cell leukemia with alternating cycles of pentostatin and recombinant leukocyte A interferon: Results of a phase II study. *Journal of Clinical Oncology* 8(4): 721–730.

McClay, E., and Mastrangelo, M. 1988. Systemic chemotherapy for metastatic melanoma. *Seminars in Oncology* 15(6): 569–577.

McGlave, P., Arthur, D., Weisdorf, D., et al. 1984. Allogeneic bone marrow transplantation as treatment for accelerating chronic myelogenous leukemia. *Blood* 63(1): 219–222.

Minasian, L., Motzer, R., Gluck, L., et al. 1993. Interferon alfa–2a in advanced renal cell carcinoma: Treatment results and survival in 159 patients with long-term follow-up. *Journal of Clinical Oncology* 11(7): 1368–1375.

Mitsuyasu, R. 1989. The enhanced potential use of recombinant alpha interferon in the treatment of AIDS-related Kaposi's sarcoma. *Oncology Nursing Forum* 16 (6 suppl): 5–7.

Mitsuyasu, R. 1988. The role of alpha interferon in the biotherapy of hematologic malignancies and AIDS-related Kaposi's sarcoma. *Oncology Nursing Forum* 15 (6 suppl): 7–12.

Mitsuyasu, R., Taylor, J., Glaspy, J., *et al.* 1986. Heterogeneity of epidemic Kaposi's sarcoma: Implications for therapy. *Cancer* 57(8): 1657–1661.

Mitsuyasu, R., and Groopman, J. 1984. Biology and therapy of Kaposi's sarcoma. *Seminars in Oncology* 11(1): 53–59.

Mitsuyasu, R., Volberding, P., Jacobs, A., *et al.* 1984. High-dose alpha–2b recombinant interferon (IFN) in the therapy of epidemic Kaposi's sarcoma (KS) in acquired immune deficiency syndrome (AIDS). *Proceedings of the American Society of Clinical Oncology* 3: 51 (abstract C196.)

Mowskowitz, S., Chin-Bow, S., and Smith, G. 1982. Interferon and cis-DPP: Combination chemotherapy for P388 leukemia in CDFI mice. *Journal of Interferon Research* 2(4): 587–591.

Mullen, M., Spicehandler, D., Davidson, M., *et al.* 1988. Phase I study of combination zidovudine (AZT) and interferon alfa–2b in patients with AIDS. *Proceedings of the American Society of Clinical Oncology* 7: 1 (abstract).

Oberg, K., Norheim, I., and Alm, G. 1989. Treatment of malignant carcinoid tumors: A randomized controlled study of steptozocin plus 5-FU and human leukocyte interferon. *European Journal of Cancer and Clinical Oncology* 25(10): 1475–1479.

Oberg, K., Norheim, I., Lind, E., *et al.* 1986. Treatment of malignant carcinoid tumors with human leucocyte interferon—long-term results. *Cancer Treatment Reports* 70(11): 1297–1304.

O'Connell, M., Colgan, J., Oken, M., *et al.* 1986. Clinical trial of recombinant leukocyte A interferon as initial therapy for favorable histology non-Hodgkin's lymphomas and chronic lymphocytic leukemia: An Eastern Cooperative Oncology Group pilot study. *Journal of Clinical Oncology* 4(2): 128–136.

Oken, M., Kyle, R., Kay, N., *et al.* 1990a. Interferon in the treatment of refractory multiple myeloma: An Eastern Cooperative Oncology Group Study. *Leukemia and Lymphoma* 1(2): 95–100.

Oken, M., Kyle, R., Greipp, P., *et al.* 1990b. Chemotherapy plus interferon (rIFN-α–2b) in the treatment of multiple myeloma. *Proceedings of the American Society of Clinical Oncology* 9: 288 (abstract).

Oken, M., Kyle, P., Greipp, N., *et al.* 1988. Alternating cycles of VBMCP with interferon in the treatment of multiple myeloma. *Proceedings of the American Society of Clinical Oncology* 7: 288 (abstract).

Olsen, E., Rosen, S., Vollmer, R., *et al.* 1989. Interferon alpha–2a in the treatment of cutaneous T-cell lymphoma. *Journal of the American Academy of Dermatology* 20: 395–407.

Olsen, E., Vollmer, R., Roenisk, H., *et al.* 1987. Interferon alfa–2a in the treatment of cutaneous T-cell lymphoma.

Proceedings of the American Society of Clinical Oncology 6: 189 (abstract).

Pazdur, R., Ajani, J., Patt, Y., *et al.* 1990. Phase II study of fluorouracil and recombinant interferon alfa–2a in previously untreated advanced colorectal carcinoma. *Journal of Clinical Oncology* 8(12): 2027–2031.

Peck, R., and Bollag, W. 1991. Potentiation of retinoid-induced differentiation of HL–60 and U937 cell lines by cytokines. *European Journal of Cancer* 27(1): 53–57.

Perillo, R., Schiff, E., Davis, G., *et al.* 1990. A randomized controlled trial of interferon alpha–2b alone and after prednisone withdrawal for the treatment of chronic hepatitis B. *New England Journal of Medicine* 323(5): 295–301.

Pestka, S. 1983. The purification and manufacture of human interferons. *Scientific American* 249(1): 37–43.

Pestka, S., Langer, J., Zoon, K. et al. 1987. Interferons and their actions. *Annual Review of Biochemistry* 56: 727–777.

Peterson B., Petroni, M., Oken, M., *et al.* 1993. Cyclophosphamide versus cyclophosphamide plus interferon alfa–2b in follicular low-grade lymphomas: A preliminary report of an intergroup trial. *Proceedings of the American Society of Clinical Oncology* 12: 366 (abstract).

Physician's Desk Reference 48th ed. 1994. Montvale, NJ: Medical Economics Data.

Pitha, P. 1990. Interferons: A new class of tumor suppressor genes? *Cancer Cells* 2(X): 215–216.

Porzolt, F. 1992. Adjuvant therapy of renal cell cancer (RCC) with interferon alfa–2a. *Proceedings of American Society of Clinical Oncology* 11: 202, (abstract).

Pyrhonen, S., Hahka-Kemppinen, M., and Muhonen, T. 1992. A promising interferon plus four-drug chemotherapy regimen for metastatic melanoma. *Journal of Clinical Oncology* 10(12): 1919–1926.

Quesada, J., Alexanian, R., Hawkins, M., *et al.* 1986. Treatment of multiple myeloma with recombinant alpha interferon. *Blood* 67(2): 275–278.

Quesada, J., Hersh, E., Manning, J., *et al.* 1986. Treatment of hairy cell leukemia with recombinant alpha interferon. *Blood* 68(2): 493–497.

Quesada, J., Talpaz, M., Rios. A., *et al.* 1986. Clinical toxicity of interferons in cancer patients: A review. *Journal of Clinical Oncology* 4(2): 234–243.

Quesada, J., Reuben, J., Manning, J., *et al.* 1984. Alpha interferon for induction of remission in hairy-cell leukemia. *New England Journal of Medicine* 310(1): 15–18.

Quesada, J., Swanson, D., Trindade, A., *et al.* 1983. Renal cell carcinoma: Antitumor effects of leukocyte interferon. *Cancer Research* 43(2): 940–947.

Ratain, M., Golomb, H., Vardiman, J., *et al.* 1988. Relapse after interferon alfa–2b therapy for hairy cell leukemia: Analysis of prognostic variables. *Journal of Clinical Oncology* 6(11): 1714–1721.

Real, F., Oettgen, H., and Krown, S. 1986. Kaposi's sarcoma and the acquired immunodeficiency syndrome:

Treatment with high and low doses of recombinant leukocyte A interferon. *Journal of Clinical Oncology* 4(4): 544–551.

Revel, M., Kimchi, A., Shulman L. *et al*. 1980. Role of interferon-induced enzymes in the antiviral and antimitogenic effects of interferon. *Annals of New York Academy of Science* 350 : 449–472.

Rios, A., Mansell, P., Newell, G., *et al*. 1985. Treatment of acquired immunodeficiency syndrome-related Kaposi's sarcoma with lymphoblastoid interferon. *Journal of Clinical Oncology* 3(4): 506–512.

Robinson, W., Kirkwood, J., Harvey, H. *et al*. 1984. Effective use of recombinant human alfa interferons in metastatic malignant melanoma: A comparison of two regimens. *Proceedings of the American Society of Clinical Oncology* 3: 60 (abstract).

Salmon, S., Durie, B., Young, L. *et al*. 1983. Effects of cloned human leukocyte interferons in the human tumor stem cell assay. *Journal of Clinical Oncology* 1(3): 217–225.

Samuels, C. 1988. Mechanisms of the antiviral action of interferons. *Progress in Nucleic Acid Research and Molecular Biology* 35: 27–72.

Saracco, G., Mazella, G., Kosina, F. *et al*. 1989. A controlled trial of human lymphoblastoid interferon in chronic hepatitis B in Italy. *Hepatology* 10(3): 336–341.

Schiffer, C. 1991. Interferon studies in the treatment of patients with leukemia. *Seminars in Oncology* 18(1): 1–6.

Sertoli, M., Bernengo, M., Ardizzoni, A., *et al*. 1989. Phase II trial of recombinant alfa–2b interferon in the treatment of metastatic skin melanoma. *Oncology* 46(2): 96–98.

Sehgal, P. 1982. The interferon gene. *Biochemistry Biophysical Acta* 695: 17–33.

Silver, R. 1990. Interferon in the treatment of myeloproliferative disorders. *Seminars in Hematology* 27 (suppl4): 6–14.

Skotnicki, A., Wolsak-Smolen, T., Bicharski, J., *et al*. 1988. Human recombinant interferon alpha–2 in the treatment of patients with hairy cell leukemia. *Cancer Detection and Prevention* 12(4): 511–522.

Slater, L., Wetzel, M., and Cesario, T. 1981. Combined interferon and antimetabolite therapy of murine L1210 leukemia. *Cancer* 48(1): 5–9.

Smalley, R., Anderson, J., Hawkins, M., *et al*. 1992. Interferon alfa combined with cytotoxic chemotherapy for patients with non-Hodgkin's lymphoma. *New England Journal of Medicine* 327(19): 1336–1341.

Speck, B., Bortin, M., Champlin, R., *et al*. 1984. Allogeneic bone-marrow transplantation for chronic myelogenous leukaemia. *Lancet* 1(8378): 665–668.

Spiers, A., Parekh, S., and Bishop, M. 1984. Hairy cell leukemia: Induction of complete remission with pentostatin (2' deoxycoformycin). *Journal of Clinical Oncology* 2(12): 1336–1342.

Sporn, M., Roberts, A., Roche, N., *et al*. 1986. Mechanism of action of retinoids. *Journal of the American Academy of Dermatology* 15: 756–764.

Springer, E., Kuzel, T., and Rosen, S. 1991. International symposium on cutaneous T-cell lymphoma. *Journal of the American Academy of Dermatology* 24: 136–138.

Stewart, W., Blalock J., Burke, D. *et al*. 1980. Interferon nomenclature (letter). *Journal of Immunology* 125(5): 2353.

Tallman, M., Hakimian, D., Variakojis, D., *et al*. 1992. A single cycle of 2-chlorodeoxyadenosine results in complete remission in the majority of patients with hairy cell leukemia. *Blood* 80: 2203–2209.

Talpaz, M., O'Brien, S., Kurzock, R., *et al*. 1992. Alpha interferon (IFN-a) and chemotherapy combination in early chronic myelogenous leukemia (CML)—A summary of three M. D. Anderson Studies. *Proceedings of The American Society of Clinical Oncology* 11: 908, (abstract).

Talpaz, M., Kantarjian, H., McCredie, K., *et al*. 1987. Clinical investigation of human alpha interferon in chronic myelogenous leukemia. *Blood* 69(5): 1280–1288.

Talpaz, M., Kantarjian, H., McCredie, K., *et al*. 1986. Hematologic remission and cytogenetic improvement induced by recombinant human interferon alpha in chronic myelogenous leukemia. *New England Journal of Medicine* 314(17): 1065–1069.

Vadhan-Raj, S., Wong, G., Gnecco, C., *et al*. 1986. Immunological variables as predictors of prognosis in patients with Kaposi's sarcoma and the acquired immunodeficiency syndrome. *Cancer* 61: 1071–1074.

Vogelzang, N., Lipton, A., and Figlin, R. 1993. Subcutaneous interleukin-2 plus interferon alfa–2a in metastatic renal cancer: An outpatient multicenter trial. *Journal of Clinical Oncology* 11(9): 1809–1816.

Volberding, P., and Mitsuyasu, R. 1985. Recombinant interferon alpha in the treatment of acquired immunodeficiency syndrome-related Kaposi's sarcoma. *Seminars in Oncology* 12(4): 2–6.

Wadler, S., Lembersky, B., Atkins, M., *et al*. 1991. Phase II trial of fluorouracil and recombinant interferon alfa–2a in patients with advanced colorectal carcinoma: An Eastern Cooperative Oncology Group study. *Journal of Clinical Oncology* 9(10): 1806–1810.

Wadler, S., and Wiernik, P. 1990. Clinical update on the role of fluorouracil and recombinant interferon alpha–2a in the treatment of colorectal carcinoma. *Seminars in Oncology* 17: 516–21 (suppl).

Wadler, S., Schwartz, E., Goldman, M., *et al*. 1984. 5-Fluorouracil and recombinant alpha–2a interferon: An active regimen against advanced colorectal carcinoma. *Journal of Clinical Oncology* 7: 1769–1775.

Wagstaff, J., Loynds, P., and Crowther, D. 1986. A Phase II study of human rDNA alpha–2 interferon in patients with lowgrade non-Hodgkin's lymphoma. *Cancer Chemotherapy and Pharmacology Journal* 18(1): 54–58.

Willemse, P., DeVries, E., Mulder, N., *et al.* 1990. Intraperitoneal human recombinant interferon alpha–2b in minimal residual ovarian cancer. *European Journal of Cancer* 26(3): 353–358.

Williams, B. 1983. Biochemical actions of interferon. In Sikora, K. (ed). *Interferon and Cancer.* New York: Plenum Press, pp. 33–52.

York, M., Greco, F., Figlin, R., et al. 1993. A randomized phase III trial comparing 5-FU with or without interferon alfa–2a for advanced colorectal cancer. *Proceedings of the American Society of Clinical Oncology* 12: 590 (abstract).

Yoshitake Y., Kishida T., Esaki K. *et al.* 1976. Antitumor effects of interferon on transplanted tumors in congenitally athymic nude mice. *Giken Journal* 19: 125–127.

CHAPTER 5 | The Interleukins

Eileen Sharp, RN, BSN, OCN

Interleukins (ILs) are cytokines or proteins that exist as natural components of the human immune system. The primary function of these proteins is the **immunomodulation** and **immunoregulation** of leukocytes. The term *interleukin* (between leukocytes) refers to the signaling and communication that occur between cells in the immune system. Most ILs have **pleiotropic** functions, that is, they are capable of inducing multiple biological activities in a variety of target cells. As a result, many of the ILs identified earlier each have several names that describe their different functions. In an effort to standardize the nomenclature, ILs are now designated by the order in which they were identified (i.e., IL–1, IL–2, IL–3, etc.). Table 5.1 summarizes the biological activities of all ILs described through 1993 (Kuby, 1992; Mulé and Rosenberg, 1992; Oettgen and Old, 1991).

Interleukins, which are produced and secreted primarily by leukocytes, activate target cells by binding to receptor sites present on the cell-surface membranes. In many cases, IL receptors are expressed specifically by cells in the immune system after antigen exposure. The binding of the IL to the membrane receptor signals the interior of the cell to alter the cell's activation level or functional capacity. Various ILs may produce autocrine, paracrine, or endocrine actions within the body. **Autocrine action** refers to the binding and activation of the same cell that produced the IL. **Paracrine action** describes the binding and activation of nearby cells; whereas **endocrine action** occurs when ILs are secreted and bind to distant cells in the body (Kuby, 1992; Dinarello and Mier, 1987). Primarily, ILs affect local or regional cells rather than distant cells as in endocrine action.

The complex balance between cellular activation and immunoregulation is orchestrated by the secretion of ILs and the resultant effects on cells of the immune system. Actions

Table 5.1   Biological activities of interleukins

Interleukin	Biological Activities
Interleukin-1	• Activates resting T cells • Mediates inflammation • Activates endothelial cells and macrophages • Functions as a cofactor for hematopoietic growth factors • Induces sleep, fever, ACTH release, acute phase response • Enhances activity of NK cells • Chemotactically attracts neutrophils and macrophages • Stimulates the synthesis of lymphokines
Interleukin-2	• Induces the synthesis and secretion of lymphokines • Induces proliferation of antigen-primed T cells • Functions as a co-factor for growth and differentiation of B cells • Augments LAK activity • Enhances NK activity
Interleukin-3	• Supports the growth of pluripotent bone marrow stem cells • Acts as a growth factor for mast cells • Stimulates histamine secretion
Interleukin-4	• Acts as a growth factor for activated B cells • Induces MHC class II antigens on B cells • Acts as a growth factor for resting T cells • Enhances cytolytic activity of cytotoxic T cells • Acts as a growth factor for mast cells • Promotes growth of melanoma TIL • Induces class switch to IgE and IgG1 • Increases phagocytic activity of macrophages
Interleukin-5	• Induces B-cell proliferation and differentiation • Induces eosinophil growth and differentiation • Acts with IL-4 to stimulate IgE production
Interleukin-6	• Increases secretion of antibodies by plasma cells • Co-stimulates T-cell activation with IL-1 • Aids in differentiation of myeloid stem cells • Induces B-cell differentiation into plasma cells
Interleukin-7	• Supports the growth of B-cell precursors • Stimulates the growth of thymocytes • Increases the expression of IL-2 and IL-2R by resting T cells
Interleukin-8	• Chemotactically attracts neutrophils • Induces adherence of neutrophils to vascular endothelial cells and aids migration to tissues
Interleukin-9	• Acts as a mitogen to induce T-helper-cell growth • Acts as a growth factor for mast cells
Interleukin-10	• Suppresses cytokine production by T-helper cell subset • Stimulates cytotoxic T-cell growth
Interleukin-11	• Enhances early hematopoietic progenitor cells • Enhances megakaryocytopoiesis with IL-3 • Inhibits lipoprotien lipase activity
Interleukin-12	• Activates NK-mediated cytotoxicity • Facilitates cytotoxic T-cell responses

produced by the ILs may by redundant, synergistic, or antagonistic. **Redundant actions** are similar actions that may be produced by different ILs. **Synergistic activity** occurs when more than one IL is essential to produce activity in a particular target cell. **Antagonistic effects** occur when an IL inhibits the target cell activity induced by another cytokine (Kuby, 1992; Paul, 1989).

This chapter will focus on IL–1, IL–2, and IL–4 and will include information on biological actions, clinical trials, regulatory approval, and future applications. Specific information about IL–3 may be found in Chapter 6 and information about IL–6, in Chapter 16.

INTERLEUKIN–1

Interleukin–1, originally was known as lymphocyte-activating factor and endogenous pyrogen, and was first described by Gery *et al.* in 1972. It is a glycoprotein molecule primarily secreted by activated macrophages in the body. Interleukin–1 is also produced by a variety of other cells, including B and T lymphocytes, neutrophils, natural killer cells, fibroblasts, endothelial cells, smooth muscle cells, and vascular tissues in response to trauma, infection, or exposure to antigens (Kuby, 1992). Two forms of the IL–1 molecule, α and β, have been identified. The two forms are related but are products of separate genes and have different amino acid sequences; however, both bind to the same cell-surface receptors and therefore share biological activities (Dinarello and Wolff, 1993; Dower *et al.*, 1986).

Biological Actions

The biological actions of IL–1 are numerous and include immunomodulation, promotion of hematopoiesis, mediation of inflammation, and mediation of disease in the body. Other activities of IL–1 include promoting bone resorption, stimulation of fibroblasts, and conferring radioprotective effects on normal tissues. These actions may benefit the human body by conveying protective or healing properties following inflammation and injury or may negatively affect the body through their pathogenic role (Dinarello and Wolff, 1993).

Immunomodulation

Immunomodulatory functions of IL–1 include the activation of T cells, natural killer (NK) cells, polymorphonuclear cells, and monocytes. Interleukin–1 also enhances B-cell growth and antibody production. Although IL–1 has little direct antitumor effect against most tumor cell lines, it enhances the antitumor effects of monocytes and NK cells (Spriggs, 1992) and induces the secretion of secondary cytokines that may possess antitumor activities (Philip and Epstein, 1986). Interleukin–1 and tumor necrosis factor (TNF) may act synergistically to enhance TNF cytotoxicity (Spriggs, 1991; Dinarello and Mier, 1987).

Promotion of Hematopoiesis

Preclinical and *in vitro* studies have demonstrated that IL–1 induces the production of hematopoietic growth factors such as granulocyte-macrophage colony-stimulating factor (GM-CSF) and macrophage colony-stimulating factor (M-CSF), and IL–6. IL–1 acts synergistically with these colony-stimulating factors to promote the proliferation and differentiation of hematopoietic progenitor cells *in vitro* (Moore, 1991). Preclinical studies showed that IL–1 could accelerate the recovery of granulocytes and platelets if given after chemotherapy or radiation, and was myeloprotective if given before (Castelli *et al.*, 1988).

Mediation of Inflammation

Interleukin–1 is an important mediator of the inflammatory response and can be detected in the circulatory system within a few hours after the onset of infection or trauma (Dinarello and Mier, 1987). Interleukin–1 induces fever, sleep, acute-phase protein synthesis and production of adrenocorticotropic hormone (ACTH), cortisol, and insulin. Interleukin–1 induces local inflammation via its effects on hematopoietic cells, fibroblasts, vascular endothelial cells, and secondary cytokine production. During an inflammatory reaction, IL–1 induces neutrophils to travel from the bone marrow through the peripheral circulatory system and then to extravasate through capillary walls to extravascular spaces and tissue sites. Both neutrophils and monocytes are activated by and chemotactically attracted to IL–1, which induces an increase in phagocytic cells during an inflammatory response (Kuby,

1992; Stroud *et al.*, 1990). Interleukin–1 also induces endocrine effects on liver hepatocytes to produce acute-phase proteins, including fibrinogen, C-reactive protein, and haptoglobin that contribute to host defense during an inflammatory response (Kuby, 1992).

Mediation of Disease

Interleukin–1 appears also to have a role as a mediator of diseases in the human body. In septic shock, IL–1 induces the synthesis and production of platelet-activating factor, prostaglandins, and nitric oxide. In laboratory animals, these mediator molecules act as potent vasodilators and produce hypotension and shock. Tumor necrosis factor, which produces similar effects, also stimulates the production of IL–1 (Dinarello and Wolff, 1993). Interleukin–1 may also play a role in autoimmune disorders such as insulin-dependent diabetes mellitus (Mandrup-Poulsen *et al.*, 1989), which is characterized by the destruction of beta cells in the islets of Langerhans. *In vitro* incubation of human and animal islet cells with IL–1 induces beta cell death. Therefore, the destruction of beta cells in patients with insulin-dependent diabetes may be caused by IL–1 that has been produced as a result of an autoimmune process within the islet cells (Dinarello and Wolff, 1993).

Interleukin–1 may also play a role in the pathogenesis of such inflammatory diseases as rheumatoid arthritis and inflammatory bowel disease. In patients with rheumatoid arthritis, IL–1 can be detected in the synovial fluid and lining. In animals, intra-articular injections of IL–1 induce leukocyte infiltration and cartilage degeneration. These findings lead to postulation of a role for IL–1 in the pathophysiology of rheumatoid arthritis (Dinarello and Wolff, 1993). In inflammatory bowel disease (ulcerative colitis and Crohn's disease), the lesions contain activated neutrophils and macrophages. In these bowel lesions, concentrations of IL–1 and IL–8 (an inflammatory cytokine whose production is stimulated by IL–1) in tissue are high. In animals, blocking the effects of IL–1 with an IL–1-receptor antagonist reduces the severity of inflammatory bowel disease (Dinarello and Wolff, 1993). This evidence links IL–1 to the pathophysiology of inflammatory bowel disease. The role of IL–1 as a direct or an indirect growth factor for both acute and chronic myelogenous leukemia also is being investigated as a result of observations that IL–1β messenger RNA can be detected in cells from patients with acute myelogenous leukemia (Rambaldi *et al.*, 1991) or in chronic granulocytic leukemia cells of the juvenile type (Bagby *et al.*, 1988). The mechanism of action by which IL–1 may stimulate myelogenous leukemia cells is similar to the action by which IL–1 stimulates the production of CSFs and serves as a cofactor for the proliferation of stem cells (Dinarello and Wolff, 1993).

Based on increased IL–1 concentrations in plasma and evidence of IL–1 gene expression in affected tissues, the pathogenic contributory role of IL–1 is being investigated to determine its role in other diseases or conditions. These conditions include atherosclerosis, psoriasis, asthma, osteoporosis, periodontal disease, transplant rejection, graft-versus-host disease, sleep disturbances, alcoholic hepatitis, and premature labor secondary to uterine infection (Dinarello and Wolff, 1993).

Clinical Trials

Theoretically, the potential for therapeutic application of the biological actions of IL–1 is great as a result of both its beneficial and harmful effects in the body. Thus there is interest in the development of both agonists and antagonists of this cytokine. Interleukin–1 may be useful in the treatment of cancer because of its ability to activate effector cells, induce production or activity of secondary cytokines, protect cells from radiation-induced injury, restore bone marrow damaged by chemotherapy, and confer anti-infective properties. Antagonists of IL–1 may be useful to reduce the production or action of IL–1 in other diseases (Starnes, 1992).

Clinical trials are under way to study the toxic and hematologic effects of IL–1 in patients with advanced malignant disease. In a phase I study, intravenous IL–1 was administered over 15 minutes every day for seven days to patients with advanced malignancies. The maximum-tolerated dose (MTD) of IL–1 was determined to be 0.3 µg/kg. Dose-limiting toxic effects included hypotension, confusion, renal insufficiency, myocardial infarction, and severe abdominal pain. Observed hematologic effects may have potential benefit. Therapy with IL–1 induced a significant dose-related increase in the total white blood cell count. Platelet counts temporarily decreased during IL–1 therapy, but there was a significant increase in the platelet count one to two weeks after therapy. Bone marrow cellularity also increased during therapy (Smith et al., 1992). Other studies have shown IL–1α to accelerate the recovery of platelets after high-dose carboplatin therapy (Vadhan-Raj et al., 1994; Smith et al., 1993). Early studies evaluating IL–1β post chemotherapy with 5-FU demonstrated fewer days of neutropenia in patients receiving 5-FU plus IL–1β, than in those patients receiving 5-FU alone. This difference, however, did not achieve statistical significance. The data did show that IL–1β had stimulatory effects in human hematopoiesis. Hypotension was a dose-limiting factor in this study (Crown et al., 1991).

Several strategies to reduce the production or action of IL–1 are also being investigated. Medications, such as corticosteroids and nonsteroidal anti-inflammatory drugs, or cytokines, such as IL–4 or IL–10, may reduce IL–1 production. Inhibition of IL–1-converting enzymes may decrease IL–1 processing and release from cells. More attention has been devoted to neutralizing IL–1 by using anti-IL–1 antibodies and soluble IL–1 receptors. Another strategy to decrease the action of IL–1 is through the use of IL–1-receptor antagonists (IL–1ra) that compete with and bind to the IL–

1 receptor sites on the target cells. (See Figure 5.1.) This naturally occurring protein was described in 1985, and subsequently expressed in recombinant form (Dinarello, 1991; Eisenberg et al., 1990). Administration of IL–1 receptor antagonist has been shown to reduce mortality among patients with septic shock syndrome (Fisher et al., 1991).

Regulatory Approval

As of June 1994, IL–1 continues to be studied in clinical trials but has not yet received approval from the Food and Drug Administration (FDA) for clinical use.

Side Effects

The most common side effects observed in patients who received IL–1 included constitutional side effects (fever, chills, headache, myalgias) and gastrointestinal side effects (nausea and vomiting). The majority of patients experienced chills followed by a monophasic temperature elevation. Chills were successfully treated by administering intravenous meperidine and covering the patient with warm blankets. Nausea and vomiting, occurring soon after therapy, was common but not severe in nature (grade 2 or less). Less common side effects of IL–1 included somnolence, abdominal pain, dyspnea, and peripheral vein phlebitis (Smith et al., 1992).

Future Directions

Future applications and clinical trials evaluating IL–1 will involve the areas of immunomodulation, inflammation, hematopoiesis, autoimmune disorders, wound healing, and radioprotection. Direct administration of IL–1 may be useful for treating patients with cancer (Johnson, 1993) and severe burns and for those who receive toxic therapies such as irradiation. Reducing the production or activity of

Figure 5.1   Interactions between interleukin-1, interleukin-1–receptor antagonist, and interleukin-1 receptors. Panel A depicts a cell with the two types of interleukin-1 receptors. The two types have similar extracellular structures, and both bind interleukin-1 (**a** or **b**) or interleukin-1–receptor antagonist. Normally, there is partial occupancy by interleukin-1 and partial occupancy by interleukin-1–receptor antagonist. In this cell, interleukin-1 is still able to trigger a response, as indicated by the arrows directed toward the nucleus (N). The cell in Panel B is exposed to a large excess of interleukin-1–receptor antagonist, so all the interleukin-1 receptors are occupied by the receptor antagonist. No stimulation occurs under these conditions, since interleukin-1 cannot bind to the interleukin-1 receptors. The cell in Panel C is exposed to soluble type I receptors and interleukin-1. The soluble type I receptors bind to interleukin-1, so interleukin-1 cannot bind to and activate its cell-surface receptors.

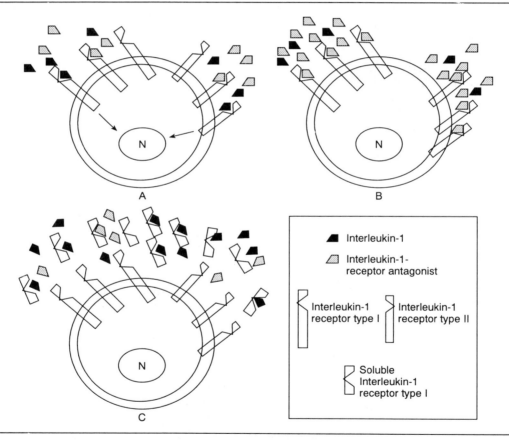

Source: Reprinted by permission, Dinarello, C., and Wolff, S. 1993. The role of interleukin-1 in disease. *The New England Journal of Medicine* 328(2): 106–113 (1993).

IL–1 may be a useful strategy in the treatment of patients who have acute or chronic inflammatory or autoimmune disorders.

INTERLEUKIN–2

Interleukin–2 is a lymphokine first described in 1976 as T-cell growth factor (Morgan *et al.*, 1976). Produced primarily by activated T-helper cells, IL–2 is a messenger regulatory molecule that has profound immunomodulatory effects in the body. The regulation of IL–2 production is dependent on the activation of T cells by antigens. This production and release of IL–2 requires two signals. First, the T-helper cell must recognize an antigen in conjunction with the major histocompatibility complex (MHC) antigens expressed on an antigen-presenting cell. Second, the T-helper cell interacts with IL–1 produced by the antigen-presenting cell. Once activated, T-helper cells begin to produce and secrete IL–2 and express IL–2 receptors. Autocrine activity is displayed by IL–2 as it binds to and activates the same cell line that secreted it (Malek and Gutgsell, 1993; Smith, 1993).

Biological Actions

The biological actions of IL–2 are critical for the generation of an immune response. The specific actions of IL–2 are numerous and complex. In addition to its primary role in the proliferation of all T-cell subpopulations, IL–2 promotes the activation of cytotoxic T-cells, NK cells, and monocytes (Boldt and Ellis, 1993). The activation of peripheral blood lymphocytes into lymphokine-activated killer (LAK) cells is induced by IL–2 (Grimm, 1993). B-cell growth and antibody production are supported by IL–2 and by the secretion of secondary cytokines (IL–4, IL–5, IL–6) induced by IL–2 that serve as B-cell growth and differentiation factors. Through the activation of target cells, IL–2 also induces the release of other cytokines such as interferon-gamma (IFN-γ), GM-CSF, and TNF. Interleukin–2 also enhances expression of the IL–2 receptor on

T-cell surfaces (Rubin, 1993; Galazka *et al.*, 1991; Lotze, 1991).

The activation of target cells by IL–2 is accomplished by the binding of the IL–2 protein molecule to the IL–2 receptor (IL–2R) located on the target cell-surface membrane. The IL–2R is composed of three separate chains: the alpha chain, the beta chain, and the recently discovered gamma chain. The IL–2R is depicted in Figure 5.2. When all three chains are expressed simultaneously, a high-affinity heterotrimeric receptor is formed. If cells display the beta chain and the gamma chain but not the alpha chain, an intermediate affinity receptor is formed. Cells that display only the alpha chain do not generate a signal when IL–2 binds. Resting T cells do not express high-affinity IL–2Rs, but when T cells are exposed to antigens, low concentrations of IL–2 will saturate high-affinity IL–2Rs and antigen-specific T-cell proliferation will occur. Withdrawal of the antigen leads to reduction of the high-affinity IL–2Rs and of T-cell clonal expansion despite the presence of IL–2 (Smith, 1993). These findings have been applied in the laboratory to increase proliferation of cytotoxic T cells for use in clinical trials with cancer.

Clinical Trials

Early studies demonstrated that native IL–2 alone or in combination with LAK cells caused tumor regressions in animal models. Production of recombinant IL–2 began when the DNA sequence coding for IL–2 was identified. Although the recombinant form of IL–2 differs slightly from its native form, the two have similar functional and biological activities (Doyle *et al.*, 1985). The recombinant form differs primarily in that the protein is not glycosylated and the amino acid serine is substituted for cysteine at amino acid position 125. Large-scale clinical trials using IL–2 were begun in 1984. Recombinant IL–2 has been used in clinical trials to treat a variety of human malignancies. Used either as a single agent or in conjunction with **LAK cells, tumor-infil-**

Figure 5.2   Schematic of interleukin-2 to its receptor.

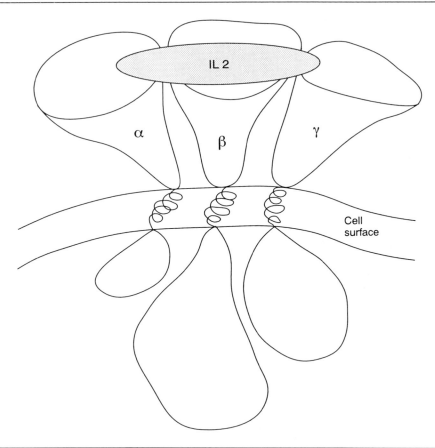

IL 2

α

β

γ

Cell
surface

Source: Reprinted with permission from Smith, K. 1993. Lowest dose interleukin-2 immunotherapy. *Blood* 81(6): 1414–1423.

trating lymphocytes (TILs), other biological response modifiers, or chemotherapy, IL–2 has induced responses against some tumors, especially renal cell carcinoma and malignant melanoma (Atkins and Mier, 1993; Dillman *et al.*, 1993; Rosenberg *et al.*, 1989).

In May 1992, the FDA licensed IL–2 for use in the treatment of adult patients with metastatic renal cell carcinoma. That approval was based on an evaluation of 255 patients treated with single-agent IL–2 at a dosage of 600,000 International Units (IU)/kg of body weight administered every 8 hours by a 15-minute intravenous bolus infusion for a total of 14 doses. After nine days of rest, the schedule was repeated. Objective responses were observed in 37 patients (15%), with 9 complete and 28 partial responses. Responses were noted in metastases to the lung, liver, lymph node, soft tissue, and renal bed. The median duration of the objective responses was 23.2 months (Chiron Corporation, 1994). At the described dose and schedule of administration, close patient monitoring was needed because many patients suffered severe side effects that often necessitated intensive care support. The most acute side effects involved the cardio-vascular, pulmonary, and renal systems, or were related to the vascular leak syndrome.

Since its approval by the FDA, IL–2 continues to be studied in clinical trials in an effort to define its activity using different doses, routes, schedules, and combination regimens that produce fewer toxic effects while maintaining efficacy. Interleukin–2 has been administered by a variety of routes, including intravenous (bolus vs. continuous infusion), subcutaneous, intra-arterial, intra-lymphatic, intraperitoneal, and inhalation routes (Huland et al., 1994).

Numerous studies are using IL–2 alone at various doses, routes, and schedules. Use of low-dose IL–2 regimens has enabled a greater number of patients to receive therapy and has allowed for prolonged exposure to IL–2. Sleijfer et al. (1992) reported a phase II study of IL–2 administered subcutaneously to outpatients with metastatic renal cell carcinoma. Interleukin–2 was administered subcutaneously in a five-days-per-week cycle for six consecutive weeks. During the first five-day cycle, the dose was 18 million international units (IU) given once daily. In subsequent weeks, the daily dose for the first two days was reduced to 9 million IU. Of the 26 patients whose disease could be evaluated for response, two achieved a complete response and four achieved a partial response (overall response rate, 23%). These results suggest that IL–2 has activity against renal cell carcinoma when administered as low-dose subcutaneous therapy. The observed response rate was similar to that observed with high-dose IL–2 with or without LAK cells. Additional studies continue, and will ultimately define the efficacy and toxic effects of low-dose IL–2 therapy. In addition, combination studies evaluating the efficacy of low-dose IL–2 therapy are in progress (Vogelzang et al., 1993).

Interleukin–2 has also been combined with adoptive cellular therapy using LAK cells or TIL. Lymphokine-activated killer cells are generated from peripheral blood lymphocytes after exposure to IL–2. These acti-vated lymphocytes are capable of lysing a variety of tumor cell lines. Studies employing IL–2 plus LAK cells yield response rates similar to those achieved with single-agent IL–2 (Dillman et al., 1991b; Dutcher et al., 1989; Fischer et al., 1988; West et al., 1987; Rosenberg et al., 1985), but the incidence of complete responses is greater in patients who received IL–2 plus LAK cells (Rosenberg et al., 1989). The impact of the addition of LAK cells on patient survival is currently being evaluated. Tumor-infiltrating lymphocytes are expanded and activated lymphocytes obtained from tumor specimens. In theory, TIL have specific activity against the tumor from which they were derived, in contrast with LAK cells, which have broader cytolytic activity (Itoh and Balch, 1993). Trials utilizing IL–2 plus TIL have focused primarily on patients with renal cell carcinoma and melanoma and have demonstrated some objective responses (Dillman et al., 1991a; Oldham et al., 1991; Rosenberg et al., 1988). Further studies are needed to evaluate the potential benefits of **adoptive cellular therapy** combined with IL–2. The toxic reactions experienced by patients who received IL–2 plus LAK cells or TIL were mainly dependent on the dose and schedule of IL–2 (Brogley and Sharp, 1990).

Interleukin–2 has been combined with chemotherapeutic agents for a variety of malignancies in an attempt to produce synergistic antitumor effects. The sequencing of the two therapies may affect their efficacy and toxicity patterns. If chemotherapy is administered first, it may prime the immune system or decrease the tumor burden. If IL–2 and chemotherapy are administered concurrently, synergistic actions may include chemo-therapy-induced damage to the tumor cell membrane or IL–2-induced intratumor capillary leak. Among theoretical reasons for administering IL–2 prior to chemotherapy is to allow IL–2 immunomodulation without immunosuppression and alteration of tumor cells by IL–2 or secondary cytokines, which would render the tumor cells more susceptible to the cytotoxic effects of chemotherapy

(Sznol and Longo, 1993). Combination regimens of IL–2 plus chemotherapy have been studied in a variety of malignancies, including melanoma, renal cell carcinoma, gastrointestinal malignancies, non-small-cell lung cancer, and head and neck cancer. Generally, these combinations have response rates equivalent to those achieved with chemotherapy alone. However, combination therapy using agents with proven activity against melanoma has generated more promising results with potential additive activity. Richards *et al.* (1992) reported a phase II study using carmustine, cisplatin, dacarbazine, IL–2, and IFN-α for melanoma. Among 36 patients who completed one treatment cycle, there was one complete response, 23 partial responses, and one minor response (overall response rate, 69%). The median duration of response was seven months, and the median survival was 11.5 months. Other investigators have studied the effects of IL–2 plus chemotherapy for metastatic melanoma. Legha *et al.* (1993) studied the effects of IL–2, IFN-α, and chemotherapy with cisplatin, vinblastine, and dacarbazine, and achieved response rates superior to those achieved with either biotherapy or chemotherapy alone. In ongoing studies, Legha and Buzaid (1993) have examined the sequence of administration of biotherapy plus chemotherapy and have observed response rates ranging from 47% (arm with biotherapy administered first) to 73% (arm with chemotherapy administered first). Toxic effects have included the standard side effects for these agents and included constitutional symptoms and myelosuppression.

Combination therapy with IL–2 plus IFN-α has been studied particularly in patients with metastatic renal cell carcinoma. (Mulé and Rosenberg, 1991). Refer to Chapter 4 for further information.

Regulatory Approval

In May 1992, the FDA approved aldesleukin, a form of human IL–2 produced by recombinant DNA technology, for the treatment of adults (18 years of age) with metastatic renal cell carcinoma. Aldesleukin is manufactured by the Chiron Corporation under the trade name Proleukin® (Chiron Corporation, 1994). Recommended dosage is as previously noted. Because adverse effects at this dosage level are frequent, often serious, and sometimes fatal, it is recommended that patients have normal cardiac, pulmonary, hepatic, and CNS function prior to initiation of therapy.

Side Effects

The side effects profile for patients who receive IL–2 therapy differs depending on the dose, route, and schedule of IL–2 (Parkinson, 1989). In general, high-dose IL–2 therapy produces more severe toxic effects (Margolin, 1993). Examples of IL–2 doses with their required levels of patient care are listed in Table 5.2. Factors such as patient performance status, major organ function, age, and tumor burden also will affect the onset, duration, and severity of the side effects. Duration of therapy also has an impact on the side effects profile. Protracted therapy with IL–2 may produce more toxic effects. Side effects generally begin shortly after the initiation of therapy and intensify over time. Once therapy has been completed, most side effects resolve within a few days. Irreversible or permanent side effects from IL–2 therapy are rare. Prior to IL–2 regimens, patients should be thoroughly screened to determine their ability to tolerate this therapy. The side effects of IL–2 have the potential to involve nearly every major organ system (Rieger, 1994; Jassak, 1993; Rieger *et al.*, 1993; Hood and Abernathy, 1991; Siegel and Puri, 1991; Jassak and Sticklin, 1986).

A major side effect experienced by patients who receive IL–2 therapy is the flu-like syndrome. Patients may experience chills or rigors followed by fevers. Other constitutional symptoms include myalgias, arthralgias, malaise, headache, and nasal stuffiness. The onset of these symptoms is usually 4 to 6 hours after initiation of therapy. Fatigue is also a signifi-

Table 5.2 Interleukin-2 dosing schedule examples

Interleukin-2 Dose	Administration Route	Care Setting
High Dose		
600,000 IU/kg Q 8 hours	Intravenous bolus	Inpatient Intensive care (potential)
Intermediate Dose		
18 million IU/m²/ Day	Intravenous continuous Infusion	Inpatient General oncology unit
Low Dose		
18 million IU/Day	Subcutaneous	Outpatient

Source: Sharpe, 1993; Tsevat *et al.* 1993; Viele and Moran, 1993.

cant side effect in patients who receive IL–2 therapy (Piper *et al.*, 1989). Interleukin–2 triggers the release of cytokines such as IL–1 and IFN-γ from target cells and that release may induce these symptoms (Rieger, 1992; Weidmann *et al.*, 1992; Sergi, 1991).

Potential cardiovascular side effects related to IL–2 therapy include tachycardia, hypotension, arrhythmias, edema, and weight gain. In part, these toxic effects result from dose-related fluid imbalances caused by a vascular leak syndrome. Release of cytokines such as IL–1, TNF, and IFN-γ may affect the permeability of vascular walls, decrease systemic vascular resistance, and allow fluid to leak from the vascular bed to the interstitial spaces (Mier, 1993b; Lee *et al.*, 1989; Gaynor *et al.*, 1988).

Potential pulmonary side effects include dyspnea and pulmonary congestion. These side effects may occur as a result of interstitial pulmonary edema related to increased vascular permeability, the migration of activated T cells to the lungs, or the release of secondary cytokines in the lungs (Sergi, 1991; Padavic-Shaller, 1988). In extreme cases, patients who receive high-dose IL–2 therapy may develop adult respiratory distress syndrome (ARDS), which can progress to severe respiratory failure requiring intubation (Gaynor and Fisher,

1993; Farrell, 1992). Patients with poor pulmonary reserve should be screened carefully prior to receiving IL–2 therapy and should be monitored closely during therapy.

Renal dysfunction, another potential side effect of IL–2 therapy, is manifested by decreased urine output and increased serum creatinine and blood urea nitrogen levels. Contributing factors include hypoperfusion of the kidneys and direct effects of IL–2 on the kidneys (Kozeny *et al.*, 1988; Belldegrun *et al.*, 1987). Patients with metastatic renal cell carcinoma who have undergone prior nephrectomy or who have impaired renal function prior to IL–2 therapy should be monitored closely.

Liver function may also be temporarily impaired during IL–2 therapy. Signs of this include elevated liver function enzymes and jaundice. The reversible cholestasis that occurs may be a result of direct effects of IL–2 or indirect effects of secondary cytokines such as TNF or IL–6 (Rieger, 1992; Fisher *et al.*, 1989). Patients who have metastatic disease in the liver should be monitored closely.

Skin changes associated with IL–2 therapy are common. Patients may experience a diffuse erythematous rash, intense pruritus, and dry skin with desquamation. The palms of the hands and the soles of the feet may peel. Results of histologic examinations of skin biopsy samples have been inconclusive (Wolkenstein *et al.*, 1993; Rieger, 1992; Gaspari *et al.*, 1987). Patients who receive subcutaneous injections of IL–2 have experienced local inflammatory responses at injection sites (Atzpodien *et al.*, 1991). Inflammation may begin 4 to 6 hours after injection and may persist for up to five days. The injection site may be painful, erythematous, and indurated. Subcutaneous nodules may also develop at injection sites. These nodules are usually small and painless but may take several months to resolve.

Gastrointestinal toxic effects are commonly experienced by patients who receive IL–2 therapy. Nausea, vomiting, diarrhea, anorexia, and mucositis are symptoms experienced by the majority of patients at all dose levels of IL–2. Nausea, vomiting, and diarrhea commonly occur within several hours after intravenous bolus IL–2 or subcutaneous IL–2. With continuous-infusion IL–2, these side effects may occur intermittently. Anorexia may be a severe side effect of long-term or repeated IL–2 therapy and may result in significant weight loss. The gastrointestinal side effects generally resolve rapidly on completion of therapy.

Neurologic changes may also occur in patients who receive therapy with IL–2 (Sparber and Biller-Sparber, 1993). Lethargy, confusion, sleep disturbances, decreased concentration, mood swings, and depression may occur. Severe neurologic changes may represent a dose-limiting toxic effect with high-dose IL–2 therapy.

Hematologic changes may occur during IL–2 therapy. Mild anemia, leukopenia, and thrombocytopenia are possible (Oleksowiez et al., 1991; Paciucci et al., 1990). With prolonged or repeated courses of IL–2, eosinophilia is common (Silberstein et al., 1989). After IL–2 has been discontinued, a marked rebound lymphocytosis occurs as activated lymphocytes circulate in the peripheral bloodstream (Boldt and Ellis, 1993; Thompson et al., 1988).

Impaired neutrophil function with resultant decreased chemotaxis is associated with IL–2 therapy. Therefore, patients with a pre-existing infection should be treated with antibiotics prior to receiving IL–2 therapy. Consideration should also be given to the use of prophylactic antibiotics in patients with indwelling central lines or long-term venous access devices (Klempner and Snydman, 1993; Pockaj et al., 1993; Bock et al., 1990; Snydman et al., 1990; Hartman et al., 1989).

An increased incidence of reactions to both ionic and nonionic radiographic CT contrast media has been reported in patients who have received therapy with IL–2. Symptoms included fever, chills, nausea, vomiting, hypotension, leukocytosis, skin rash, and elevation in serum creatinine (Choyke et al., 1992; Abi-aad et al., 1991; Fishman et al., 1991; Oldham and Brogley, 1990; Zukiwski et al., 1990).

Because the risk of contrast media reactions may be greater early after IL–2 therapy, the use of contrast agents should be avoided during this time (Shulman et al., 1993).

Future Directions

A continuing area of interest and investigation is the use of IL–2 after chemotherapy in patients undergoing bone marrow transplantation. Interleukin–2 produces immunologic effects and increased NK and LAK activity that may eliminate minimal residual disease. In addition, a short course of high-dose IL–2 may diminish graft-versus-host disease without diminishing the graft-versus-leukemia effect of allogeneic T cells (Fefer et al., 1993; Sykes et al., 1993).

Interleukin–2 is also being investigated in the treatment of patients with human immunodeficiency virus (HIV) infections and acquired immunodeficiency syndrome (AIDS) (Smith, 1993; Schwartz et al., 1991; Schwartz and Merigan, 1990). The goal of such therapy is to increase the numbers of lymphocytes as well as their functional capacity. Studies have demonstrated that a temporary increase in T-cell numbers can be achieved with two to three weeks of low-dose IL–2 therapy. The full impact of this therapy and the potential risks of promoting HIV transcription or viral entry into healthy activated cells has yet to be determined.

Because of its profound effects as an immunostimulant, IL–2 is being tested as a proactive anti-infective agent. Low doses of IL–2 administered to patients with lepromatous leprosy led to a significant reduction in the bacterial load in those patients. With this observation, consideration is being given to the use of IL–2 for treating bacterial, fungal, viral, and parasitic infections and for preventing infections in burn patients (Smith, 1993).

Another area of interest is the reduction of IL–2-induced toxic effects, especially hypotension and the vascular leak syndrome. Since these hemodynamic effects of IL–2 are related to secondary cytokines such as TNF and IL–1, strategies are being employed to use other agents to interfere with the secretion of these cytokines. Pentoxifylline, an agent that suppresses TNF synthesis, has been shown to reduce IL–2 toxicity in mice while preserving antitumor efficacy (Edwards *et al.*, 1992). Preliminary studies also indicate that the presence of pentoxifylline does not inhibit human LAK cytotoxicity (Thompson *et al.*, 1993). Clinical trials are currently under way in an attempt to deliver higher doses of IL–2 without severe toxic effects. Other agents being considered for use with IL–2 include dexamethasone (initial studies have shown blockage of all IL–2 effects) (Vetto *et al.*, 1987), anti-TNF antibodies, soluble TNF receptors, platelet-activating factor antagonists, and IL–1-receptor antagonists (Mier, 1993a). It has yet to be determined what effect these agents may have on the potential antineoplastic activity of IL–2. Although there is interest in decreasing IL–2 toxicity so that higher doses of it may be given, there is also interest in delivering low doses of IL–2 that bind to high-affinity IL–2Rs and signal the target cell without triggering secondary cytokine production (Smith, 1993).

Future investigations of IL–2 will involve combination regimens that include other cytokines, activated lymphocytes, vaccines, and chemotherapeutic agents for a variety of malignancies and other diseases. Doses, routes of administration, and schedules will be altered to attempt to achieve greater efficacy with less toxic effects. As more complex therapies are delivered to outpatients, IL–2 therapy will be applied in that setting (Fisher, 1993).

INTERLEUKIN–4

Interleukin–4, initially described as B-cell growth factor in 1982, is a cytokine produced primarily by activated T cells (Howard *et al.*, 1982). Antigens, antigen-presenting cells, or antibodies in conjunction with T cells induce production of IL–4. It exerts its functional activity by binding to receptors on the cell-surface membranes of target cells (Paul, 1991).

Biological Actions

Like most cytokines, IL–4 displays pleiotropic functions. It exerts different effects on resting and activated B cells. Interleukin–4 stimulates the growth of resting B cells by increasing cell numbers and by enhancing the expression of class II histocompatibility antigens. Following antigen activation, IL–4 serves as a B-cell growth factor by stimulating the B cell to replicate its DNA. Interleukin–4 also promotes the differentiation of antibody-stimulated B cells; it is therefore known as a B-cell growth and differentiation factor. As a "switch factor," IL–4 is a major regulator of immunoglobulin (Ig) isotope expression, inducing IgE and IgG1 production (Oppenheim *et al.*, 1991; Feldmann and Male, 1989).

Interleukin–4 also induces T-cell growth and enhances production of IL–2 (Paul, 1991). Interleukin–4 increases the expression of the IL–2R to increase T-cell stimulation by IL–2 (Galazka *et al.*, 1991). The proliferation and differentiation of cytotoxic T cells are enhanced by IL–4. *In vitro*, the combination of IL–2 and IL–4 has synergistic effects on the growth and lytic activity of cytotoxic T cells but may inhibit LAK activity. Induction of LAK activity may be mediated by IL–4. When lymphocytes are exposed to suboptimal doses of IL–2, IL–4 may stimulate LAK activity (Higuchi *et al.*, 1989). In addition, IL–4 promotes the growth of TIL cytotoxic to human melanoma (Lotze *et al.*, 1992; Kawakami *et al.*, 1988). IL–4 also acts synergistically with IL–2 to enhance the expansion of activated CD4+ cells while inhibiting nonspecific cytotoxicity (Tso *et al.*, 1992). In summary, IL–4 has a variety of effects on cytotoxic cells depending upon the phenotype of the cells, the presence of other cytokines, and the state of activation of the cells (Atkins et al., 1992).

In addition to stimulating B and T cells, IL–4 also activates granulocytes, macrophages, megakaryocytes, thymocytes, and mast cells

(Snoeck *et al.*, 1993). It also serves as a co-stimulant with G-CSF, GM-CSF, and erythropoietin for the production of progenitor cells (Oppenheim *et al.*, 1991). Conflicting data exist on the effects of IL–4 on macrophages. Increased phagocytic activity and cytotoxicity may be stimulated in macrophages for certain tumor cells (Dawson 1991; Jansen *et al.*, 1990; Ohara, 1989; Crawford *et al.*, 1987) while IL–4 has also been shown to inhibit the growth of macrophages (Jansen *et al.*, 1989).

Clinical Trials

Phase I clinical trials have been conducted using IL–4. It has been administered alone or with IL–2 by intravenous bolus injection, continuous intravenous infusion, or subcutaneous injection. In a phase I study by Atkins *et al* (1992) the MTD was determined to be 10 μg/kg/dose when administered by intravenous bolus every eight hours on days 1 to 5 and days 15 to 19. No tumor responses were observed (Atkins *et al.*, 1992). When administered by daily subcutaneous injection, dose limiting toxicity was reached at a dose of 5 μg/kg/day (Gilleece *et al.*, 1992). Escalating doses of IL–4 up to 360 μg/m^2/day administered by continuous intravenous infusion for seven had not yet reached dose limiting toxicity (Sosman *et al.*, 1992). Based on the premise that IL–4 may activate cytotoxic effector cells most effectively following IL–2, phase I studies have also incorporated the use of continuous intravenous infusion of IL–4 followed by IL–2. In addition, IL–4 has also been administered simultaneously with IL–2. Subcutaneous IL–2 (9 million IU/m^2/dose) and IL–4 were administered simultaneously for 5 days/week for 3 weeks followed by a one-week rest period. The beginning dose of IL–4 was 100 μg/m^2/dose with plans to escalate to 400 μg/m^2/dose. The MTD has not been determined at the current dosage level of 300 μg/m^2/dose (Whitehead *et al.*, 1992). No antitumor responses were noted with IL–4 alone and combination trials with IL–2 and IL–4

have shown no increase in response rates in melanoma or other tumors when compared to IL–2 alone.

Phase II trials have been conducted using TIL whose proliferation has been increased *in vitro* by IL–2 and IL–4 administration. The TIL were administered in conjunction with IL–2 to patients with metastatic renal cell carcinoma. Although a few tumor responses were observed, the response rate was not greater than that noted with IL–2 alone. The toxic effects were those expected with combined IL–2 plus TIL therapy (Puri and Siegel, 1993; Bukowski *et al.*, 1992).

Regulatory Approval

As of June 1994, IL–4 continues in clinical trials and has not yet received approval by the Food and Drug Administration (FDA).

Side effects

The most common side effects observed in patients receiving single-agent IL–4 included fever, nasal congestion, headache, nausea/vomiting, diarrhea, anorexia, fatigue, capillary leak syndrome, weight gain, and dyspnea. Asymptomatic elevations in liver function tests have also occurred but were transient. In a review of 73 patients with advanced malignancies who were treated with either single agent IL–4 or combination therapy with IL–2 and IL–4, Rubin and Lotze (1992) reported that 12 of 84 courses of therapy were associated with the development of gastroduodenal erosion or ulceration. Transfusions were required in 3 of these courses and no treatment-related deaths occurred. In studies evaluating the administration of IL–2 plus IL–4 stimulated TIL cells, the side effect profile is similar to that observed with IL–2 alone.

Future Directions

Although IL–4 appears to demonstrate antitumor activity in animal models, it has yet to produce useful antitumor responses in man.

The role of IL–4 in the activation of cytolytic T cells and TIL cells continues to be studied in an attempt to develop clinical applications for this cytokine.

Another possible application of IL–4 lies in its ability to induce class switch in immunoglobulin production to IgE and IgG1. Control of Ig synthesis could prevent or minimize IgE-mediated allergic conditions. Strategies to neutralize IL–4, block the production of IL–4 or inhibit the activity of IL–4 may be explored.

SUMMARY

The interleukins are pivotal in maintaining the complex balance of the human immune system. Interleukins provide the communication network between T cells, B cells, macrophages, hematopoietic cells, and antigen-presenting cells. Knowledge about the roles and functions of the ILs has expanded greatly during the past decade, and this information has afforded opportunities for the clinical application of these powerful cytokines.

References

Abi-aad, A., Figlin, R., Belldegrun, A., et al. 1991. Metastatic renal cell cancer: Interleukin–2 toxicity induced by contrast agent injections. *Journal of Immunotherapy* 10: 292–295.

Atkins, M., Vachino, G., Tilg, H., et al. 1992. Phase I evaluation of thrice-daily intravenous bolus interleukin–4 in patients with refractory malignancy. *Journal of Clinical Oncology* 10(11): 1802–1809.

Atkins, M., and Mier, J. (eds). 1993. *Therapeutic Application of Interleukin–2*. New York: Marcel Dekker, pp. 3–476.

Atzpodien, J., Poliwoda, H., and Kirchner, H. 1991. Alpha-interferon and interleukin–2 in renal cell carcinoma: Studies in nonhospitalized patients. *Seminars in Oncology* 18(5 Suppl 7): 108–112.

Bagby, G., Dinarello, C., Neerhout, R., et al. 1988. Interleukin 1-dependent paracrine granulopoiesis in chronic granulocytic leukemia of the juvenile type. *Journal of Clinical Investigations* 82: 1430–1436.

Belldegrun, A., Webb, D., Austin, H., et al. 1987. Effects of interleukin–2 on renal function in patients receiving immunotherapy for advanced cancer. *Annals of Internal Medicine* 106(6): 817–822.

Bock, S., Lee, R., Fisher, B., et al. 1990. A prospective randomized trial evaluating prophylactic antibiotics to prevent triple-lumen catheter-related sepsis in patients treated with immunotherapy. *Journal of Clinical Oncology* 8(1): 161–169.

Boldt, D., and Ellis, T. 1993. Biologic effects of interleukin–2 administration on the immune system. In Atkins, M., and Mier, J. (eds). *Therapeutic Applications of Interleukin–2*. New York: Marcel Dekker, pp. 73–91.

Brogley, J., and Sharp, E. 1990. Nursing care of patients receiving activated lymphocytes. *Oncology Nursing Forum* 17(2): 187–193.

Bukowski, R., Rayman, P., Gibson, V., et al. 1992. Treatment of human metastatic renal cell carcinoma with IL2/IL4-grown tumor-infiltrating lymphocytes (TIL) and rIL2. *Proceedings of the Annual Meeting of the American Association of Cancer Resesarch* 33: A1941, p. 325.

Castelli, M., Black, P., Schneider, M., et al. 1988. Protective, restorative, and therapeutic properties of recombinant human IL–1 in rodent models. *Journal of Immunology* 140: 3830–3837.

Chiron Corporation 1994. Proleukin® (aldesleukin) package insert. Emeryville, CA: Chiron Corporation.

Choyke, P., Miller, D., Lotze, M., et al. 1992. Delayed reactions to contrast media after IL–2 therapy. *Radiology* 183(1): 111–114.

Crawford, R., Finbloom, D., Ohara, J., et al. 1987. BSF–1: A new macrophage activation factor: B cell stimulatory factor–1 (interleukin–4) activates macrophages for increased tumoricidal activity and expression in Ia antigens. *Journal of Immunology* 139(1): 135–141.

Crown, J., Jakubowski, A., Kemeny, N., et al. 1991. A phase I trial of recombinant human interleukin–1β alone and in combination with myelosuppressive doses of 5-fluorouracil in patients with gastrointestinal cancer. *Blood* 78(6): 1420–1427.

Dawson, M. (ed). 1991. *Lymphokines and Interleukins*. Boca Raton: CRC Press.

Dillman, R., Church, C., Oldham, R., et al. 1993. Inpatient continuous-infusion interleukin–2 in 788 patients with cancer. *Cancer* 71(7): 2358–2370.

Dillman, R., Oldham, R., Barth, N., et al. 1991a. Continuous interleukin–2 and tumor-infiltrating lymphocytes as treatment of advanced melanoma. *Cancer* 68(1): 1–8.

Dillman, R., Oldham, R., Tauer, K., et al. 1991b. Continuous interleukin–2 and lymphokine-activated killer cells for advanced cancer. *Journal of Clinical Oncology* 9(7): 1233–1240.

Dinarello, C. 1991. Interleukin–1 and interleukin–1 antagonism. *Blood* 77(8): 1625–1652.

Dinarello, C., and Wolff, S. 1993. The role of interleukin–1 in disease. *New England Journal of Medicine* 328(2): 106–113.

Dinarello, C., and Mier, J. 1987. Current concepts: Lymphokines. *New England Journal of Medicine* 317(15): 940–945.

Dower, S., Kronheim, S., March, C., *et al.* 1986. The cell surface receptors for interleukin 1-alpha and interleukin 1-beta are identical. *Nature* 324(6094): 266–269.

Doyle, M., Lee, M., and Fong, S. 1985. Comparison of the biologic activities of human recombinant interleukin–2 and native interleukin–2. *Journal of Biological Response Modifiers* 4(1): 96–109.

Dutcher, J., Creekmore, S., Weiss, G., *et al.* 1989. A phase II study of interleukin–2 and lymphokine-activated killer cells in patients with metastatic malignant melanoma. *Journal of Clinical Oncology* 7(4): 477–485.

Edwards, M., Heniford, B., Klar, E., *et al.* 1992. Pentoxifylline inhibits interleukin–2-induced toxicity in C57BL/6 mice but preserves antitumor efficacy. *Journal of Clinical Investigations* 90(2): 637–641.

Eisenberg, S., Evans, R., Arend, W., *et al.* 1990. Primary structure and functional expression from complementary DNA of a human interleukin–1 receptor antagonist. *Nature* 343: 341–346.

Farrell, M. 1992. The challenge of adult respiratory distress syndrome during interleukin–2 immunotherapy. *Oncology Nursing Forum* 19(3): 475–480.

Fefer, A., Benyunes, M., Massumoto, C., *et al.* 1993. Interleukin–2 therapy after autologous bone marrow transplantation for hematologic malignancies. *Seminars in Oncology* 20(6 Suppl 9): 41–45.

Feldmann, M., and Male, D. 1989. Cell cooperation in the antibody response. In Roitt, I., Brostoff, J., and Male, D. (eds). *Immunology*. Philadelphia: J. B. Lippincott, pp. 8.1–8.12.

Fisher, R. (ed). 1993. Interleukin–2: Advances in clinical research and treatment. *Seminars in Oncology* 20(6 Suppl 9): 1–59.

Fisher, B., Keenan, A., Garra, B., *et al.* 1989 Interleukin–2 induces profound reversible cholestasis: A detailed analysis in treated cancer patients. *Journal of Clinical Oncology* 7(12): 1852–1862.

Fisher, C., Slotman, G., Opal, S., *et al.* 1991. Interleukin–1 receptor antagonist reduces mortality in patients with sepsis syndrome. *Annual Meeting of the American College of Chest Physicians*, San Francisco, Abstract.

Fisher, R., Coltman, C., Doroshow, J., *et al.* 1988. Metastatic renal cancer treated with interleukin–2 and lymphokine-activated killer cells. *Annals of Internal Medicine* 108: 518–523.

Fishman, J., Aberle, D., Moldawer, N., *et al.* 1991. Atypical contrast reactions associated with systemic interleukin–2 therapy. *AJR American Journal of Roentgend* 156(4): 833–834.

Galazka, A., Weiner, J., Barth, N., *et al.* 1991. Lymphokines and cytokines. In Oldham, R. (ed). *Principles of Cancer Biotherapy* 2nd ed. New York: Marcel Dekker, pp. 327–361.

Gaspari, A., Lotze, M., Rosenberg, S., *et al.* 1987. Dermatologic changes associated with interleukin–2 administration. *JAMA* 258(12): 1624–1629.

Gaynor, E., and Fisher, R. 1993. Hemodynamic and cardiovascular effects of interleukin–2. In Atkins, M., and Mier, J. (eds). *Therapeutic Applications of Interleukin–2*. New York: Marcel Dekker, pp. 381–388.

Gaynor, E., Vitek, L., Sticklin, L., *et al.* 1988. The hemodynamic effects of treatment with interleukin–2 and lymphokine-activated killer cells. *Annals of Internal Medicine* 109(12): 953–958.

Gery, I., Gershon, R., and Waksman, B. 1972a. Potentiation of the T-lymphocyte response to mitogens, I. The responding cell. *Journal of Experimental Medicine* 136(1): 128–142.

Gery, I., Gershon, R., and Waksman, B. 1972b. Potentiation of the T-lymphocyte response to mitogens, II. The cellular source of potentiating mediators. *Journal of Experimental Medicine* 136(1): 143–155.

Gilleece, M., Scarffe, J., Ghosh, A., *et al.* 1992. Recombinant human interleukin–4 (IL–4) given as daily subcutaneous injections—A phase I dose toxicity trial. *British Journal of Cancer* 66(1): 204–210.

Grimm, E. 1993. Properties of IL–2-activated lymphocytes. In Atkins, M. and Mier, J. (eds). *Therapeutic Applications of Interleukin–2*. New York: Marcel Dekker, pp. 27–38.

Hartman, L., Urba, W., Steis, R., *et al.* 1989. Use of prophylactic antibiotics for prevention of intravascular catheter-related infections in interleukin–2-treated patients. *Journal of the National Cancer Institute* 81(15): 1190–1193.

Higuchi, C., Thompson, J., Lindgren, C., *et al.* 1989. Induction of lymphokine-activated killer activity by interleukin–4 in human lymphocytes preactivated by interleukin–2 *in vivo* or *in vitro*. *Cancer Research* 49(23): 6487–6492.

Hood, L., and Abernathy, E. 1991. Biological response modifiers. In Baird, S., McCorkle, R., and Grant, M. (eds). *Cancer Nursing: Comprehensive Textbook*. Philadelphia: W. B. Saunders, pp. 321–343.

Howard, M., Farrar, J., Hilfiker, M., *et al.* 1982. Identification of a T-cell derived B-cell growth factor distinct from interleukin–2. *Journal of Experimental Medicine* 155(3): 914–923.

Huland, E., Heinzer, H., and Huland, H. 1994. Inhaled interleukin–2 in combination with low dose systemic interleukin–2 and interferon alpha in patients with pulmonary metastatic renal cell carcinoma: effectiveness and toxicity of mainly local treatment. *Journal of Cancer Research and Clinical Oncology* 120(4): 221–228.

Itoh, K., and Balch, C. 1993. Properties of human tumor-infiltrating lymphocytes. In Atkins, M., and Mier, J. (eds). *Therapeutic Applications of Interleukin–2*. New York: Marcel Dekker, pp. 39–48.

Jansen, J., Fibbe, W., Willemze, R., *et al.* 1990. Interleukin–4: A regulatory protein. *Blut* 60: 269–274.

Jansen, J., Wientjens, G., Fibbe, W., *et al.* 1989. Inhibition of human macrophage colony formation by interleukin–4. *Journal of Experimental Medicine* 170(2): 577–588.

Jassak, P. 1993. Biotherapy. In Groenwald, S., Frogge, M., Goodman, M., and Yarbro, C. (eds). *Cancer Nursing: Principles and Practice* 3rd ed. Boston: Jones and Bartlett, pp. 366–392.

Jassak, P., and Sticklin, L. 1986. Interleukin–2: An overview. *Oncology Nursing Forum* 13(6): 17–22.

Johnson, C. 1993. Interleukin–1: Therapeutic potential for solid tumors. *Cancer Investigation:* 11(5): 600–608.

Kawakami, Y., Rosenberg, S., and Lotze, M. 1988. Interleukin–4 promotes the growth of tumor infiltrating lymphocytes cytotoxic for human autologous melanoma. *Journal of Experimental Medicine* 168(6): 2183–2191.

Klempner, M., and Snydman, D. 1993. Infectious complications associated with interleukin–2. In Atkins, M., and Mier, J. (eds). *Therapeutic Applications of Interleukin–2.* New York: Marcel Dekker, pp. 409–424.

Kozeny, G., Nicolas, J., Creekmore, S., et al. 1988. Effects of interleukin–2 immunotherapy on renal function. *Journal of Clinical Oncology* 6(7): 1170–1176.

Kuby, J. 1992. Cytokines. In Kuby, J. (ed). *Immunology.* New York: W. H. Freeman, pp. 245–270.

Lee, R., Lotze, M., Skibber, J., et al. 1989. Cardiorespiratory effects of immunotherapy with interleukin–2. *Journal of Clinical Oncology* 7(1): 7–20.

Legha, S., Ring, S., Bedikian, A., et al. 1993. Biochemotherapy using interleukin–2 + interferon alpha–2a (IFN) in combination with cisplatin (C), vinblastine (V) and DTIC (D) in patients with metastatic melanoma. *Third International conference on Melanoma: Abstracts 3:* 32–33.

Legha, S., and Buzaid, A. 1993. Role of recombinant interleukin–2 in combination with interferon-alpha and chemotherapy in the treatment of advanced melanoma. *Seminars in Oncology* 20(6 Suppl 9): 27–32.

Lotze, M. 1991. Interleukin–2: Basic principles. In DeVita, V., Hellman, S. and Rosenberg, S. (eds). *Biologic Therapy of Cancer.* Philadelphia: J.B. Lippincott, pp. 123–141.

Lotze, M., Zeh, H., Elder, E., et al. 1992. Use of T-cell growth factors (interleukins 2, 4, 7, 10, and 12) in the evaluation of T-cell reactivity to melanoma. *Journal of Immunotherapy* 12(3): 212–217.

Malek, T., and Gutgsell, N. 1993. IL–2 and its receptor: Structure, function, and regulation of expression. In Atkins, M., and Mier, J. (eds). *Therapeutic Applications of Interleukin–2.* New York: Marcel Dekker, pp. 3–25.

Mandrup-Poulsen, T., Helqvist, S., Molvig, J., et al. 1989. Cytokines as immune effector molecules in autoimmune endocrine diseases with special reference to insulin-dependent diabetes mellitus. *Autoimmunity* 4(3): 191–218.

Margolin, K. 1993. The clinical toxicities of high-dose interleukin–2. In Atkins, M., and Mier, J. (eds). *Therapeutic Applications of Interleukin–2.* New York: Marcel Dekker, pp. 331–362.

Mier, J. 1993a. Abrogation of interleukin–2 toxicity. In Atkins, M., and Mier, J. (eds). *Therapeutic Applications of Interleukin–2.* New York: Marcel Dekker, pp. 455–475.

Mier, J. 1993b. Pathogenesis of the interleukin–2-induced vascular leak syndrome. In Atkins, M. and Mier, J. (eds). *Therapeutic Applications of Interleukin–2.* New York: Marcel Dekker, pp. 363–379.

Moore, M. 1991. Clinical implications of positive and negative hematopoietic stem cell regulators. *Blood* 78: 1–19.

Morgan, D., Ruscetti, F., and Gallo, R. 1976. Selective *in vitro* growth of T lymphocytes from normal human bone marrows. *Science* 193(4257): 1007–1008.

Mulé, J., and Rosenberg, S. 1992. Catalogue of cytokines. *Biologic Therapy of Cancer Updates* 2(1): 1–11.

Mulé, J., and Rosenberg, S. 1991. Combination cytokine therapy: experimental and clinical trials. In DeVita, V., Hellman, S., and Rosenberg, S. (eds). *Biologic Therapy of Cancer.* Philadelphia: J.B. Lippincott, pp. 393–416.

Oettgen, H., and Old, L. 1991. The history of cancer immunotherapy. In DeVita, V., Hellman, S., and Rosenberg, S. (eds). *Biologic Therapy of Cancer.* Philadelphia: J.B. Lippincott, pp. 87–119.

Ohara, J. 1989. Interleukin–4: Molecular structure and biochemical characteristics, biological function and receptor expression. In Cruse, J., and Lewis, R. (eds). *The Year in Immunology. Immunoregulatory Cytokines and Cell Growth* Vol. 5. Switzerland: Basel Karger, pp. 126–159.

Oldham, R., and Brogley, J. 1990. Contrast medium "recalls" interleukin–2 toxicity. *Journal of Clinical Oncology* 8(5): 942.

Oldham, R., Dillman, R., Yannelli, J., et al. 1991. Continuous infusion interleukin–2 and tumor-derived activated cells as treatment of advanced solid tumors. *Molecular Biotherapy* 3(2): 68–73.

Oleksowicz, L., Paciucci, P., Zuckerman, D., et al. 1991. Alterations of platelet function induced by interleukin–2. *Journal of Immunotherapy* 10(5): 363–370.

Oppenheim, J., Ruscetti, F., and Faltynek, C. 1991. Cytokines. In Stites, D., and Terr, A. (eds). *Basic and Clinical Immunology.* Norwalk, Connecticut: Appleton and Lange, pp. 78–100.

Paciucci, P., Mandeli, J., Oleksowicz, L., et al. 1990. *American Journal of Medicine* 89(3): 308–312.

Padavic-Shaller, K. 1988. IL–2: Nursing applications in a developing science. *Seminars in Oncology Nursing* 4(2): 142–150.

Parkinson, D. 1989. The role of interleukin–2 in the biotherapy of cancer. *Oncology Nursing Forum* 16(6 Suppl): 16–20.

Paul, W. 1991. Interleukin–4: A prototypic immunoregulatory lymphokine. *Blood* 77(9): 1859–1870.

Paul, W. 1989. Pleiotropy and redundancy: T cell-derived lymphokines in the immune response. *Cell* 57(4): 521–524.

Philip, R., and Epstein, L. 1986. Tumor necrosis factor as immunomodulator and mediator of monocyte cytotoxicity induced by itself, gamma-interferon and interleukin–1. *Nature* 328(6083): 86–89.

Piper, B., Rieger, P., Brophy, L., et al. 1989. Recent advances in the management of biotherapy-related side effects: Fatigue. *Oncology Nursing Forum* 16(6 Suppl): 27–34.

Pockaj, B., Topalian, S., Steinberg, S., et al. 1993. Infectious complications associated with interleukin–2 administration: A retrospective review of 935 treatment courses. *Journal of Clinical Oncology* 11(1): 136–147.

Puri, R., and Siegel, J. 1993. Interleukin–4 and cancer therapy. *Cancer Investigation* 11(4): 473–486.

Rambaldi, A., Torcia, M., Bettoni, S., et al. 1991. Modulation of cell proliferation and cytokine production in acute myeloblastic leukemia by interleukin–1 receptor antagonist and lack of its expression by leukemic cells. *Blood* 78: 3248–3253.

Richards, J., Mehta, N., Ramming, K., et al. 1992. Sequential chemoimmunotherapy in the treatment of metastatic melanoma. *Journal of Clinical Oncology* 10(8): 1338–1343.

Rieger, P. 1994. Biotherapy. In Otto, S. (ed). *Oncology Nursing* 2nd ed. St. Louis: Mosby Yearbook, pp. 526–560.

Rieger, P. 1992. The pathophysiology of selected symptoms associated with BRM therapy. *Biologic Response Modifiers: Perspectives for Oncology Nurses*. Monograph. Emeryville, CA: Cetus Corporation, pp. 4–10.

Rieger, P., Weatherly, B., and Rumsey, K. 1993. Clinical update: Strategies for caring for patients receiving IL–2 therapy. *Nursing Interventions in Oncology* 5: 23–30.

Rosenberg, S., Lotze, M., Yang, J., et al. 1989. Experience with the use of high-dose interleukin–2 in the treatment of 652 cancer patients. *Annals of Surgery* 210(4): 474–485.

Rosenberg, S., Packard, B., Aebersold, P., et al. 1988. Use of tumor-infiltrating lymphocytes and interleukin–2 in the immunotherapy of patients with metastatic melanoma. *New England Journal of Medicine* 319(25): 1676–1680.

Rosenberg, S., Lotze, M., Muul, L., et al. 1985. Observations on the systemic administration of autologous lymphokine-activated killer cells and recombinant interleukin–2 to patients with metastatic cancer. *New England Journal of Medicine* 313(23): 1485–1492.

Rubin, J. 1993. Interleukin–2: Its biology and clinical application in patients with cancer. *Cancer Investigation* 11(4): 460–472.

Rubin, J., and Lotze, M. 1992. Acute gastric mucosal injury associated with the systemic administration of interleukin–4. *Surgery* 111(3): 274–280.

Schwartz, D. and Merigan, T. 1990. Interleukin–2 in the treatment of HIV disease. *Biotherapy* 2(2): 119–136.

Schwartz, D., Skowron, G., and Merigan, T. 1991. Safety and effects of interleukin–2 plus zidovudine in asymptomatic individuals infected with human immunodeficiency virus. *Journal of Acquired Deficiency Syndromes* 4(1): 11–23.

Sergi, J. 1991. The physiology of the flu-like syndrome and the cardiopulmonary and renal symptoms associated with BRM therapy. *Biologic Response Modifiers: Perspectives for Oncology Nurses*. Monograph. Emeryville, CA: Cetus Corporation, pp. 4–10.

Sharp, E. 1993. Case management of the hospitalized patient receiving interleukin–2. *Seminars in Oncology Nursing* 9(3 Suppl 1): 14–19.

Shulman, K., Thompson, J., Benyunes, M., et al. 1993. Adverse reactions to intravenous contrast media in patients treated with interleukin–2. *Journal of Immunotherapy* 13(3): 208–212.

Siegel, J., and Puri, R. 1991. Interleukin–2 toxicity. *Journal of Clinical Oncology* 9(4): 694–704.

Silberstein, D., Schoof, M., Rodrick, M., et al. 1989. Activation of eosinophils in cancer patients treated with IL–2 and IL–2-generated lymphokine-activated killer cells. *Journal of Immunology* 142(6): 2162–2167.

Sleijfer, D., Janssen, R., Buter, J., et al. 1992. Phase II study of subcutaneous interleukin–2 in unselected patients with advanced renal cell cancer on an outpatient basis. *Journal of Clinical Oncology* 10(7): 1119–1123.

Smith, K. 1993. Lowest dose interleukin–2 immunotherapy. *Blood* 81(6): 1414–1423.

Smith, J., Longo, D., Alvord, W., et al. 1993. The effects of treatment with interleukin–1α on platelet recovery after high-dose carboplatin. *New England Journal of Medicine* 328(11): 756–761.

Smith, J., Urba, W., Curti, B., et al. 1992. The toxic and hematologic effects of interleukin–1 alpha administered in a phase I trial to patients with advanced malignancies. *Journal of Clinical Oncology* 10(7): 1141–1152.

Snoeck, H., Lardon, F., Bockstaele, D., et al. 1993. Effects of interleukin–4 (IL–4) on myelopoiesis: Studies of highly purified CD34+ hematopoietic progenitor cells. *Leukemia* 7(4): 625–629.

Snydman, D., Sullivan, B., Gill, M., et al. 1990. Nosocomial sepsis associated with interleukin–2. *Annals of Internal Medicine* 112(2): 102–107.

Sosman, J., Ellis, T., Bodner, B., et al. 1992. A phase IA/IB trial of continuous infusion (CI) interleukin–4 alone and following interleukin–2 in cancer patients. *Proceedings of the Annual Meeting of the American Association of Cancer Research* 33: A2070, p. 347.

Sparber, A., and Biller-Sparber, K. 1993. Immunotherapy and neuropsychiatric toxicity. *Cancer Nursing* 16(3): 188–192.

Spriggs, D. 1991. Tumor necrosis factor: Basic principles and preclinical studies. In DeVita, V., Hellman, S., and Rosenberg, S. (eds). *Biologic Therapy of Cancer*. Philadelphia: J.B. Lippincott, pp. 354–392.

Starnes, H. 1991. Biological effects and possible clinical applications of interleukin–1. *Seminars in Hematology* 29(2 Suppl 2): 34–41.

Stroud, M., Swindell, B., and Bernard, G. 1990. Cellular and humoral mediators of sepsis syndrome. *Critical Care Nursing Clinics of North America* 2(2): 151–160.

Sykes, M., Abraham, V., Harty, M., *et al.* 1993. IL–2 reduces graft-versus-host disease and preserves a graft-versus-leukemia effect by selectively inhibiting CD4+ T cell activity. *Journal of Immunology* 150(1): 197–205.

Sznol, M., and Longo, D. 1993. Chemotherapy drug interactions with biological agents. *Seminars in Oncology* 20(1): 80–93.

Thompson, J., Lindgren, C., Benyunes, J., *et al.* 1993. The effects of pentoxifylline on the generation of human lymphokine-activated killer cell cytotoxicity. *Journal of Immunotherapy* 13(2): 84–90.

Thompson, J., Lee, D., Lindgren, C., *et al.* 1988. Influence of dose and duration of infusion of interleukin–2 on toxicity and immunomodulation. *Journal of Clinical Oncology* 6(4): 669–678.

Tsevat, J., Kappler, K., and Martin, R. 1993. Nursing management of patients receiving high-dose IL-2 therapy. In Atkins, M., and Mier, J. (eds.). *Therapeutic Applications of Interleukin–2*. New York: Marcel Dekker, pp. 425–438.

Tso, C., Duckett, J., deKernion, J., *et al.* 1992. Modulation of tumor-infiltrating lymphocytes derived from human renal cell carcinoma by interleukin–4. *Journal of Immunotherapy* 12(2): 82–89.

Vadhan-Raj, S., Kudelka, A., Garrison, L., *et al.* 1994. Effects of interleukin–1α on carboplatin-induced thrombocytopenia in patients with recurrent ovarian cancer. *Journal of Clinical Oncology* 12(4): 707–714.

Vetto, J., Papa, M., Lotze, M., *et al.* 1987. Reduction of toxicity of interleukin–2 and lymphokine activated killer cells in humans by the administration of corticosteroids. *Journal of Clinical Oncology* 5: 496–503.

Viele, C., and Moran, T. 1993. Nursing management of the nonhospitalized patient receiving recombinant interleukin–2. *Seminars in Oncology Nursing* 9(3 Suppl 1): 20–24.

Vogelzang, N., Lipton, A., and Figlin, R. 1993. Subcutaneous interleukin–2 plus interferon alfa–2a in metastatic renal cancer: An outpatient multicenter trial. *Journal of Clinical Oncology* 11(9): 1809–1816.

Weidmann, E., Bergmann, L., Stock, J., *et al.* 1992. Rapid cytokine release in cancer patients treated with interleukin–2. *Journal of Immunotherapy* 12(2): 123–131.

West, W., Tauer, K., Yannelli, J., *et al.* 1987. Constant-infusion recombinant interleukin–2 in adoptive immunotherapy of advanced cancer. *New England Journal of Medicine* 316(15): 898–905.

Whitehead, R., Friedman, K., and Clark, D. 1992. A phase I trial of SC interleukin–2 and interleukin–4. *Proceedings of the Annual Meeting of the American Association of Cancer Resesarch* 33: A1381, p. 231.

Wolkenstein, P., Chosidow, O., Wechsler, J., *et al.* 1993. Cutaneous side effects associated with interleukin–2 administration for metastatic melanoma. *Journal of the American Academy of Dermatology* 28(1): 66–70.

Zukiwski, A., David, C., Coan J., *et al.* 1990. Increased incidence of hypersensitivity to iodine containing radiographic contrast media after interleukin–2 administration. *Cancer* 65(2): 1521–1524.

CHAPTER 6 | Hematopoietic Growth Factors

Debra Wujcik, RN, MSN, OCN

Hematopoietic growth factors (HGF) constitute a large family of glycosylated proteins that interact with specific receptors to regulate the reproduction, maturation, and functional activity of blood cells (Crosier and Clark 1992; Williams and Quesenberry, 1992). These proteins attach to receptors on the surface membrane of the target cell, and in response, the cell proliferates, differentiates, and matures. Although some HGFs stimulate a single response, others stimulate a cascade effect. Because HGFs are produced only in minute amounts in humans, study of their effects was difficult until recombinant technology made it possible for HGFs to be cloned, reproduced in large quantities, and made available for clinical trials.

Hematopoietic growth factors were first identified through **colony assays** in the laboratory (Metcalf and Morstyn, 1991; Golde and Gasson, 1988). Bone marrow cells, which included **pluripotent stem cells**, were added to culture dishes containing **feeder layers** consisting of various types of leukocytes and semi-solid medium. Colonies of leukocytes formed in response to incubation. When the feeder layers were varied, different types of colonies formed, suggesting that the cells grew in response to specific growth factors. A number of these growth factors have now been identified (Metcalf and Morstyn, 1991).

Originally discovered in the 1950s, HGFs are hormone-like proteins that mediate intracellular communication. Although similar to hormones, there are differences. First, HGFs may be produced by several different types of cells, whereas hormones are produced only by specialized cells. Second, HGFs usually have only a local effect rather than effects on distant organs as hormones do (Metcalf and Morstyn, 1991). Historically these factors were named colony-stimulating factors (CSFs) due to their ability to induce growth and maturation of specific colonies of cells *in vitro*. The four clas-

Table 6.1   Side effects of approved and investigational hematopoietic growth factors

	HGF	Generic Name (Trade Name)	Manufacturer	Side Effects
Approved	Epo	epoetin-alfa (Epogen®)	Amgen	Flu-like symptoms with arthralgias and myalgias.
		epoetin-alfa (Procrit®)	Ortho Biotech	Occasional headache and bloodshot eyes.
	G-CSF	filgrastim (Neupogen®)	Amgen	Bone pain in areas of high bone marrow reserve. Rare allergic reactions with rash, urticaria, facial edema, dyspnea, hypotension, tachycardia.
	GM-CSF	sargramostim (Leukine®)	Immunex	Fever. Dose-related fluid retention, dyspnea, myalgias, joint pain, bone pain.
Investigational		molgrastim (Leucomax®)	Sandoz/Schering	Fever. Fluid retention, dyspnea, myalgias, joint pain, bone pain.
	M-CSF	M-CSF (Macstim®) (Macrolim®)	Genetics Institute/ Sandoz/Schering Chiron Therapeutics	Fever, rash, headache, facial flushing, myalgias, photophobia. (May have thrombocytopenia, chest tightness, wheezing with *E. coli* product.)
	IL-3		Sandoz	Dose-related fever, chills, headache, bone pain, facial flushing, nausea, and vomiting.
	SCF		Amgen Systemix	Local injection site reaction; dermatologic reactions, occasional cough, sore throat, throat tightness and hypotension.
	PIXY321 (GM-CSF/IL-3 fusion protein)	GM-CSF + IL-3 (Pixikine)	Immunex	Local injection site reaction, headache, chest pain, asthenia.

Abbreviations: Epo, erythropoietin; G-CSF, granulocyte colony-stimulating factor; GM-CSF, granulocyte-macrophage colony-stimulating factor; M-CSF, macrophage colony-stimulating factor; IL-3, interleukin-3; SCF, stem cell factor.

sic CSFs are granulocyte colony-stimulating factor, granulocyte-macrophage colony-stimulating factor, macrophage colony-stimulating factor and interleukin–3 (multipotential colony-stimulating factor). These CSFs are the major regulatory molecules controlling the formation of neutrophils and monocyte-macrophages and are part of a large family of specific hematopoietic regulators known as HGFs.

Three HGFs have been approved by the Food and Drug Administration (FDA) for use while others remain under evaluation (see Table 6.1). The efficacy of **granulocyte colony-stimulating factor** (G-CSF) and **granulocyte-macrophage colony stimulating factor** (GM-CSF) in minimizing the myelosuppression of chemotherapy is well established. **Erythropoietin** (Epo) was initially indicated for patients with anemia due to chronic renal failure who are dependent on transfusions, but recently another indication was added, the treatment of anemia resulting from cancer chemotherapy. Other HGFs such as **interleukin–3** (IL–3), **macrophage colony-stimulating factor** (M-CSF), and **stem cell factor** (SCF) are in clinical trials (Bockheim and Jassak, 1993).

There are several clinical applications for HGFs (See Table 6.2). They are used most frequently in patients who are receiving che-

Table 6.2 Clinical applications for hematopoietic growth factors

- Decrease chemotherapy-induced myelosuppression
- Stimulate hematopoiesis in marrow failure
- Promote cellular differentiation
- Support peripheral stem cell harvesting
- Enhance antibiotic therapy

motherapy. In bone marrow transplantation, HGFs are used to hasten engraftment after autologous transplant and for those with delayed engraftment after allogeneic transplants. Additional indications such as differentiation therapy and peripheral blood stem cell harvesting are still under investigation. Combinations of HGFs are being studied in attempts to maximize their effectiveness. Some HGFs such as G-CSF or M-CSF may be useful in treating patients with infection.

CLASSIFICATION

Classification of HGFs is based on the type of mature cells that grow in the colonies produced in response to these proteins. Class I HGFs are **multilineage,** acting on the pluripotent and immature progenitors. Class II HGFs act on more mature progenitor cells and are **lineage restricted** (See Table 6.3).

Lineage-Restricted Hematopoietic Growth Factors

The lineage-restricted HGFs include G-CSF, M-CSF, and Epo. Granulocyte colony-stimulating factor stimulates neutrophil production and maturation (Crosier and Clark, 1992; Wujcik, 1992). The effect occurs further along in the differentiation cascade on maturing progenitor cells (See section on hematopoiesis). Granulocyte colony-stimulating factor enhances the function of mature neutrophils as well.

Erythropoietin is produced in response to decreased levels of oxygen in the blood circulating through the kidneys. The presence of Epo allows a proliferating pool of committed erythroid progenitors to be maintained, permits erythroblast differentiation, and recruits immature progenitors (Spivak, 1989).

Macrophage colony-stimulating factor activates monocytes, prompting macrophage production. It also stimulates enhanced cytotoxicity against fungi.

Multilineage Hematopoietic Growth Factors

The class I, or multilineage, HGFs include GM-CSF, IL–3, and SCF. Granulocyte-macrophage colony-stimulating factor preferentially supports neutrophil, eosinophil, and macrophage development and interacts with earlier progenitors than G-CSF (Leary et al., 1987; Sieff et al., 1987). It has both direct and indirect cellular effects. Direct effects on mature cells include inhibition of neutrophil migration, degranulation, changes in receptor expression and effects on cytoskeleton and cell shape (Gasson et al., 1990). Indirect effects have been referred to as priming effects because they enhance the ability of neutrophils to respond to secondary triggering signals and allow amplification of the immune response (Crosier and Clark, 1992). This includes enhancing the phagocytic function of neutrophils, macrophages, and eosinophils and increasing antibody-dependent cell-mediated cytotoxicity toward tumor cells.

Interleukin–3 causes stem cells to differentiate into granulocytes, macrophages, megakaryocytes, erythrocytes, and lymphocytes. Stem cell factor works at the earliest level of commitment and may affect the pluripotent stem cell.

SOURCE CELLS

Hematopoietic growth factors are synthesized by a wide variety of cells (See Table 6.3). Activated T lymphocytes produce IL–3 whereas G-CSF and GM-CSF are secreted by fibroblasts, endothelial cells, and macrophages.

Table 6.3 Source and function of hematopoietic growth factors

HGF	Classification	Source	Function
Epo	Lineage-restricted	Kidney, liver	Stimulates erythrocyte progenitors.
G-CSF	Lineage-restricted	Macrophages, fibroblasts, endothelial cells	Simulates neutrophil progenitors.
M-CSF	Lineage-restricted	Many cell types	Stimulates progenitors of monocytes/macrophages.
GM-CSF	Multilineage	T lymphocytes, macrophages, endothelial cells, fibroblasts	Stimulates progenitors of neutrophils, eosinophils, monocytes, basophils.
IL-3	Multilineage	T lymphocytes	Stimulates early progenitors for neutrophils, monocytes, platelets, eosinophils, basophils, and stem cells.
SCF	Multilineage	Bone marrow stroma, many cell types	Stimulates pluripotent stem cell and progenitors for all cell lines.

Abbreviations: Epo, erythropoietin; G-CSF, granulocyte colony-stimulating factor; GM-CSF, granulocyte-macrophage colony-stimulating factor; M-CSF, macrophage colony-stimulating factor; IL-3, interleukin-3; SCF, stem cell factor.

Macrophage colony-stimulating factor is produced by activated macrophages, fibroblasts, and endothelial cells (Bajorin et al., 1991).

BIOLOGICAL ACTIONS

Hematopoietic growth factors are usually given in supraphysiologic dosages. However, a basic understanding of the role of HGFs in normal **hematopoiesis** is required in order to understand the clinical role of HGFs.

Hematopoiesis

The process of hematopoiesis or blood cell production begins with the pluripotent stem cell (PPSC) and culminates with the production of fully functional circulating cells (See Figure 6.1) (Metcalf and Morstyn, 1991; Appelbaum, 1989; Erslev and Weiss, 1983). The PPSC is an uncommitted cell with the potential to become any cell of the blood. Although PPSCs are small in number within the marrow (1 to 2 million or 0.1% of marrow cells), they possess a unique characteristic. Each PPSC produces two daughter cells, one that enters a differentiation pathway and another that returns to a resting pool of cells. This allows self-renewal of the stem cell pool and provides a supply of cells to replace dying mature cells of the periphery. Production of PPSC can be in-creased by stress, infection, hemorrhage, or bone marrow depletion.

Hematopoiesis occurs in the extravascular spaces. The PPSC grow and develop in sinusoidal spaces surrounded by bone marrow stroma which consists of endothelial cells, fibroblasts, adipocytes, and macrophages that produce collagen and adhesive proteins. The **progenitor** cells stick to the collagen and adhesive proteins, ensuring maturation and development in the presence of the appropriate growth factors. Many of the HGFs necessary for hematopoiesis are produced by these stromal cells (Erslev and Weiss, 1983).

Committed progenitors

Once a cell leaves the stem cell pool, it begins the commitment process. The first level of commitment is to the myeloid or lymphoid lineage. These cells are somewhat pluripotent as they can commit to one of several cell lineages. The cells become more differentiated as they change from pluripotent to unipotent cells, that is, more committed to a single cell line.

The lymphoid stem cells mature first into pre-B and pre-T progenitor cells, eventually maturing to B and T lymphocytes. Myeloid stem cells, under the influence of HGFs, become the multilineage colony-forming unit (CFU-GEMM) that can produce granulocytes, erythrocytes, macrophages, and megakaryocytes.

Figure 6.1   Hematopoietic cascade. (PPSC, pluripotent stem cells; BFU, burst-forming unit; CFU, colony-forming units; CSF, colony-stimulating factor; GM, granulocyte-macrophage; GEMM, granulocyte, erythrocyte, macrophage, megakaryocyte; Epo, erythropoietin; IL, interleukin; SCF, stem cell factor.)

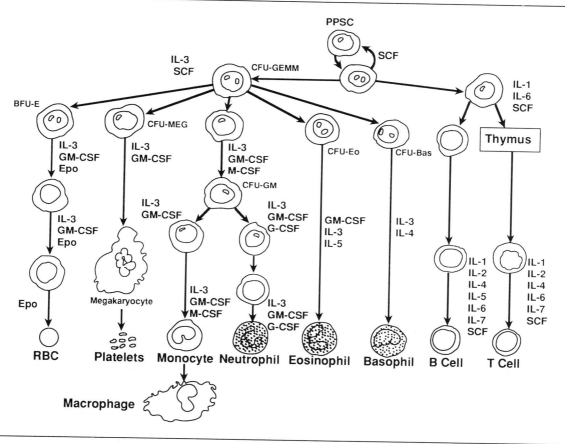

Source: Reprinted with permission from: Wujick, D. 1993. Infection control in oncology patients. *Nursing Clinics of North America* 28(3): 639–650.

Each of the cell lineages that produces a mature functioning cell follows the same maturation process: from progenitor cell to precursor cell to mature cell. Progenitors are the earliest committed cells in each lineage. **Precursors** are immature forms. As the cells mature, the proliferative capacity becomes progressively restricted (Metcalf and Morstyn, 1991).

Neutrophils

Granulocytes, which include neutrophils, eosinophils, and basophils, constitute the body's main defense against bacterial infection. Of these three cell types, the neutrophils are the most numerous, accounting for 50% to 70% of the total white blood cell count (WBC). Neutrophils go through six stages of maturation. The first three, the myeloblasts, promyelocytes, and myelocytes, undergo cellular division over four to five days. At the metamyelocyte level, cells are no longer capable of mitosis, but maturation continues for approximately six more days. Mature cells are released into the peripheral blood where one-half circulate freely and the other half adhere to vessel walls. Neutrophils remain in the circulation 6 to 8 hours, then move into the tissues where they survive for two to three days.

Neutrophils are mature white blood cells containing neutrophil granules that attack and destroy bacteria. They are the first and most numerous cells to arrive at any area of disease or tissue injury. Because there are usually three times as many stored in the bone marrow as are circulating, a reserve pool is always ready. In times of serious injury, the total life span of a neutrophil decreases to several hours.

Eosinophils

Eosinophils, another type of granulocyte, comprise up to 4% of the total WBC. The committed eosinophil progenitor, colony-forming unit-eosinophil (CFU-Eo), descends from the CFU-GEMM. There are three immature forms (eosinophilic myeloblast, promyelocyte, and myelocyte) and the mature eosinophil. Eosinophils circulate for around 8 hours, then migrate into the tissue. Eosinophils ingest bacteria and release factors that alter the inflammatory response. The eosinophil level is generally increased in parasitic infections and allergic responses.

Basophils

Basophils differentiate in a manner parallel to that of eosinophils: colony-forming unit-basophil (CFU-Bas), basophilic myeloblast, promyelocyte, myelocyte, metamyelocyte, and basophil. Unlike neutrophils and eosinophils, basophils do not phagocytize bacteria. Rather they release substances (including heparin and histamine) following stimulation, contributing to hypersensitivity reactions. Basophils account for up to 0.05% of

the WBC and may be elevated in patients with asthma, allergies, and some carcinomas.

Monocytes/Macrophages

Monocytes and neutrophils share a common progenitor cell, colony-forming unit-granulocyte-macrophage (CFU-GM). Upon stimulation by certain HGFs, these cells produce monoblasts. Further maturation results in promonocytes and monocytes. The mature monocyte is released into the blood stream, where it circulates for one to three days. After entering the tissue, the monocyte matures into a macrophage, which provides nonspecific immunity against parasitic, protozoan, and fungal infections. Normal monocyte levels are 6% to 8% of the WBC.

Erythrocytes

Erythrocyte development begins with the burst forming unit-erythroid (BFU-E). The proliferating immature forms are proerythroblast and erythroblast. The normoblast, or next level of differentiation, loses the ability to divide. The **reticulocyte** is released into the bloodstream, where it circulates for one to two days until a fully matured erythrocyte. The function of the erythrocyte is to transport oxygen to the tissues and carry carbon dioxide from the tissues to the lungs via the hemoglobin molecule.

Thrombocytes

The committed megakaryocyte progenitor cell is the colony-forming unit-megakaryocyte (CFU-Meg). The earliest thrombocyte progenitor detected in the bone marrow is the megakaryoblast. The next level of differentiation is the megakaryocyte, which releases many platelets. Through a complex process, platelets form hemostatic plugs at the site of injured blood vessels. They also release factors that initiate clotting. Thrombocytes usually survive seven to eight days in the blood.

Lymphocytes

Lymphocytes account for 30% to 35% of the total WBC. The lymphoid stem cell arises from the PPSC and differentiates into one of two cell lineages, B or T lymphocytes. Pre-T lymphocytes mature in the thymus into prothymocytes, lymphoblasts, and T lymphocytes. T lymphocytes mediate cellular immunity, circulating freely between tissue and peripheral blood. When stimulated by specific antigens, T lymphocytes produce many cytokines that regulate the specific immune response.

Pre-B lymphocytes migrate to lymph tissue, such as the spleen and lymph nodes, to mature. The B lymphoblast, responding to the antigen-antibody binding on its surface, matures into the B lymphocyte. This cell eventually matures into a plasma cell capable of secreting specific antibodies (*i.e.,* immunoglobulins). B lymphocytes comprise 20% to 25% of the lymphocyte count.

Hematopoietic Growth Factors in Hematopoiesis

The entire process of hematopoiesis is controlled by a complex feedback system. The HGFs regulate hematopoiesis by stimulating the cells to divide and mature in an orderly manner. Some HGFs have a specific influence on precursor and mature cells, while others affect cell differentiation and proliferation at the progenitor level (Crosier and Clark, 1992).

In the patient with infection, HGF levels increase to stimulate neutrophil production and activity. When the T-cell receptor is activated by an antigen, one of the major responses is the production of multiple cytokines, including IL–2, IL–3, IL–4, IL–5, and IL–9; GM-CSF; tumor necrosis factor (TNF); and interferon gamma (IFN-γ) (Crosier and Clark, 1992). Monocytes and macrophages respond to bacteria, bacterial cell wall products, and other cytokines by releasing other cytokines such as IL–1 and IL–6, TNF, G-CSF, M-CSF and GM-CSF (Wimperis *et al.,* 1989). As infection resolves, HGF levels return to normal.

In vivo studies have shown that endogenous levels of G-CSF are high in persons with chemotherapy-induced neutropenia and decline as the neutrophil count recovers (Layton *et al.,* 1989; Watari *et al.,* 1989). It has been shown that M-CSF and IL–6 are also elevated in patients who are febrile and neutropenic.

Cell Surface Receptors

Hematopoietic growth factors work at the cellular level by binding to specific cell surface membrane receptors. Each receptor appears to receive only a single type of HGF, but receptors for more than one type of growth factor may be expressed on a given cell. The direct actions of HGFs are initiated by the binding of the particular HGF to cell surface receptors. After binding to its specific receptor, the protein and its receptor are internalized into the cell and direct the cell to divide or mature. The remaining cell surface receptors specific for the HGF are internalized or inactivated.

Moreover, the HGF can act indirectly on cells. The protein product released from the initial action can bind to a different cell and stimulate it, initiating a secondary cytokine cascade. For example, GM-CSF stimulates the release of macrophages, TNF, and IFN-γ. These cytokines are known to cause symptoms such as fever and chills (Traynor, 1992). Individual cells express more than one receptor. There are relatively few receptors on the cells (a few hundred per cell), and the biological effects are elicited with low levels of receptor occupancy around 10% (Metcalf and Morstyn, 1991; Nicola, 1989). Receptors are present on both mature and immature cells.

Genetics

Genes that encode for three HGFs (GM-CSF, M-CSF, and IL–3) have been localized to a closely clustered region of the distal long arm of chromosome 5. Of interest is that this chromosome region is frequently deleted in patients with myelodysplastic syndromes. Designated the 5q- syndromes, they are also the chromosomal abnormalities seen most frequently in acute myeloid leukemia secondary to radiation exposure. The gene that encodes G-CSF has been mapped to chromosome 17 (Van Leeuwan et al., 1989; Yang et al., 1988; Kanda et al., 1987; Simmers et al., 1987).

Once the genes for specific HGFs were identified, researchers were able to use recombinant techniques to produce HGFs in large quantities. Specific genes are isolated and combined with a DNA strand from another organism which then serves as a factory, continuing to produce DNA identical to that in the original molecule (Jaramilla, 1992).

ANIMAL STUDIES

Preclinical studies with G-CSF began with intraperitoneal administration in mice (Kobayashi et al., 1987; Fujisawa et al., 1986). When given alone, G-CSF induced neutrophilia. When given after 5-fluorouracil and total body irradiation, neutrophil recovery was accelerated.

A study in which monkeys received subcutaneously administered G-CSF for 28 days resulted in neutrophilia with marrow hypercellularity and extramedullary hematopoiesis in lymph nodes (Welte et al., 1987). When administered after cyclophosphamide and continued for 14 days, G-CSF restored neutrophil levels to pretreatment levels within 10 days. After the G-CSF was discontinued, the neutrophil levels remained higher than those in the control group for another week. When G-CSF was also given before and concomitantly with the cyclophosphamide, the neutropenia was more severe than in the control group, but neutrophil recovery was not affected. It was postulated that the G-CSF recruited responsive cells into the cell cycle, causing them to be more sensitive to the cytotoxic effects of the chemotherapy (Welte et al., 1987).

Murine studies with GM-CSF demonstrated multilineage response that included neutrophils, macrophages, and eosinophils in addition to erythrocyte and megakaryocyte precursors (Metcalf et al., 1986; Metcalf, 1980;

Metcalf et al., 1980). This factor has activity at both the progenitor level (CFU-GEMM) and in the differentiation of mature cells.

Further studies in monkeys showed an acute and sustained rise in leukocytes in response to intravenous infusion of GM-CSF. Leukocytosis occurred within 24 to 72 hours following the initiation of the infusion, and bone marrow cellularity was increased by day 7 (Donahue et al., 1986). Further studies demonstrated dose-dependent leukocytosis. Dosages have ranged from 4 to 300 µg/kg/day (Demetri and Antman, 1992). Two early studies on primates demonstrated a nadir that occurred sooner than expected after chemotherapy, and combinations of HGFs were more effective than single HGFs in producing cellular response (Bonilla et al., 1987; Donahue et al., 1987). Positive results in these studies led to clinical trials evaluating the effectiveness of HGFs in patients.

CLINICAL TRIALS

Clinical trials with HGFs began in 1986. Phase I studies sought to identify adverse effects and to define a dose-response relationship. Phase II studies endeavored to optimize the dose needed to achieve the desired biological effect. For example with G- and GM-CSF the dose needed to reduce neutropenia following chemotherapy. Phase III studies attempted to measure not only the biological effects of the HGFs, but also to confirm clinical benefits.

Erythropoietin

Erythropoietin was first identified in 1906, isolated in 1977, and is now produced by recombinant technology (Metcalf and Morstyn, 1991). Because the kidneys produce 90% of endogenous erythropoietin, patients with chronic renal failure suffer from decreased erythropoietin production and subsequent chronic anemia. Initial clinical trials with Epo demonstrated that administration of Epo stimulated erythropoiesis in these patients, usually increasing the reticulocyte count within 10 days and increasing the hematocrit two to six weeks after beginning therapy. Patients with renal failure typically became independent of transfusions on dosages of 50 to 300 units/kg three times weekly (Eschbach, et al., 1987).

Subsequent studies demonstrated that patients who are infected with the human immunodeficiency virus (HIV) also responded to Epo according to their serum level of endogenous erythropoietin prior to treatment (Eschbach et al., 1987). Patients with erythropoietin levels less than or equal to 500 mUnits/ml generally responded to Epo therapy while those with ≥ 500 mUnits/ml did not seem to respond.

In patients with cancer, anemia may be related to the disease process itself or to the myelosuppressive effects of chemotherapy. A series of clinical trials evaluated 131 anemic patients who were receiving cyclic chemotherapy containing cisplatin or therapies that did not include cisplatin (Doweiko and Goldberg, 1991; Means and Krantz, 1991; Platanias et al., 1991). Patients with lower endogenous erythropoietin levels responded to the therapy as demonstrated by increased hematocrit levels and decreased transfusion requirements.

Granulocyte-Macrophage Colony-Stimulating Factor

Early clinical trials of GM-CSF were conducted in patients with acquired immunodeficiency syndrome (AIDS), myelodysplastic syndromes (MDS) and in patients who were receiving myelosuppressive chemotherapy. Receiving HGFs allowed patients with AIDS to continue to receive therapeutic but myelosuppressive drugs such as zidovudine, gancyclovir, or pentamidine. Groopman et al. (1987) administered GM-CSF in an intravenous bolus and as a continuous infusion to patients with AIDS. Increased WBC counts were documented along with edema, weight

gain, and myalgias. Baldwin et al. (1987) demonstrated an increased number and function of circulating neutrophils in these patients when GM-CSF was administered intravenously.

Granulocyte-macrophage colony-stimulating factor was used to induce differentiation of dysplastic cells in MDS. In 1987, Vadhan-Raj (1987) administered GM-CSF to patients with MDS and noted an increase in neutrophil levels and a subsequent decrease in the incidence of infections and transfusions in these patients. A later study (Thompson et al., 1989) verified the increased neutrophil levels, but noted that the increase was temporary. Patients experienced fever and flu-like symptoms. Demetri and Antman (1992) reviewed 11 studies of GM-CSF in MDS. Overall, there was an increase in leukocyte levels in 50% to 75% of patients, but 10% to 25% of patients had concurrent increases in peripheral blood blast counts (Demetri and Antman, 1992). No significant risk of HGF-induced transformation to acute leukemia has been documented.

In early studies of HGFs administered following chemotherapy, patients with sarcoma who received MAID (mesna, doxorubicin, ifosfamide, and dacarbazine) received intravenous GM-CSF for 5 to 14 days after the first course of therapy (Antman et al., 1987). The response of the WBC to this regimen was compared to that after the second cycle when no HGF was given. The WBC was higher and the nadir period was shorter by 4 days in the first cycle than in the second. This study has been criticized because a longer nadir period is expected after the second cycle of therapy. At doses of 4 to 32 μg/kg/day, side effects were mild, but at 64 μg/kg/day, fluid retention and pericardial and pleural effusions were reported.

In studies with GM-CSF, a dose-response leukocytosis has reliably been achieved with continuous intravenous infusion, bolus intravenous infusion, and subcutaneous injection. In placebo-controlled randomized studies of patients who were receiving myelosuppressive chemotherapy, the number of days of neutropenic fever, days of treatment of infection with antibiotics, and days of hospitalization were reduced with this factor (Herrmann *et al.*, 1990; Antman *et al.*, 1988).

The use of GM-CSF has also been evaluated after high-dose chemotherapy followed by autologous bone marrow transplant BMT (Nemunaitis *et al.*, 1990b; 1988a). The period of neutropenia was reduced in these patients from 18 days to 12 days, but platelet recovery did not seem to occur earlier. The initial studies of GM-CSF in BMT were conducted with patients with lymphoid malignancies due to hypothetical concern that GM-CSF would stimulate growth of neoplastic myeloid cells. Aurer reviewed eight autologous BMT studies and summarized the findings. Neutrophil recovery after BMT was accelerated by 7 days in those receiving GM-CSF although the interval before neutrophils appeared in the peripheral blood after BMT was the same for both patients receiving GM-CSF and the control group. In addition, patients receiving GM-CSF had less days of fever, decreased number of platelet transfusions, and less days in the hospital after BMT. These benefits do not hold true in patients receiving marrow purged with 4 hydroperoxycyclophosphamide and anti-T or anti-B cell antibodies (Singer, 1992; Blazer *et al.*, 1989). There is no acceleration of neutrophil recovery by GM-CSF. This seems to demonstrate a need to preserve adequate numbers of colony-forming units (CFUs) in order to have a response to GM-CSF (Blazer *et al.*, 1989).

Granulocyte-macrophage colony-stimulating factor used in allogeneic BMT is also well tolerated (Mertelsmann *et al.*, 1990). Another theoretical concern was that GM-CSF would increase graft versus host disease (GVHD) due to release of IL–1 and TNF which stimulate T lymphocytes. This has not been demonstrated and there is no increase in acute GVHD. The use of GM-CSF is more effective in patients who receive GVHD prophylaxis with cyclosporine (CSA) and prednisone

versus CSA and methotrexate (Singer, 1992). Patients with matched unrelated donor (MUD) BMT have an increased risk of GVHD and graft failure. In a study using yeast derived GM-CSF in 40 patients receiving a MUD BMT, there was no significant effect on neutrophil recovery but there was decreased risk of infection (8% versus 24%). Although there was no difference in overall incidence of GVHD, there was decreased risk of more severe grade III and IV GVHD (Singer *et al.*, 1990). Graft failure, defined as no engraftment of cells by day 28 after BMT, occurs in about 10% of BMT patients. The use of GM-CSF in patients with graft failure stimulates marrow recovery with no increase in the incidence of GVHD (Nemunaitis *et al.*, 1988b).

Both G-CSF and GM-CSF have been effective in promoting neutrophil recovery after chemotherapy for acute myelogenous leukemia (AML) without evidence of CSF-induced blast cell acceleration (Buchner *et al.* 1991; Ohno *et al.* 1990). Granulocyte-macrophage colony-stimulating factor has been administered to a high-risk population of elderly patients who were newly diagnosed with AML in an attempt to decrease the period of neutropenia. Although the period of absolute neutropenia was six to nine days shorter in the group treated with GM-CSF, two patients experienced rapid regrowth of leukemic cells. This leukemia cell growth slowed in one patient after discontinuation of the HGF. Studies have been conducted in which growth factors were used to recruit AML blast cells into the S phase of the cell cycle, followed immediately by high-dose chemotherapy. This therapy significantly increased cell kill (Estey *et al.*, 1990; Cannistra *et al.*, 1989).

Clinical trials are now beginning to address the issue of whether the use of HGFs will allow for administration of dose-intensified therapy, and thereby contribute to improved patient survival. Logothetis and colleagues (1990) treated 32 patients with metastatic urothelial tumors who were refractory to standard therapy with MVAC (methotrexate, vinblastine, doxorubicin, and cisplatin). The use of unglycosylated recombinant human GM-CSF (rhGM-CSF) allowed for escalation of chemotherapy doses even in heavily pretreated patients. In phase II trials, 40% of the treated patients responded, 23% achieving a complete remission. Demitri and Antman (1992) treated patients with metastatic breast cancer who were receiving cyclophosphamide, doxorubicin, and 5-fluorouracil (CAF). Support with GM-CSF allowed increases in the dosages of cyclophosphamide and doxorubicin.

Granulocyte Colony-Stimulating Factor

Patients with MDS treated with intravenous G-CSF also had rapid increases in peripheral leukocyte and marrow granulocyte precursor levels with no increase in blast cell level (Kobayashi et al., 1989). When subcutaneous G-CSF was used in patients with MDS (Negrin et al., 1989), 10 of 12 patients had increases in neutrophil counts of 5-fold to 40-fold. No patient had converted to acute leukemia and several had some differentiation of granulocyte precursors.

Gabrilove et al. (1988) administered G-CSF subcutaneously to patients with bladder cancer who were being treated with MVAC (methotrexate, vincristine, doxorubicin, and cyclophosphamide). The HGF was given on days 4 through 11 at a dosage of 200 $\mu g/m^2$. In addition to a shorter, less severe nadir period, Gabrilove et al. noted a decreased incidence of mucositis. Transient bone pain was reported.

Crawford et al. (1991) described a study of 211 patients who received G-CSF or placebo after chemotherapy for small-cell lung cancer. The chemotherapy regimen, considered standard therapy for this disease, consists of cyclophosphamide, doxorubicin, and etoposide given for six cycles. The incidence of febrile neutropenia was 57% in the study group re-

ceiving placebo and 28% in the group receiving G-CSF. The G-CSF group had a 47% reduction in the number of days on antibiotics and spent 45% less time in the hospital.

In another classic study, patients with advanced cancer who received a continuous subcutaneous infusion of G-CSF or GM-CSF experienced less myelosuppression than control patients (Morstyn et al., 1989a). The subcutaneous route was shown to be more effective than intravenous bolus infusion.

A dose-response leukocytosis is also achieved with continuous intravenous infusion (Bronchud et al., 1987), bolus intravenous infusion (Gabrilove et al., 1988; Morstyn et al., 1988) and subcutaneous infusion (Morstyn et al., 1989b) of G-CSF. In placebo-controlled randomized studies of patients who were receiving myelosuppressive chemotherapy, the number of days of neutropenic fever, days of treatment of infection with antibiotics, and days of hospitalization were reduced with G-CSF (Crawford et al., 1991; Neidhart et al., 1989; Gabrilove et al., 1988; Morstyn et al., 1988; Bronchud et al., 1987).

G-CSF has also been evaluated after high-dose chemotherapy followed by autologous bone marrow transplant (Taylor et al., 1989; Kodo et al., 1988). A study by Sheridan et al. (1989) showed tendencies toward shorter hospital stays, fewer days of fever, shorter periods of total parenteral nutrition, and fewer days in a protected environment in patients who received the CSF, but none of these differences achieved statistical significance.

Granulocyte colony-stimulating factor has been shown to increase levels of circulating peripheral blood stem cells (PBSC). These cells are harvested by leukopheresis and used as an alternative to bone marrow for hematopoietic rescue after high-dose chemotherapy (To et al., 1987). Hematopoietic growth factors can be used to predictably increase the number of progenitor cells for harvesting. One study demonstrated that the number of PBSC collected increased by a median of 83 times (Sheridan et al., 1990). Patients who received

PBSC and HGFs had periods of neutrophil recovery similar to those of the control group who received bone marrow transplantation and G-CSF or GM-CSF, but significantly faster platelet recovery.

Several studies have demonstrated the impact of G-CSF on chemotherapy dose intensification (Neidhart *et al.*, 1989; Bronchud *et al.*, 1987). Bronchud *et al.* (1989) increased the dosage and frequency of doxorubicin administration to two to three times the normal dosages in patients with advanced breast or ovarian cancer. Administration of G-CSF allowed the cytotoxic drugs to be administered at 14-day intervals. The dose-limiting toxic effects were mucositis and skin toxicity.

REGULATORY APPROVAL

Approved Agents

Granulocyte Colony-Stimulating Factor
Granulocyte colony-stimulating factor (Filgrastim) was approved by the FDA for commercial use in 1991 to decrease the incidence of infections in patients with non-myeloid malignancies receiving myelosuppressive chemotherapy. The recommended starting dose is 5 μg/kg/day administered as a daily subcutaneous injection. If the desired response is not seen, the dosage may be doubled after the next course of chemotherapy. In 1994 it was approved for use post BMT in non-myeloid malignancies.

This agent may be given intravenously, but is given over at least 30 minutes and must be diluted to less than 2 μg/ml. Filgrastim is diluted with 5% dextrose and is not compatible with saline. Because levels of neutrophils decrease by about 50% in the first 24 hours after the G-CSF is discontinued, G-CSF must be administered past the expected nadir (Figure 6.2). It is administered daily past the expected nadir for up to two weeks or until the absolute neutrophil count exceeds 10,000 cells/mm^3.

Monitoring recommendations include a baseline and then twice weekly complete

blood count and platelet count. Uric acid levels should be monitored in patients with malignancies associated with high uric acid levels.

Granulocyte-Macrophage Colony-Stimulating Factor
Granulocyte-macrophage colony-stimulating factor was approved by the FDA in 1991 under the generic name sargramostim and is indicated to accelerate myeloid recovery in selected patients who are undergoing autologous bone marrow transplant. These are patients with non-Hodgkin's lymphoma, Hodgkin's disease, or acute lymphocytic leukemia.

Granulocyte-macrophage colony-stimulating factor is available in a powdered form along with diluent in a 250-μg or 500-μg size. The recommended dose is 250 μg/m^2/day, given as a daily infusion over 2 hours. The length of administration is 21 days or until myeloid recovery is achieved. Administration of GM-CSF is discontinued when the absolute neutrophil count exceeds 20,000 cells/mm^3 or the platelet count exceeds 500,000 cells/mm^3. This factor is compatible with saline or 5% dextrose in water if concentrations are greater than or equal to 10 μg/ml (Immunex, 1992). Human serum albumin must be added to solutions with dilutions less than 10 μg/ml.

Monitoring includes baseline then twice weekly complete blood count and differential, platelet and reticulocyte counts. Patients with pre-existing renal and/or hepatic dysfunction require monitoring of liver enzymes and creatinine.

Recombinant GM-CSF is expressed in yeast, bacteria, and mammalian cells. The GM-CSF expressed by yeast, sargramostim, is most like native GM-CSF, as both are glycosylated (that is, attached to a sugar molecule). Molgrastim is nonglycosylated and is produced by *E. coli* and remains investigational. Although the natural and recombinant products are similar, there are differences in pharmacokinetics, biological activity and immunogenicity. Dorr (1993) recently reviewed 32 clinical trials to compare frequency of

Figure 6.2 Infection risk and prophylaxis in a patient who was receiving myelosuppressive chemotherapy. (A) Chemotherapy is administered with varying numbers and combinations of drugs. (B) In response to interrupted blood cell production, the absolute neutrophil count (ANC) begins to decrease (solid line). (C) The nadir, or lowest ANC, usually occurs 10 to 14 days after chemotherapy begins. (D) Recovery of ANC is seen 3 to 4 weeks after chemotherapy begins. (E) Prophylactic antibiotics may be given to protect the patient throughout the period of neutropenia. (F) Colony-stimulating factors (CSFs) may be administered daily beginning 24 hours after therapy ends. (G) A rise in the ANC was due to the release of reserve cells from the marrow (broken line). (H) The nadir occurs earlier than expected, is of a shorter duration and is less severe, and the ANC recovers rapidly. The CSF therapy is discontinued when the ANC exceeds 10,000/mm³. (I) The ANC decreases by half in 24 hours after discontinuation; the patient continues to produce neutrophils at normal levels.

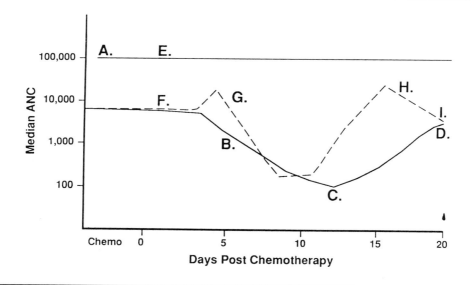

Source: Reprinted with permission from: Wujick, D. 1993. Infection control in oncology patients. *Nursing Clinics of North America* 28(3): 639–650.

adverse events in patients who received *E. coli*-derived GM-CSF and those who received yeast-derived GM-CSF and concluded that the *E. coli* product is associated with more side effects (Table 6.1).

Erythropoietin

Erythropoietin (epoetin alfa) was approved by the FDA in 1989 (Epogen®, Procrit®) for chronic renal failure requiring dialysis and HIV infection requiring myelosuppressive therapy. Administration of Epo allows these patients to become independent of transfusions or to continue therapy, respectively. The dose for renal failure is 50-100 U/kg administered subcutaneously three times per week. Recently, an additional indication was added for Procrit®, the treatment of anemia due to cancer chemotherapy. The recommended dosage for this indication is 150 U/kg subcutaneously three times weekly.

SIDE EFFECTS

For a complete review of side effects seen with HGF administration, see Table 6.1.

Granulocyte colony-stimulating factor is usually well tolerated. In Phase II/III studies, bone pain was reported in 20% to 24% of patients. It was described as mild to moderate, brief, and easily controlled with non-narcotic analgesia. The most common sites of bone pain were sternum, back, pelvis, and limbs— all bones with large marrow reserves. The pain typically occurs two to three days after administration of G-CSF begins and right before the counts begin to rise, suggesting an association with rapid myelopoiesis.

Common side effects seen with GM-CSF administration include low grade fever and bone pain. The dose-limiting toxic effects, pericarditis, and atrial arrhythmias, were identified at doses of ≥ 20 $\mu g/kg/day$ of GM-CSF. At doses ranging from 30 to 64 $\mu g/kg/day$, pulmonary emboli, severe weight gain with pleural and pericardial effusions, and capillary leak syndrome were reported (Hartmann and Edmonson, 1990; Antman et al., 1988; Brandt et al., 1988). Dosages of 2 to 20 $\mu g/kg/day$ were associated with milder side effects such as skin rashes, anorexia, fevers with chills, arthralgias, myalgias, and headaches. A "first dose" reaction has been described with IV bolus administration that includes flushing, hypotension, transient hypoxia, and tachycardia. Subsequent administrations do not generally elicit this same response.

Erythropoietin is well tolerated, although blood pressure must be controlled prior to therapy and iron supplements may be needed to maintain iron stores in patients who receive this agent over long periods.

CLINICAL ISSUES
Timing

It is recommended that HGFs be administered no sooner than 24 hours after chemotherapy. There is concern that increasing the number of divisions of the neutrophil progenitors, then destroying them with the chemotherapy, will result in severe myelosuppression. Timing of CSF administration has been explored by Crawford et al. (1992). In patients with lung cancer who were receiving cyclophosphamide, doxorubicin, and etoposide, G-CSF was administered at day 4, 6, or 8. It is not yet clear whether it is better to start earlier or later. The results remain controversial.

Morstyn et al. (1989a) gave G-CSF before melphalan and was unable to prove that the HGF gave an advantage. One study showed that G-CSF could be delayed up to 7 days after chemotherapy and administered for a short period (days 8 through 13 after chemotherapy) and still shorten the nadir period. Meropol et al. (1992) administered G-CSF along with 5-fluorouracil and leucovorin and found that patients who received G-CSF experienced more severe neutropenia. Vadhan-Raj et al (1992) evaluated the dose, schedule and timing of GM-CSF administered with Cy-ADIC (cyclophosphamide, doxorubicin, and dacarbazine) chemotherapy. The modified schedule which allowed for earlier administration of GM-CSF, immediately following discontinuation of chemotherapy, improved the beneficial effects of GM-CSF by enhancing myeloprotection and permitting dose-intensification of chemotherapy.

Length of Therapy

The optimal length of HGF therapy remains unclear. The optimal absolute neutrophil count (> 1000, 5000, or 10,000/mm³) is not apparent. In dose-intensive regimens, stopping at 10,000 mm³ does not always ensure counts will not drop lower. A priming effect has been observed: neutropenia is less severe in some patients during the second and subsequent cycles of chemotherapy (Crawford et al., 1991).

Dose Intensification

HGFs have demonstrated the ability to reduce morbidity and make more tolerable present chemotherapy regimens. However, an even greater question exists of whether the use of HGFs will allow for dose-intensification of therapy that would ultimately translate into improved patient survival. Initial studies exploring this question have been reviewed above. Currently, results are far from definitive. Additional studies utilizing randomized trials will be necessary to answer this question (Canellos and Demetri, 1993).

INVESTIGATIONAL AGENTS

Stem Cell Factor

Stem cell factor is an HGF that acts on the earliest progenitors, and possibly the PPSC. It is also known as Steel factor, so named because it is the HGF missing in Steel mutant mice, which have an aberrant hematopoietic process (Bernstein and Kufe, 1992). This HGF was simultaneously identified and named by other investigators as kit ligand (Williams *et al.*, 1990b), mast cell growth factor (Anderson *et al.*, 1990; Huang *et al.*, 1990) and stem cell factor (Zsebo *et al.*, 1990).

Stem cell factor interacts with the most primitive cell forms and supports growth of various colonies when used in combination with other HGFs (Anderson *et al.*, 1990). When compared to GM-CSF and IL–3, SCF produces a greater number of cell colonies and greater colony sizes (Bernstein *et al.*, 1991). However, exposure of bone marrow cultures to SCF alone does not result in significant colony formation. When administered in combination with G-CSF, GM-CSF, or IL–3, both colony size and number increase. (Bernstein *et al.*, 1991; McNiece *et al.*, 1991)

Several questions remain to be answered about SCF. It is not clear whether SCF acts on a common lymphoid/myeloid progenitor or on separate lymphoid and/or myeloid progenitor cells. Does SCF stimulate the self-renewal process of daughter cell formation or influence the postcommitment divisions? Does the SCF interact with the bone marrow microenvironment?

There are several potential clinical applications for SCF. Expansion of a progenitor population that is responsive to a later, more lineage restricted hematopoietin represents one possibility. Use of SCF may decrease the dosage of a second growth factor needed to stimulate an appropriate number of colonies. Another potential application is to accelerate marrow regeneration in bone marrow transplantation. It has been proposed that if SCF does stimulate the PPSC, a single stem cell could be selected, stimulated with SCF, and used for bone marrow transplantation.

Macrophage Colony-Stimulating Factor

Macrophage colony-stimulating factor is a lineage-specific HGF that supports proliferation and activation of monocytes and their committed progenitors. It has been shown in animal studies to stimulate the numbers and sizes of monocytes (Stoudemire and Garnick, 1991; Garnick and Stoudemire, 1990). In a phase I study, patients with metastatic melanoma received 7-day infusions of M-CSF ranging from 12 to 120 μg/kg/day; increased numbers of circulating monocytes were noted. There was also a decrease in platelet counts that reversed upon drug cessation. One patient showed tumor regression. Overall, the M-CSF was well tolerated.

Macrophage colony-stimulating factor has been given with IFN-γ to induce proliferation of peripheral monocytes and differentiation into circulating macrophages. It was administered by continuous intravenous infusion for 14 days at dosages from 10 to 140 μg/kg/day along with subcutaneous IFN-γ on days 8 through 14 (Weiner *et al.*, 1993). Some tumor regression was noted in 3 of 28 patients and all had increased levels of macrophages.

Monocytes stimulated by M-CSF have greater cytotoxicity in fungal infections than normal monocytes. Macrophage colony-stimulating factor has been shown to be useful in treating fungal infections refractory to amphotericin B therapy (Nemunaitis *et al.*, 1990a). A phase I/II trial of recombinant M-CSF explored the use of this HGF in patients with invasive fungal infections. Sixteen patients were treated, 13 who had had bone marrow transplants and 3 who were too ill to undergo bone marrow transplantation. The 3 very ill patients had complete resolution of infection. Ten of the 13 BMT patients had improvement or resolution (Nemunaitis *et al.*, 1993).

Interleukin–3

Interleukin–3 is also known as multi-CSF. This HGF is multilineage and acts on early progenitors (Lindemann and Mertelsmann, 1993). Alone it is the most effective cytokine in supporting CFU-GEMM colony formation in humans and, specifically, is a more potent stimulator of megakaryocytopoiesis than other HGFs. Interleukin–3 produces a multilineage response, with increases in leukocytes, platelets, and reticulocytes. The response is delayed in platelets and erythrocytes, probably indicating that IL–3 should be administered continuously for prolonged periods.

Interleukin–3 has been studied in patients with advanced malignancy, patients with prolonged myelosuppression secondary to chemotherapy or radiotherapy, and patients with MDS or aplastic anemia (Hoelzer *et al.*, 1991; Ganser *et al.*, 1990a; Ganser *et al.*, 1990b). Treatment consisted of dosages of 30 to 500 $\mu g/m^2$ given as a subcutaneous bolus injection daily for 15 days. The first doses were given intravenously over 5 minutes. The intravenous injection produced a rise of neutrophils within 30 minutes that reached a peak level at 4 to 6 hours.

The toxic effects of subcutaneous IL–3 were mild. Seventy percent of patient had fever: the fever was more pronounced during the first few days of therapy and was associated with higher dosages. Headache, chills, and bone pain were also reported.

COMBINATIONS OF HEMATOPOIETIC GROWTH FACTORS

There is synergistic enhancement of early progenitors *in vitro* when early and late acting HGFs are combined (Brugger *et al.*, 1992a; Brugger *et al.*, 1992b). The factors G-CSF and Epo prevented anemia and neutropenia in AIDS patients who were receiving zidovudine (Miles *et al.*, 1991). Other combinations of HGFs, such as IL–3 and GM-CSF have been studied. Preclinical studies indicate that sequential administration produces better results than simultaneous administration. Molecules administered simultaneously may compete for the same receptors, altering the number of functional receptors for each CSF (Brugger *et al.*, 1992a; Hoelzer *et al.*, 1991; Park *et al.*, 1989a; Park *et al.*, 1989b).

Fusion Molecules

Growth factors can be fused together using molecular techniques. Interleukin–3 and GM-CSF have been combined into a molecule, PIXY321, that has greater bioactivity than either IL–3 or GM-CSF alone (Williams *et al.*, 1990a). It is 10-fold to 20-fold more potent on a weight basis than GM-CSF or IL–3, alone or together. This molecule is administered subcutaneously once or twice daily or intravenously over 2 hours. It is unknown whether the fusion protein provides a better therapeutic response than sequential administration of the two CSFs (Bernstein *et al.*, 1991).

Three studies of PIXY321 in patients who were receiving myelosuppressive chemotherapy were recently reported. In one study, patients with sarcoma treated with cyclophosphamide, doxorubicin, and dacarbazine received PIXY321 subcutaneously twice daily before the first dosages of chemotherapy and after the second cycle of chemotherapy (Vadhan-Raj *et al.*, 1994). A dosage of 750 μg/m² was determined to be optimal for decreasing myelosuppression and reducing cumulative thrombocytopenia. Local skin reactions and mild constitutional symptoms were the only side effects reported. Other studies are evaluating PIXY321 in patients with breast cancer who are receiving doxorubicin and thiotepa (Reptis *et al.*, 1993) and with high-dose carboplatin in patients with advanced cancer (Miller *et al.*, 1993).

FUTURE DIRECTIONS

Many clinical issues remain in determining the optimal use of HGFs. Several hematopoietic and nonhematopoietic cell lines have receptors for HGFs. Colonic adenocarcinoma (Berdel *et al.*, 1989), small cell lung cancer (Avalos *et al.*, 1990), breast cancer, osteosarcoma (Baldwin *et al.*, 1989; Berdel *et al.*, 1989) and leukemia cells have been identified as having receptors for HGFs. A clinical implication is that these factors may stimulate rather than retard growth of malignant cells, but this has not yet been known to occur.

Dosing schedules continue to be evaluated. Dosage increases are recommended if the time to response by WBC or the magnitude of neutrophil response is unacceptable, for example, in patients who are heavily pretreated, patients with prior radiotherapy to bone marrow areas, patients who have had bone marrow transplant, and patients whose doses have been intensified. Thus far, the maximum tolerated dosage has not been identified. Patients have received up to 115 μg/kg/day of G-CSF.

In spite of dramatic neutrophil response to G-CSF and GM-CSF, platelet recovery after chemotherapy remains delayed. Thus, the patient may no longer be neutropenic but still requires platelet transfusions. Interleukin–6 has been shown to have multiple biological effects. One important effect is thrombopoietic activity, the ability to stimulate platelet production (Asano *et al.*, 1990; Ishibashi *et al.*, 1989). Preclinical testing of this effect is currently underway.

The use of fusion products leads researchers to wonder about the possibility of HGF cocktails that combine specific HGFs to elicit a specific response. Some speculate that neutralizing antibodies may develop secondary to an immune response to the synthetic genetic linkage (Bernstein and Kufe, 1992).

Clinicians continue to evaluate which patients undergoing specific protocols will benefit from use of HGFs. To date, HGFs have not been evaluated with drugs that cause delayed myelosuppression, such as the nitrosureas or mitomycin C. Cost and quality of life remain important issues to consider when using HGFs in the therapy of the patient with cancer.

References

Anderson, D., Lyman, S., Baird, A., *et al.* 1990. Molecular cloning of mast cell growth factor, a hematopoietin that is active in both membrane bound and soluble forms. *Cell* 63(1): 235–243.

Antman, K., Griffin, J., Elias, A., *et al.* 1987. Use of rhGM-CSF to ameliorate chemotherapy-induced myelosuppression in sarcoma patients. *Blood* 70(5 Suppl 1): 129a (abstract 372).

Antman, K., Griffin, J., Levine, J., *et al.* 1988. Effect of recombinant human GM-CSF on chemotherapy-induced myelosuppression. *New England Journal of Medicine* 319(10): 593–598.

Appelbaum, F. 1989. The clinical use of hematopoietic growth factors. *Seminars in Hematology* 26 (3 Suppl 3): 7–13.

Asano, S., Okano, A., Ozawa, K., *et al.* 1990. *In vivo* effects of recombinant human interleukin–6 in primates: Stimulated production of platelets. *Blood* 75 (8): 1602–1605.

Aurer, I., Ribas, A., Gale, R., *et al.*, 1990. What is the role of recombinant colony-stimulating factors in bone marrow transplantation? *Bone Marrow Transplantation* 6: 79–87.

Avalos, B., Gasson, J., Hedvat, C., *et al.* 1990. Human granulocyte colony-stimulating factor: Biologic activities and receptor characterization on hematopoietic cells and small cell lung cancer cell lines. *Blood* 75(4): 851–857.

Bajorin, D., Nai-Kong, V., and Houghton, A. 1991. Macrophage colony-stimulating factor: Biological effects and potential applications for cancer therapy. *Seminars in Hematology* 28(2 Suppl 2): 42–48.

Baldwin, G., Gasson, J., Kaufman, S., et al. 1989. Nonhematopoietic tumor cells express functional GM-CSF receptors. *Blood* 73(2): 1033–1037.

Baldwin, G., Gasson, J., Quan, S., et al. 1987. GM-CSF enhances neutrophil function in AIDS patients. *Blood* 70(5 Suppl 1): 130a (abstract).

Berdel, W., Danhauser-Riedl, S., Steinhauser, G., et al. 1989. Various human hematopoietic growth factors (interleukin–3, GM-CSF, G-CSF) stimulate clonal growth of nonhematopoietic tumor cells. *Blood* 73(1): 80–83.

Bernstein, I., Andrews, R., and Zsebo, K. 1991. Recombinant human stem cell factor enhances the formation of colonies by CD34+ and CD34+ lin-cells, and the generation of colony-forming cell progeny from CD34+ lin-cells cultured with IL–3, G-CSF, or GM-CSF. *Blood* 77(7): 2316–2321.

Bernstein, S., and Kufe, D. 1992. Future of basic/clinical hematopoiesis research in the era of hematopoietic growth factor availability. *Seminars in Oncology* 19(4): 441–448.

Blazer, B., Kersy, J., McGlave, P., et al., 1989. In vivo administration of recombinant human granulocyte-macrophage colony-stimulating factor in acute lymphoblastic leukemia patients receiving purged autografts. *Blood* 73: 849–857.

Bockheim, C., and Jassak, P. 1993. The expanding world of colony-stimulating factors. *Cancer Practice* 1(3): 205–216.

Bonilla, M., Gillio, A., Porter, G., et al. 1987. Effects of recombinant human granulocyte colony-stimulating factor and granulocyte-macrophage colony-stimulating factor on cytopenias associated with repeated cycles of chemotherapy in primates. *Blood* 70(5): 377a (abstract).

Brandt, S., Peters, W., Atwater, S., et al. 1988. Effect of recombinant human GM-CSF on hematopoietic reconstitution after high-dose chemotherapy and autologous bone marrow transplantation. *New England Journal of Medicine* 318(14): 869–876.

Bronchud, M., Howell, A., Crowther, D., et al. 1989. The use of granulocyte colony-stimulating factor to increase the intensity of treatment with doxorubicin in patients with advanced breast and ovarian cancer. *British Journal of Cancer* 60(1): 121–125.

Bronchud, M., Scargge, J., Thatcher, N., et al. 1987. Phase I/II study of recombinant human G-CSF in patients receiving intensive chemotherapy for small cell lung cancer. *British Journal of Cancer* 56(6): 809–813.

Brugger, W., Frisch, J., Schultz, G., et al. 1992a. Sequential administration of interleukin–3 and granulocyte-macrophage colony-stimulating factor following standard dose combination chemotherapy with etoposide, ifosfamide, and cisplatin. *Journal of Clinical Oncology* 18(9): 1452–1459.

Brugger, W., Klaus-J, B., Lindemann, A., et al. 1992b. Role of hematopoietic growth factor combinations in experimental and clinical oncology. *Seminars in Oncology* 19(2 Suppl 4): 8–15.

Buchner, T., Hidemann, W., Koenigsmann, M., et al. 1991. Recombinant human granulocyte-macrophage colony-stimulating factor after chemotherapy in patients with acute myeloid leukemia at higher age or after relapse. *Blood* 78(5): 1190–1197.

Canellos, G., and Demetri, G. 1993. Myelosuppression and "conventional" chemotherapy: What price, what benefit? *Journal of Clinical Oncology* 11(1): 1–2.

Cannistra, S., Groshek, P., and Griffin, J. 1989. Granulocyte-macrophage colony-stimulating factor enhances the cytotoxic effects of cytosine arabinoside in acute myeloblastic leukemia and in the myeloid blast crisis phase of chronic myeloid leukemia. *Leukemia* 3(5): 328–334.

Crawford, J., Ozer, H., Stoller, R., et al. 1991. Reduction by granulocyte colony-stimulating factor of fever and neutropenia induced by chemotherapy in patients with small-cell lung cancer. *New England Journal of Medicine* 325(3): 164–170.

Crawford, J., Streisman, H., Garewal, H., et al. 1992. A pharmacodynamic investigation of the recombinant human granulocyte colony-stimulating factor (r-met HuG-CSF) schedule variation in patients with small-cell lung cancer (SCLC) given CAE chemotherapy. *Proceedings of American Society of Clinical Oncology* 11: 299 (abstract 1005).

Crosier, P., and Clark, S. 1992. Basic biology of the hematopoietic growth factors. *Seminars in Oncology* 19(4): 349–361.

Demetri, G., and Antman, K. 1992. Granulocyte-macrophage colony-stimulating factor (GM-CSF): Preclinical and clinical investigations. *Seminars in Oncology* 19(4): 362–385.

Donahue, R., Seehra, J., Norton, C., et al. 1987. Stimulation of hematopoiesis in primates with human interleukin–3 and granulocyte-macrophage colony stimulating factor. *Blood* 70(5): 133a (abstract).

Donahue, R., Wang, E., Stone, D., et al. 1986. Stimulation of hematopoiesis in primates by continuous infusion of recombinant human GM-CSF. *Nature* 321(6037): 872–875.

Dorr, R. 1993. Clinical properties of yeast-derived versus *Escherichia coli*-derived granulocyte-macrophage colony-stimulating factor. *Clinical Therapeutics* 15(1): 19–29.

Doweiko, J., and Goldberg, M. 1991. Erythropoietin therapy in cancer patients. *Oncology* 5(8): 31–37.

Erslev, A., and Weiss, L. 1983. Structure and function of marrow. In Williams, W., Beutler, E., Erslev, A., et al. (eds). *Hematology* 3rd edition. New York: McGraw-Hill, pp. 75–81.

Eschbach, J., Egrie, J., Downing, M., et al. 1987. Correction of the anemia of end-stage renal disease with recombinant human erythropoietin. *New England Journal of Medicine* 316 (2): 73–78.

Estey, E., Dixon, D., Hagop, M., *et al.* 1990. Treatment of poor-prognosis, newly diagnosed acute myeloid leukemia with Ara-C and recombinant granulocyte-macrophage colony-stimulating factor. *Blood* 75(5): 1766–1769.

Fujisawa, M., Kobayashi, Y., Okabe, T., *et al.* 1986. Recombinant human granulocyte colony-stimulating factor induces granulocytosis *in vivo*. *Japanese Journal of Cancer Research* 77(9): 866–869.

Gabrilove, J., Jakubowski, A., Scher, H., *et al.* 1988. Effect of G-CSF on neutropenia and associated morbidity due to chemotherapy for transitional-cell carcinoma of the urothelium. *New England Journal of Medicine* 318(22): 1414–1422.

Ganser, A., Lindemann, A., Seipelt, G., *et al.* 1990a. Effects of recombinant human interleukin–3 in patients with normal hematopoiesis and in patients with bone marrow failure. *Blood* 76(4): 666–676.

Ganser, A., Lindemann, A., Seipelt, G., *et al.* 1990b. Effects of recombinant human interleukin–3 in aplastic anemia. *Blood* 76 (7): 1287–1292.

Garnick, M. and Stoudemire, J. 1990. Preclinical and clinical evaluation of recombinant human macrophage colony-stimulating factor (rhM-CSF). *International Journal of Cell Cloning* 8(Suppl 1): 356–371.

Gasson, J., Baldwin, G., Sakamoto, K., *et al.* 1990. The biology of human granulocyte-macrophage colony-stimulating factor (GM-CSF). *Progress in Clinical and Biological Research* 352: 375–384.

Golde, D., and Gasson, J. 1988. Hormones that stimulate the growth of blood cells. *Scientific American* 259(1): 62–70.

Groopman, J., Mitsuyasu, R., DeLeo, M., *et al.* 1987. Effects of recombinant human granulocyte-macrophage-colony-stimulating factor in patients on myelopoiesis in the acquired deficiency syndrome. *New England Journal of Medicine* 317(10): 1545–1552.

Hartmann, L., and Edmonson, J. 1990. Atrial fibrillation during treatment with granulocyte-macrophage colony stimulating factor (GM-CSF). *Proceedings of the American Society of Clinical Oncology* 9: 194 (abstract).

Herrmann, F., Schultz, G., Wieser, M., *et al.* 1990. Effect of GM-CSF in neutropenia and related morbidity induced by myelotoxic chemotherapy. *American Journal of Medicine* 88: 619–624.

Hoelzer, D., Seipelt, G., Ganser, A. 1991. Interleukin–3 alone and in combination with GM-CSF in the treatment of patients with neoplastic disease. *Seminars in Hematology* 28(2 Suppl 2): 17–24.

Huang, E., Nocka, K., Beier, D., *et al.* 1990. The hematopoietic growth factor KL is encoded at the S1 locus and is the ligand of the c-kit receptor, the gene product of the W locus. *Cell* 63(1): 255–233.

Immunex Corporation. 1992. Leukine package insert. Seattle, WA: Immunex Corporation.

Ishibashi, T., Kimura, H., Shikama, Y., *et al.* 1989. Interleukin–6 is a potent thrombopoietic factor *in vivo* in mice. *Blood* 74: 1241–1244.

Jaramilla, J. 1992. Biotechnology overview. *Pharmacology and Therapeutics* 17: 1372–1377.

Kanda, N., Fukushige, S., Murotsu, T., *et al.* 1987. Human gene coding for granulocyte-colony stimulating factor is assigned to the q21–q22 region of chromosome 17. *Somatic Cell and Molecular Genetics* 13(6): 679–684.

Kobayashi, Y., Okabe, T., Urabe, A., *et al.* 1989. Treatment of myelodysplastic syndromes with recombinant human granulocyte colony-stimulating factor: a preliminary report. *American Journal of Medicine* 86(2): 178–181.

Kobayashi, Y., Okabe, T., Urabe, A., *et al.* 1987. Human granulocyte colony-stimulating factor shortens the period of granulocytopenia induced by irradiation in mice. *Japanese Journal of Cancer Research* 78(8): 763–766.

Kodo, H., Tajika, K., Takahashi S., *et al.* 1988. Acceleration of neutrophil granulocyte recovery after bone-marrow transplantation by administration of recombinant human granulocyte colony-stimulating factor. *Lancet* 2(8601): 38–39.

Layton, J., Hockman, J., Sheridan, W., *et al.* 1989. Evidence for a novel *in vivo* control mechanism of granulopoiesis: Mature cell-related control of a regulatory growth factor. *Blood* 74 (4): 1303–1307.

Leary, A., Yang, Y.-C., Clark, S., *et al.* 1987. Recombinant gibbon interleukin–3 supports formation of human multilineage colonies and blast cell colonies in culture: Comparison with recombinant human granulocyte-macrophage colony-stimulating factor. *Blood* 70(5): 1343–1348.

Lindemann, A., and Mertelsmann, R. 1993. Interleukin–3: Structure and function. *Cancer Investigation* 11(5): 609–623.

Logothetis, C., Dexeus, F., Sella, A., *et al.* 1990. Escalated therapy for refractory urothelial tumors: methotrexate-vinblastine-doxorubicin-cisplatin plus unglycosylated recombinant human granulocyte-macrophage colony-stimulating factor. *Journal of the National Cancer Institute* 82(8): 667–672.

McNiece, J., Langley, K., Zsebo, K., *et al.* 1991. Recombinant human stem cell factor synergized with GM-CSF, G-CSF, IL–3 and Epo to stimulate human progenitor cells of the myeloid and erythroid lineages. *Journal of Experimental Hematology* 19(3): 226–231.

Means, R., and Krantz, S. 1991. Erythropoietin in cancer therapy. *Biologic Therapy of Cancer Updates* 1(4): 1–7.

Meropol, N., Miller, L., Korn, E., *et al.* 1992. Severe myelosuppression resulting from concurrent administration of G-CSF and cytotoxic chemotherapy. *Journal of the National Cancer Institute* 84(15): 1201–1203.

Mertelsmann, R., Herrmann, F., Hecht, T., *et al.*, 1990. Hematopoietic growth factors in bone marrow transplantation. *Bone Marrow Transplantation* 6: 73–77.

Metcalf, D. 1980. Clonal analysis of proliferation and differentiation of paired daughter cells; Action of granulocyte-macrophage colony-stimulating factor on granulocyte-macrophage precursors. *Proceedings of the National Academy of Sciences* 77: 5327–5330.

Metcalf, D., Johnson, G., and Burgess, A. 1980. Direct stimulation of purified GM-CSF on the proliferation of multipotential and erythroid precursor cells. *Blood* 55(2): 138–147.

Metcalf, D., Burgess, A., Johnson, G., et al. 1986. *In vitro* actions on hematopoietic cells of recombinant murine GM-CSF purified after production in *Escherichia coli:* Comparison with purified native GM-CSF. *Journal of Cellular Physiology* 128(3): 421–431.

Metcalf, D., and Morstyn, G. 1991. Colony-stimulating factors: General biology. In DeVita, V., Hellman, S., Rosenberg, S. (eds). *Biologic Therapy of Cancer* Philadelphia: J.B. Lippincott, pp. 417–444.

Miles, S., Mitsuyasu, R., and Moreno, J. 1991. Combined therapy with recombinant granulocyte colony-stimulating factor and erythropoietin decreases hematologic toxicity from zidovudine. *Blood* 77(10): 2109–2117.

Miller, L., Smith, J., Urba, W., et al. 1993. A phase I study of an IL–3/GM-CSF fusion protein (PIXY321) and high dose carboplatin (CBCDA) in patients with advanced cancer. *Proceedings of the American Society of Clinical Oncology* 12: 353 (abstract).

Morstyn G., Campbell, L., Lieschke, G., et al. 1989a. Treatment of chemotherapy induced neutropenia by subcutaneously administered granulocyte colony-stimulating factor (G-CSF) with optimization of dose and duration of therapy. *Journal of Clinical Oncology* 7(10): 1554–1562.

Morstyn, G., Lieschke, G., Sheridan, W., et al. 1989b. Clinical experience with recombinant human granulocyte colony-stimulating factor and granulocyte-macrophage colony-stimulating factor. *Seminars in Hematology* 26(2 Suppl 2.): 9–13.

Morstyn, G., Campbell, L., Souza, L., et al. 1988. Effect of G-CSF on neutropenia induced by cytotoxic chemotherapy. *Lancet* 1(8587): 667–672.

Negrin, R., Haueber, D., Nagler, A., et al. 1989. Treatment of myelodysplastic syndrome with recombinant human granulocyte colony stimulating factor: A phase I–II trial. *Annals of Internal Medicine* 110(12): 967–984.

Neidhart, J., Mangalik, A., Kohler, W., et al. 1989. Granulocyte colony-stimulating factor stimulates recovery of granulocytes in patients receiving dose-intensive chemotherapy without bone marrow transplantation. *Journal of Clinical Oncology* 7(11): 1685–1692.

Nemunaitis, J., Meyers, J., Buckner, C., et al. 1993. Phase I/II trial of recombinant human macrophage colony-stimulating factor (M-CSF) in patients with invasive fungal infection. *Proceedings of the American Society of Clinical Oncology* 12: 159 (abstract).

Nemunaitis, J., Meyers, J., Buckner, C., et al. 1990a. Phase I/II trial of recombinant macrophage colony stimulating factor (M-CSF) in patients with invasive fungal infection. *Blood* 76(10 Suppl 1): 159a.

Nemunaitis, J., Singer, J., Buckner, C., et al. 1990b. Use of recombinant human granulocyte-macrophage colony-stimulating factor in graft failure after bone marrow transplantation. *Blood* 76(1): 245–253.

Nemunaitis, J., Singer, J., Buckner, C., et al. 1988a. Use of recombinant human granulocyte-macrophage colony-stimulating factor in autologous marrow transplantation for lymphoid malignancies. *Blood* 72(2): 834–836.

Nemunaitis, J., Singer, J., Buckner, C., et al., 1988b. The use of rHuGM-CSF for graft failure in patients after autologous, allogeneic, or syngeneic bone marrow transplantation (BMT). *Blood* 72(Suppl 1): 398a (abstract #1503).

Nicola, N. 1989. Hemopoietic cell growth factors and their receptors. *Annual Review of Biochemistry* 58: 5–77.

Ohno, R., Tomonoaga, M., and Kogayashi, T. 1990. Effect of G-CSF after intensive induction therapy in relapsed or refractory acute leukemia. *New England Journal of Medicine* 323(13): 871–877.

Park, L., Friend, D., Price, V., et al. 1989a. Heterogeneity in human interleukin–3 receptors. A subclass that binds human GM-CSF. *Journal of Biological Chemistry* 264(10): 5420–5427.

Park, L., Waldron, P., Friend, D, et al. 1989b. Interleukin–3, GM-CSF and G-CSF receptor expression on cell lines and primary leukemia cells: Receptor heterogeneity and relationship to growth factor responsiveness. *Blood* 74(1): 56–65.

Platanias, L., Miller, C., Mick, R., et al. 1991. Treatment of chemotherapy-induced anemia with recombinant human erythropoietin in cancer patients. *Journal of Clinical Oncology* 9(11): 2021–2026.

Reptis, G., Gilewski, T., Gabrilove, J., et al. 1993. Evaluation of PIXY321 (PIXY) as a myeloprotective agent in patients (pts) with metastatic breast cancer receiving doxorubicin and thiotepa. *Proceedings of the American Society of Clinical Oncology* 12: 235 (abstract).

Sheridan, W., Juttner, C., Szer, J., et al. 1990. Granulocyte colony-stimulating factor (G-CSF) in peripheral blood stem cell (PBSC) and bone marrow (BM) transplantation. *Blood* 76(5 Suppl 1): 565a (abstract).

Sheridan, W., Morstyn, G., Wolf, M., et al. 1989. Granulocyte colony-stimulating factor and neutrophil recovery after high-dose chemotherapy and bone marrow transplantation. *Lancet* 2(8668): 891–895.

Sieff, C., Niemeyer, C., Nathan, D., et al. 1987. Stimulation of human hematopoietic colony formation by recombinant gibbon multi-CSF or IL–3. *Journal of Clinical Investigation* 80(3): 818–823.

Simmers, R., Webber, L., Shannon, M., et al. 1987. Localization of the G-CSF gene on chromosome 17 proximal to the breakpoint in the t(15;17) in acute promyelocytic leukemia. *Blood* 70(1): 330–332.

Singer, J. 1992. Role of colony-stimulating factors in bone marrow transplantation. *Seminars in Oncology* 19(3 Suppl): 27–31.

Singer, J., Nemunaitis, J., Bianco, J., et al., 1990. RhGM-CSF following allogeneic bone marrow transplantation from unrelated marrow donors: A phase II study. *Blood* 76(Suppl): 566a (abstract).

Spivak, J. 1989. Erythropoietin. *Blood Reviews* 3(20): 130–135.

Stoudemire, J., and Garnick, M. 1991. Effects of recombinant human macrophage colony-stimulating factor on plasma cholesterol levels. *Blood* 77(4): 750–755.

Taylor, K., Jagannath, S., Spitzer, G., *et al.* 1989. Recombinant human granulocyte colony-stimulating factor hastens granulocyte recovery after high-dose chemotherapy and autologous bone marrow transplantation in Hodgkin's disease. *Journal of Clinical Oncology* 7(12): 1791–1799.

Thompson, J., Lee, D., Kidd, P., *et al.* 1989. Subcutaneous granulocyte-macrophage colony-stimulating factor in patients with myelodysplastic syndrome: Toxicity, pharmacokinetics and hematological effects. *Journal of Clinical Oncology* 7(5): 629–637.

To, L., Dyson, P., Branford, A., *et al.* 1987. Peripheral blood stem cells collected in very early remission produce rapid and sustained autologous hematopoietic reconstitution in acute non-lymphoblastic leukaemia. *Bone Marrow Transplantation* 2(1): 103–108.

Traynor, B. 1992. The cytokine network. In International Society of Nurses in Cancer Care (ed). *Proceedings of the 7th International Conference on Cancer Nursing* Vienna, Austria August 1992, pp. 6–10.

Vadhan-Raj, S., Papadoupoulos, N., Burgess, M., *et al.* 1994. Effects of PIXY321, a granulocyte-macrophage colony-stimulating factor/interleukin–3 fusion protein, on chemotherapy-induced multilineage myelosuppression in patients with sarcoma. *Journal of Clinical Oncology* 12(4): 715–724.

Vadhan-Raj, S., Broxmeyer, H., Hittelman, W., *et al.*, 1992. Abrogating chemotherapy-induced myelosuppression by recombinant granulocyte-macrophage colony-stimulating factor in patients with sarcoma: Protection at the progenitor cell level. *Journal of Clinical Oncology* 10(8): 1266–1277.

Vadhan-Raj, S., Keating, M., LeMaistre, A., *et al.* 1987. Effects of recombinant human granulocyte-macrophage colony-stimulating factor in patients with myelodysplastic syndrome. *New England Journal of Medicine* 17(25): 1545–1552.

van Leeuwen B., Martinson M., Webb, G., *et al.* 1989. Molecular organization of the cytokine gene cluster, involving the human IL–3, IL–4, IL–5, and GM-CSF genes, on chromosome 5. *Blood* 73(5): 1142–1148.

Watari, K., Asano, S., Shirafuji, N., *et al.* 1989. Serum granulocyte colony-stimulating factor levels in healthy volunteers and various disorders estimated by enzyme immunoassay. *Blood* 73(1): 117–122.

Weiner, L., Li, W., Catalano, R., *et al.* 1993. Phase I trial of recombinant macrophage colony-stimulating factor (M-CSF) and recombinant gamma-interferon (γ-IFN): Peripheral blood mononuclear phagocyte proliferation and differentiation. *Proceedings of the American Society of Clinical Oncology* 12: 291 (abstract 947).

Welte, K., Bonilla, M., Gillio, A., *et al.* 1987. Recombinant human granulocyte colony-stimulating factor. Effects on hematopoiesis in normal and cyclophosphamide-treated primates. *Journal of Experimental Medicine* 165(4): 941–948.

Williams, D., Broxmeier, H., Curtis, B., *et al.* 1990a. Enhanced biological activity of a human GM-CSF/IL–3 fusion protein. *Experimental Hematology* 18(2): 256a (abstract).

Williams, D., Eisenman, J., Baird, A., *et al.* 1990b. Identification of a ligand for the c-kit proto-oncogene. *Cell* 63(1): 167–174.

Williams, M., and Quesenberry, P. 1992. Hematopoietic Growth Factors. *Hematologic Pathology* 6(3): 105–124.

Wimperis, J., Niemeyer, C., Sieff, C., *et al.* 1989. Granulocyte-macrophage colony-stimulating factor and interleukin–3 mRNAs are produced by a small fraction of blood mononuclear cells. *Blood* 74(5): 1525–1530.

Wujcik, D. 1992. Overview of colony-stimulating factors: Focus on the neutrophil. In Carroll-Johnson, R. (ed). *A Case Management Approach to Patients Receiving G-CSF* Pittsburgh, PA: Oncology Nursing Society, pp. 8–11.

Yang, Y.-C., Kovacic, S., Kriz, R., *et al.* 1988. The human genes for GM-CSF and IL-3 are closely linked in tandem on chromosome 5. *Blood* 71(4): 958–961.

Zsebo, K., Wypych, J., McNiece, I., *et al.* 1990. Identification, purification, and biological characterization of hematopoietic stem cell factor from Buffalo rat liver-conditioned medium. *Cell* 63(1): 195–201.

CHAPTER 7 | Monoclonal Antibodies

Janet E. DiJulio, RN, MSN
Tina Marie Liles, RN, BSN

Antibodies are naturally occurring proteins that are elicited in response to foreign antigens to protect the host. The immune system is able to develop antibodies that are unique to any antigen encountered by the host. The theory that **passive antibody therapy** could be used for controlling and eradicating tumors has been speculated on for decades, but testing this theory has been fraught with problems. Early studies of passive antibody therapy used heterologous antisera that were either obtained from animals or humans immunized with whole tumor cells or cell extracts. Unfortunately, immunization in this fashion resulted in a mixture of antibodies **(polyclonal),** many of which were not specific for tumor antigens. Not surprisingly, early attempts at passive immunotherapy showed little promise (Rosenberg and Terry, 1977).

In the mid-1970s, Nobel prize winners Köhler and Milstein (1975) developed a technique to fuse mouse antibody-producing cells with a myeloma cell line; resulting in an "immortal" hybrid cell that produced a single antibody recognizing a single antigen. This **hybridoma** technique made it possible to produce unlimited amounts of pure monoclonal antibody (MAB) which varied little from batch to batch and were highly specific for a single **antigenic determinant** (Benjamini and Leskowitz, 1988). Because of this discovery, researchers can now develop MABs from a variety of sources to essentially any antigen they choose, but the primary source is the mouse (Lotze and Rosenberg, 1988).

The search for tumor-specific antigens to use as targets for the antibodies however has proved troublesome. Most of the monoclonal antibodies tailored to specific tumors have been targeted to **oncofetal antigens** or **differentiation antigens**, proteins that are present on all cells, but in higher concentrations on malignant cells (Lotze and Rosenberg, 1988). An exception is in B-cell lymphomas. Because this tumor arises from an antibody producing cell, the immunoglobulin produced by this cell line is usually present on the cell surface. The binding region unique for each immunoglobulin, or **idiotype**, can be used as a specific target for the antibody. In essence, the idiotype is a truly "tumor specific" antigen since it is unique to each B cell tumor (Maloney et al., 1992b). Molecular biologists have also identified cell surface receptors that are products of cellular oncogenes and several of these receptors are for growth factors including platelet derived growth factor and epidermal growth factor. These receptor sites have been used as targets for antibodies (LoBuglio and Saleh, 1992).

The naming of MABs may cause confusion to health professionals if they have not been involved with the early clinical trials of these products. Often, the naming of the antibody relates to the antigen for which it is targeted, the specific clone from which it originated, or the corporation that developed it. Frequently this consists of only numbers and letters. It is helpful to remember that there are at least five different types of tumor associated antigens against which MABs may be targeted. These include oncofetal antigens, differentiation antigens, tissue-specific antigens, growth factor receptors, oncogene products and idiotypes (Schlom, 1991).

MABs are used now in the diagnosis of many diseases including autoimmune disease, cancer, and myocardial infarction. They are also used in the treatment of cell-mediated rejection in organ transplant patients and in the treatment of gram negative sepsis with an antibody targeted against bacterial endotoxin. This chapter will cover the technology of manufacturing antibodies and the multiple uses for MABs in the diagnosis and treatment of malignancies and other selected diseases. Clinical trials of MABs conjugated to drugs, toxins, and isotopes will be reviewed and common toxicities involved in the use of these therapies will be discussed. How these biologicals differ from other drugs in the FDA approval process will be identified. Finally, the obstacles to successful treatment and future directions for the use of this unique biological therapy will be presented.

HYBRIDOMA TECHNOLOGY

Köhler and Milstein (1975) were able to capitalize on the properties of two different murine cell populations, antibody-forming B lymphocytes and malignant plasma cells. If one attempts to develop a specific antibody by immunizing a mouse and harvesting the antibody-forming lymphocytes, the cells can be maintained in culture for only a very short time, and the antibody yield is low. If, on the other hand, that cell line is fused with a malignant plasma cell that is a poor antibody producer but possesses the malignant property of immortality, the cell culture can be maintained for years. Figure 7.1 is a schematic representation of Köhler and Milstein's hybridoma technology. The mouse is first immunized with the desired antigen and an antibody response is allowed to develop. The mouse's spleen is harvested and the lymphocytes from the spleen are placed in solution with myeloma cells selected from a culture that is deficient in the enzyme hypoxanthine phosphoribosyl transferase (HPRT). Because myeloma cells need this enzyme to survive, they fuse with the mouse lymphocytes which contain this necessary enzyme and the desired antibody. Successfully fused cells are selected and grown in a medium containing hypoxanthine, aminopterin and thymidine (HAT). Any surviving enzyme-deficient (unfused) malignant cells will die in this culture medium. The selected cells are assayed for antibody production, and only those cells that are producing antibody are cloned. These cells constitute the hybridoma. At this point several options are available. The hybridoma may be frozen for future use, or grown in mass cultures and used to produce large quantities of antibody. Alternatively, a myeloma tumor may be induced in the mouse that will produce antibodies in ascitic fluid (Benjamini and Leskowitz, 1988; Köhler and Milstein, 1975).

Figure 7.1   Schematic representation of hybridoma technique for the production of monoclonal antibodies. The mouse is immunized with the desired antigen and an antibody response is allowed to develop. The mouse's spleen is harvested and the lymphocytes from the spleen are placed in solution with myeloma cells from a culture that is deficient in the enzyme hypoxanthine phosphoribosyl transferase (HPRT). Only the fused cells will survive in the HAT media. Assay for antibody production is done and those cells producing antibody are cloned. The hybridoma may be frozen for future use, it may be grown in mass culture, or it may be used to induce a tumor in the mouse that results in antibody production.

HYBRIDOMA TECHNOLOGY

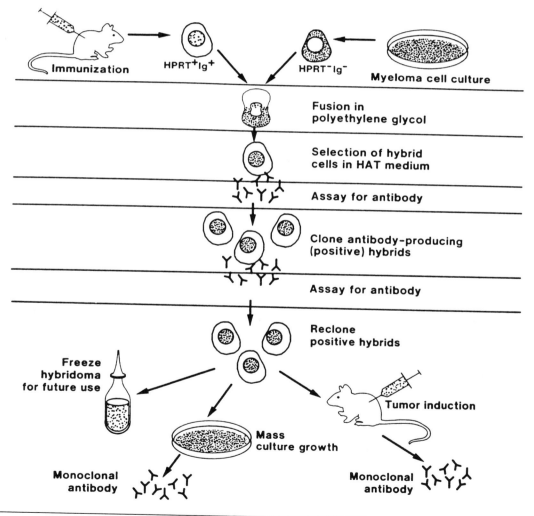

Source: Reprinted with permission from DiJulio, J. 1988. Treatment of B-cell and T-cell lymphomas with monoclonal antibodies. *Seminars in Oncology Nursing,* 4: 103.

More recently, molecular techniques have been developed to speed up the production of the antibody. The first part of the process is identical to that shown in Figure 7.1, but instead of culturing the hybridomas, a technology called **polymerase chain reaction (PCR)** is used to amplify the specific genes that code for the variable region of the mouse antibody. The two strands of DNA are separated, and the separated strands serve as a template for building a complementary strand of DNA. Continuous repetitions of the process allow production of more than two million copies of the desired gene in a matter of hours (Overmyer, 1990; Cooper and Flaum, 1988).

BIOLOGICAL ACTIONS

Native MABs, those that are not bound to drugs, toxins, or isotopes, have been used to treat human malignancies since 1981. Tumors treated with MABs include the B-cell lymphomas, chronic lymphocytic leukemia, cutaneous T-cell lymphoma, acute lymphocytic leukemia, neuroblastoma, lung malignancies, gastrointestinal malignancies (including colon), and melanoma (Houghton *et al.*, 1991; Levy and Miller, 1991; Mulshine *et al.*, 1991; Waldman, 1991). How the antibody alone kills tumor cells requires a discussion of structure and function of antibodies. The antibody consists of four polypeptide chains, two heavy and two light . Each chain is made up of a constant region and a variable region. It is the variable region that gives the antibody its uniqueness and the potential to react with an infinite number of different antigens.

The antibody structure can be separated by enzymatic treatment into three fragments. Two of the fragments retain the antibody's ability to bind antigen and are referred to as **Fab (fragment antigen binding)**. The third fragment is called **Fc (fragment crystallization)** because it can be crystallized out of solution. The Fc cannot bind antigens but is responsible for the biological functions of the molecule once the antigen has been bound to the Fab of the intact molecule (Benjamini and

Leskowitz, 1988). See Figure 7.2 for a schematic diagram of an antibody.

Two mechanisms have been identified that may trigger antibody tumor cell destruction. The first is via activation of the complement cascade, the second is **antibody-dependent cell-mediated cytotoxicity.** Some classes of antibody have the ability to firmly fix the complement subcomponent **C1q.** Once this protein is bound, the antibody-C1q complexes may trigger phagocytosis of the tumor cells via the host's reticuloendothelial system. A bond between the antibody and C1q also induces the remaining steps in the complement cascade, which causes cell lysis by disruption of the cell membrane. The Fc portion of the antibody may mediate recruitment of effector cells by binding to the malignant cell. Antibody-dependent cell-mediated cytotoxicity occurs when the Fc portion of antibody-coated cells joins by specific receptors with the host's effector cells. The cellular components include natural killer cells, killer T cells, and macrophages. Antibody-coated cells are engulfed by the phagocytic cells in the reticuloendothelial system (Benjamini and Leskowitz, 1988; Lotze and Rosenberg, 1988). Different antibody classes mediate the complement cascade. For example, IgM appears to be a better activator of complement than IgG^2a or IgG^2b (Lotze and Rosenberg, 1988).

For the antibody to locate and destroy the tumor, several critical factors must come into play. First, it is important that the antibody does not have cross-reactivity with normal tissue, and that the surface membrane antigens on the tumor are distributed in high density. The antibody should possess a high affinity for the antigen target and the antigen should remain on the surface of the tumor providing a specific target for the antibody. Optimally, there should be little circulating antigen to react with the antibody before it reaches the tumor. It is also important that the tumor be highly vascularized so that the antibody can be delivered to the site. Tumor size and tumor burden also must be considered, because there may be more volume than the dose or

Figure 7.2   Schematic diagram of an immunoglobulin molecule. The antigen-binding sites are formed by the juxtaposition of the VL and VH domains. The locations of complement and Fc receptor-binding sites within the heavy chain constant regions are approximations. S--S refers to intrachain and interchain disulfide bonds; N and C refer to amino and carboxy termini of the polypeptide chains.

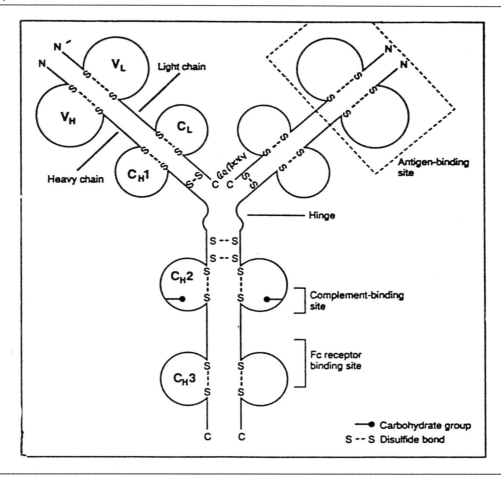

Source: Reprinted with permission from Abbas, A., Lichtman, M., and Prober, J. 1991. Antibodies and antigens. In *Cellular and Molecular Immunology.* Philadelphia: Saunders, p. 51.

doses of antibody can handle. A related problem in using monoclonal antibody therapy is that of human antiglobulin response. Since the MAB is derived from the mouse, individuals who are immunocompetent may develop a **human anti-mouse antibody (HAMA)** response. Once this occurs, the anti-tumor response may be negated. There is concern that with continued use of the MAB, immune complexes could form resulting in rapid clearance and possible tissue damage. These problems will be addressed in detail later in the chapter.

CLINICAL STUDIES

Unconjugated Antibodies

Hematologic Malignancies

The majority of studies with unconjugated MAB have occurred in patients with leukemia or lymphoma. The surface antigen T–65, present on mature T lymphocytes and on certain subsets of T and B malignancies, has been studied in several therapeutic trials. Patients with T-cell lymphoma, T-cell leukemia, and chronic lymphocytic leukemia (a B-cell malignancy) received antibodies directed against the surface antigen T–65 (Dillman et al., 1985; Foon et al., 1983; Miller et al., 1983; Dillman et al., 1982; Foon et al., 1982). Although clinical responses varied, there was transient clearing of cells in patients with chronic B-cell lymphocytic leukemia (Lowder et al., 1985). Observable tumor responses also occurred in the patients with T-cell lymphoma. Responses lasted from 1.4 to 4 months, but many of the responses were interrupted by the development of human anti-mouse antibody (HAMA) (Lowder et al., 1985).

In B-cell malignancies, the immunoglobulin produced by the tumor provides an ideal tumor marker. The antibody binding site, also called the idiotype, serves as a tumor specific marker on the surface of the B-cell. Taking advantage of the unique nature of these malignancies, investigators have developed MABs against the variable region or idiotype. These antibodies are called **anti-idiotypes.** Miller et al. (1982) reported the first study with a "tailor made" antibody for each patient. These "private" antibodies have been studied extensively in vivo (Maloney et al., 1992b). Brown et al. (1989b) reported on 16 evaluable patients, 15 of whom had low-grade lymphoma and 1 of whom had prolymphocytic leukemia. Three patients converted to intermediate- or high-grade lymphoma by the time of treatment. Thirteen of the 16 had been treated with chemotherapy. Table 7.1 summarizes the responses of these patients. In this first trial the 16 patients were treated with antibody tailored to their specific idiotype.

They received between 400 and 1600 mg of antibody. A continuation of this work by Maloney et al. (1992b) shows two patients who have had durable complete remissions now continuing over 62 months. Patient 1 had an initial complete response that lasted 72 months. A localized recurrence that developed in a lower extremity remained idiotype positive. The site was treated with local radiation and the remission has continued for another 3.5 years. The second patient remains in complete remission more than 5 years following therapy. Six patients had a partial remission ranging from 1 to 12 months, and 2 patients had minor responses of short duration. The remaining 6 patients had no response. Interestingly, despite the presence of disease, these patients did not require immediate therapy. In one case therapy was not required for 20 months. These studies established that anti-idiotype antibodies are active therapeutic agents in both heavily treated patients and patients who have progressed to higher grade lymphomas.

Shared Anti-Idiotype Antibodies (SIDs) Because an anti-idiotype MAB has to be custom made for each patient, both the time factor for developing the antibody and the expense are major drawbacks. Fortunately, researchers found that it is possible to identify **shared idiotypes (SIDs)** that are reactive to lymphoma cells from more than one patient (Maloney et al., 1992b; Miller et al., 1989). IDEC Pharmaceutical Corporation (San Diego, CA) has now produced 15 anti-idiotype antibodies that react with the tumors of 20% of the patients with B-cell lymphoma (Maloney et al., 1992b). The ability to use SIDs overcomes many of the problems with private anti-idiotypes. They are available for immediate use and may be used to treat many different patients. Clinical trials evaluating therapeutic efficacy have been conducted in patients with both relapsed lymphoma and untreated low-grade lymphoma with the goal of determining therapeutic efficacy and improving clinical responses. To date, 18 patients have been

Table 7.1

Antibody Trial	Patient	Clinical Responses	Freedom from Progression (months)	Time to Next Therapy (months)
Monoclonal anti-idiotype antibody alone	PK	CR	72	80
	CC	CR	62+	62+
	KC	PR	12	24
	JC (2)	PR	6	6
	RD	PR	5	7
	PE	PR	4	8
	EL (2)	PR	10	15
	CJ	PR	1	3
	CG	MR	3	14
	BJ	MR	1	1
	EL (1)	NR	0	1
	CP	NR	0	20
	TG	NR	0	1
	JC (1)	NR	0	8
	EW	NR	0	4
	BL	NR	0	3
Monoclonal anti-idiotype antibody and alpha-interferon	BL (2)	CR	61+	61+
	BR (2)	CR	58+	58+
	DT	CR	61+	61+
	MW	PR	9	10
	BE (1)	PR	7	7
	RW (1)	PR	5	8
	BR (1)	PR	3	5
	PC	PR	3	6
	JC (3)	PR	2	5
	RT	MR	6	11
	KB	MR	5	35
	RV	NR	0	3
Monoclonal anti-idiotype antibody and pulse chlorambucil	RB	CR	31	52+
	CD	PR	14	16
	AI	PR	12	27+
	RCS	PR	7	12
	KG	PR	5	12
	BE (2)	PR	5	6
	RS	PR	4	4
	LV	PR	4	6
	RW (2)	PR	3	4
	ID	MR	7	21
	RF	MR/SD	6	18
	TL	NR	3	3
	SG	NR	1	4

Source: Reprinted with permission from Maloney, D., Levy, R., and Miller, R. 1992. Monoclonal anti-idiotype therapy of B-cell lymphoma. In DeVita, V., Hellman, S., and Rosenberg, S. (eds.). *Biologic Therapy of Cancer Updates.* 2(6). Philadelphia: J.B. Lippincott, 1992, pp.1–10.

treated at Stanford University Medical Center in Palo Alto. Responses have included 1 complete remission, 3 partial remissions, and 2 minor responses with varying duration, the longest remission lasting 36 months (Maloney et al., 1992b).

Unlike the responses to chemotherapy or radiotherapy, the onset of response with MAB therapy in the B-cell lymphoma trials is generally one to two months following therapy, although some patients can exhibit regression many months following therapy (Maloney et al., 1992b). This suggests that the treatment induced an immune response in the patient against the tumor. In a summary of the anti-idiotype trials there has been an overall complete response rate of 18% and a 50% partial remission rate. It appears that if patients can enter a complete remission, they will remain disease free for an extended period of time (Maloney et al., in press).

Solid Tumors
Monoclonal antibodies have also been studied in the treatment of solid tumors with the focus being primarily on colorectal carcinoma and malignant melanoma (LoBuglio and Saleh, 1992). The antibody 17–1A is directed against a surface antigen present on gastrointestinal and other adenocarcinomas. LoBuglio and Saleh summarized four studies where over one hundred patients collectively with colorectal carcinoma were treated with 17–1A. The overall response rate was approximately 5% (Saleh et al., 1990; Khazaeli et al., 1988; LoBuglio et al., 1988; Sears et al., 1982). Monoclonal antibody therapy of malignant melanoma has been attempted with a variety of antibodies. Partial responses have been reported with the use of R24, Me36.1, 3F8, 14G2a and human L7 (Murray et al., 1994; Bajorin et al., 1992; Licten et al., 1988; Vadhan-Raj et al., 1988; Irie and Morton, 1986; Cheung et al., 1987).

Although the treatments are usually well tolerated, several obstacles to treatment exist. Human immune responses are frequent (HAMA) and tumor-cell kill is limited despite the presence of the antibody at the tumor site.

When responses are obtained, they are generally not of a lasting duration.

Bone Marrow Purging
Monoclonal antibodies have been used in vitro to perform immunologic purging of bone marrow following high-dose ablative therapy. Once purged, the marrow is then used for autologous bone marrow transplantation. The use of this technique in the management of advanced cancers is increasing, but the tumor groups in which the technique has been studied include primarily the leukemias and lymphomas (Gribben et al., 1991; Ball et al., 1990; Freedman et al., 1990). Gribben et al. attempted to determine whether the removal of residual tumor cells from the bone marrow prolongs disease-free survival. It is frequently difficult to determine whether occult lymphoma cells remain in the marrow after purging. These investigators use PCR to detect the 14:18 chromosome translocation observed in 85% of follicular lymphomas and 30% of diffuse lymphomas. This method is sensitive enough to detect one lymphoma cell in one million normal cells. In their study, Gribben et al. purged bone marrow ex vivo with a cocktail of three B-cell antibodies. Rabbit complement was added to enhance tumor cell destruction. Residual lymphoma cells were detected by PCR in the bone marrow of all of the patients prior to immunologic purging. Following the purging, no lymphoma cells were detected in 57 of the 114 treated patients. Disease-free survival was significantly longer ($p < 0.00001$) in these patients than in the patients whose marrow still had detectable lymphoma cells after treatment (Gribben et al., 1991).

Negrin et al. (1991) confirmed the usefulness of PCR in detecting minimal residual disease before and after bone marrow purging. In an ex vivo study they used mixtures of either 4 B-cell antibodies or 8 T-cell antibodies combined with rabbit complement. They also noted an increased efficacy of purging with monoclonal antibodies.

Press et al. (1989) purged autologous bone marrow with the MAB anti-CD20 1F5 and complement prior to treatment with I^{131} radiolabeled antibody in a trial of refractory non-Hodgkin's lymphoma. The purged marrow is cryopreserved and held for potential reinfusion. Of the five patients treated in this study thus far, 2 have required reinfusion of their marrow for severe bone marrow toxicity. The investigators anticipate that more patients will require rescue with the purged marrow as the dose of I^{131} escalates. In a current trial of radiolabeled antibodies at Stanford University Medical Center, harvested bone marrow is treated with a mixture of four antibodies and complement.

Combination Therapy

Because the most encouraging results and the most extensive testing so far has involved non-Hodgkin's lymphoma and anti-idiotype antibody therapy, the next generation of clinical trials has involved combining MABs with other cytotoxic agents and biological agents. As previously discussed, the private anti-idiotype antibodies have produced favorable responses in a small subset of patients, irrespective of prior treatment or histology. Building on these trials, Brown *et al.* (1989a) studied the effect of interferon-alpha in combination with private anti-idiotype antibodies. Interferon-alpha was chosen because of its independent tumor activity and its synergistic effect in combination with monoclonal anti-idiotype antibodies (Basham *et al.*, 1986). The addition of interferon was an attempt to overcome idiotype-negative variance of tumor cells that had been observed in their earlier trial. In that trial, tumor cells were present that did not contain the idiotype protein on their surface and thus rendered them invisible as targets for the antibody. Twelve patients received antibody doses ranging from 1.6 g to 8.4 g. Interferon-alpha was administered intramuscularly at a dose of 12 MIU before antibody infusion and subsequently 3 times per week for a total of 8 weeks. Of the 12 patients treated, 3 experienced complete remissions, all of which have now lasted longer

than 61 months. Partial remissions, with a shorter duration (up to 9 months), were noted in 6 patients. Two minor responses lasted 6 months. Only 1 patient had no response to treatment. Investigators were able to conclude that with the addition of interferon-alpha, significant anti-tumor effects were observed. However, idiotype-negative variance was still a problem (Brown *et al.*, 1989a). Table 7.1 provides a summary of patients treated in this study.

Further studies have tested the combination of pulse-dose chlorambucil with anti-idiotype antibodies (Maloney *et al.*, 1992a). The addition of the alkylating agent, chlorambucil, was chosen to overcome the emergence of idiotype negative cells. Chlorambucil is an active agent in the treatment of lymphoma and it was thought that if the idiotype negative cells were proliferating at a more rapid rate, they would be more susceptible to a cell cycle specific agent. Patients received 2 courses of anti-idiotype therapy. Concurrent with the second course patients received a 5-day pulse of chlorambucil. Antibody doses ranged from 3.4 g to 11.4 g. Thirteen patients were treated: 1 had a complete remission, 8 had a partial remission, 2 had a minor response, and 2 were without a response. The patient in complete remission has remained so for over 52 months. Again, the durations of partial remission were variable: they ranged from 4 to 27 months. This trial also failed to prevent the emergence of idiotype-negative cells. Maloney *et al.* (1992a) were not surprised by this finding, since tumor cell analysis revealed that the idiotype-negative tumor cells did not have an increased rate of proliferation. Table 7.1 provides a summary of patients treated in this study.

The antitumor effects of interleukin–2 (IL–2) have also been tested in combination with anti-idiotype antibodies. Because this trial is not yet complete, only the rationale behind the use of this combination therapy will be discussed. IL–2 is a lymphokine produced by activated helper T cells and has a role in activating different cells of the immune system. In a murine model, Berinstein and Levy (1987) demonstrated synergy between IL–2 and anti-idiotype antibodies. They showed that IL–2 increased the cellular response of T cells and natural killer cells. Furthermore, they showed an antitumor effect associated with antibody-dependent cell mediated cytotoxicity. In a follow-up study, Berinstein *et al.* (1988) showed that IL–2 potentiated antibody-directed tumor lysis. The treatment was powerful enough to reduce tumor size and even cure some established tumors.

MABs have also been combined with chemotherapy and biological agents in solid tumors such as melanoma. Interleukin–2 has been combined with MABs in an attempt to augment ADCC mediated by antibodies. Interferon-alpha can modulate the expression of cell surface antigens, thus enhancing tumor targeting by the MAB. Other trials have evaluated antimelanoma MABs in combination with chemotherapy, such as dacarbazine, known to be effective in treating melanoma. Thus far, these combination trials remain at an early stage with only a few minor or partial responses seen (Houghton *et al.*, 1991).

Conjugate Technology

In an attempt to utilize the unique targeting properties of MABs, investigators have coupled antibodies with therapeutic agents such as alpha-, beta-, and gamma-emitting radionuclides; with protein toxins such as ricin, pseudomonas, and diphtheria; and with chemotherapeutic drugs such as doxorubicin and methotrexate (Lotze and Rosenberg, 1988; Redwood *et al.*, 1984; Pimm *et al.*, 1982; Thorpe and Ross, 1982; Vitetta *et al.*, 1982; Houston and Nowinski, 1981). These agents, known as **immunoconjugates**, are frequently viewed as "magic bullets" and are currently undergoing clinical trials. Advantages of the use of radioisotopes for immunoconjugates are that they radiate beyond a single cell and generally do not require internalization by the target cell. There are numerous radioisotopes that can be used in this fashion. Toxins make an excellent

choice for conjugates in that they are extremely potent and have well-defined chemistry. Antineoplastic drugs have a proven record in cancer therapy, their toxicity and maximum tolerated dose are well known. A primary disadvantage of immunoconjugates thus far has been in stability of the binding between the **conjugate** and the antibody. This is particularly troublesome when using toxins because damage to normal tissue can occur if the toxin is freed prior to reaching the tumor site. Both toxins and drugs must be internalized by the cell to cause cell death (Vitetta and Thorpe, 1991).

Isotope Immunoconjugates

Radioimmunodetection Conjugates of monoclonal antibodies with isotopes have been developed both as a treatment modality and as a method of imaging tumors. Use of these antibodies in imaging has proven useful in such solid tumors as melanoma; lymphomas; and tumors of the lung, ovaries, and breast. The term most commonly associated with this technique is **radioimmunodetection (RAID)**. Since the ideal tumor antigen has not yet been identified, the RAID technique utilizes markers that are quantitatively increased in malignancies. The first group of immunoconjugates included polyclonal and monoclonal antibodies against oncofetal antigens, carcinoembryonic antigen (CEA) (Goldenberg, 1978; Goldenberg *et al.*, 1978; Gold and Freedman, 1965) found in gastrointestinal and other diverse malignancies, and alpha-fetoprotein (AFP) found in germ cell and hepatocellular carcinomas (Goldenberg *et al.*, 1987; Goldenberg *et al.*, 1980a). Another antigen that proved useful for imaging was human chorionic gonadotropin (HCG) in germ cell and trophoblastic tumors (Goldenberg *et al.*, 1981; Goldenberg *et al.*, 1980b). The number of available MABs targeted to cell surface antigens has grown over the past decade.

The optimal radioisotopes used with antibodies are chosen on the basis of their high photon energy, with the desired level between

100 and 200 keV; minimal particulate radiation to maximize safety; adequate half-life; low expense, and availability. The 5 principle isotopes now in use include indium–111 (^{111}In), iodine–131 (^{131}I), iodine–123 (^{123}I), technetium–99m (^{99m}Tc) and Yttrium-90 (Goldenberg and Larson, 1992). Currently only 1 radiolabeled imaging agent has been approved by the Food and Drug Administration, OncoScint® CR/Ov-In, or ^{111}In-labeled satumomab pendetide (Hoppszallern, 1993). This agent is used for determining the extent and location of extrahepatic malignant disease in patients with a diagnosis of colon or ovarian carcinoma. It is not indicated as a screening test for either of these malignancies.

In an attempt to overcome problems with the development of HAMA, investigators have developed human immunoglobulins that do not elicit a significant human anti-human antibody response (HAHA). An example of a human immunoglobulin (IgG class) labeled with TEchnetium-99 is 88BV59, which targets an intracellular tumor associated antigen termed CTA. Early trials with this antibody in 36 patients with colorectal carcinoma showed that the radiolabeled antibody was more sensitive than CT scan in detecting abdominal and pelvic tumors ($p<0.05$). The authors state that the absence or weak immunogenicity of this antibody make it a good candidate for radioimmunodetection and radioimmunotherapy (DeJagar et al., 1993).

Radiotherapy The historical basis of using radionuclides for therapy of malignancies has been well established by the use of phosphorus–32 and iodine–131. The next step in this therapy is to link the radionuclides with MABs to deliver a lethal dose to the tumor site. The lymphomas are an ideal group of malignancies to study radiolabeled antibodies because they are radiosensitive and MABs with relative specificity for these tumors already exist. In studies of non-Hodgkin's lymphomas and Hodgkin's disease, investigators have shown that these tumors respond to radioimmunoconjugates (Press et al., 1989; De-

Nardo et al, 1987; Rosen et al., 1987). Bone marrow toxicity is the most significant problem, however an approach used to circumventing this toxicity is to harvest autologous bone marrow prior to treatment and reinfuse it if necessary (Press et al., 1989).

When using radioimmunoconjugates, there are several critical issues in the application of radioimmunoconjugates that must be addressed. First is the biodistribution of the radiolabeled antibody. Since the antibody is usually cleared by the liver, it is imperative that the dosage not cause liver toxicity and damage. Second, stability of radioimmuno-conjugates in vivo has been a problem. Occasionally, the MAB and the radionuclide separate before reaching the intended target (Eary et al., 1990). This has been especially true for radioiodine which is readily cleaved from the antibody. Third is the ability of the MAB to reach the intended target. Despite the specificity of MABs, only a small fraction of the radiolabeled antibody reaches the tumor. Fourth, the antibody must be freshly labeled and exposure to radiation controlled, making it inconvenient to use in an outpatient treatment setting and potentially hazardous for the health care worker (Larson et al., 1991).

The radioisotope most frequently used in phase I trials has been iodine–131. Its antitumor activity has been demonstrated in lymphoma with the ^{131}I-labeled antibody Lym–1 (DeNardo et al., 1987) and with ^{131}I-labeled LL2 (EPB–2) (Goldenberg et al., 1991). The antimelanoma antibody 96.5 labeled with ^{131}I had limited clinical effect although good tumor localization was achieved (Larson et al., 1983). Ovarian tumors treated with intraperitoneal ^{131}I-labeled HMGF1 (antibody targeted to epithelial tumor associated antigen) had favorable response with one complete remission lasting longer than 3 years (Epenetos, 1985; Epenetos et al., 1987). Limited clinical effect has also been seen in the treatment of breast or colorectal cancers with ^{131}I labeled MABs (Murray, in press; Murray et al., 1994).

Most trials use high doses of radioisotopes conjugated to MABs (232–608 millicuries of iodine–131). In contrast to the above-mentioned trials, Kaminski *et al.* (1993) have shown promising results with low dose therapy using doses of 34—66 mCi of iodine–131 per dose in patients with B-cell lymphoma. The MAB used targeted the CD20 antigen, and they documented responses in 6 of 9 patients. Four patients had complete remissions lasting 8 to 11 months, and 2 patients had partial remissions lasting up to 5 months. They theorize that the "low dose" radiation induced **apoptosis** (programmed cell death) in lymphoid cell lines and that binding of the MAB was synergistic in inducing this effect. (Kaminski *et al.*, 1993). They also noted that the anti-CD20 may be a superior targeting agent for B-cell lymphomas. These results are encouraging and offer new insight into the use of radiolabeled antibodies.

Yttrium–90 is currently being used in treatment of patients with B-cell lymphoma (LoBuglio and Saleh, 1992). In a group of patients with refractory Hodgkin's disease, complete remissions were observed in 30% of evaluable patients treated with ^{90}Y-labeled polyclonal antiferritin Ig (Vriesendorp *et al.*, 1991).

Chemoimmunoconjugates

Because MABs are able to target tumors, linking chemotherapeutic drugs with the antibody **(chemoimmunoconjugates)** is a logical step in achieving the "magic bullet" approach to killing tumors. Although a number of agents, such as doxorubicin, methotrexate, chlorambucil, vinca alkaloids, and mitomycin have been conjugated with MABs, no significant responses have been observed in clinical trials (LoBuglio and Saleh, 1992). Of the 23 patients with a variety of tumors treated by Oldham (1991) with doxorubicin-antibody conjugates, only a few had minor responses. The instability of the conjugate appears to be the greatest obstacle. In a phase I study of patients with non-small-cell-lung cancer, the murine antibody MAB KS1/4 and the MAB KS1/4-methotrexate immunoconjugate were administered. Of the 5 patients receiving the

Figure 7.3   Pathway of immunotoxin entry. The figure illustrates receptor-mediated endocytosis. The antibody component of the IT binds to antigen on the cell surface. The entire complex then diffuses laterally in the cell membrane to a coated pit. The coated pit gives rise to an endocytic vesicle (receptosome) which moves away from the cell surface by saltatory motion and fuses with another organelle, the TR Golgi. A sorting process that occurs in the Golgi, and much of the IT is sent on to lysosomes to be degraded, some is released into the extracellular fluid, and a small amount escapes in the cytosol. Within the cytosol, the IT acts on its substrates-inactivating either elongation-factor 2 or ribosomes. The fate of the antigen is not shown. Conceivably it is also degraded in the lysosomes resulting in "down-regulation," or else it is returned to the cell surface to associate with other IT molecules.

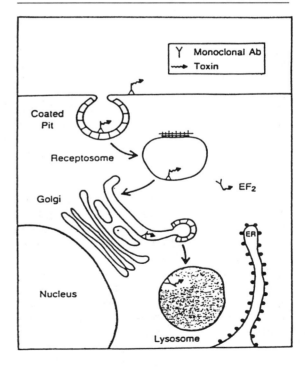

Source: Reprinted with permission from Pastan, D., Willingham, M., Fitzgerald, D. 1986. Immunotoxins. *Cell* 47: p. 643. Copyright held by Cell Press.

immunoconjugate, 1 had a minor response (Elias *et al.*, 1990). This and other studies have demonstrated that there is deposition of the antibody onto tumor cells and that **antigen modulation** does occur (LoBuglio and Saleh, 1992).

Protein Toxin-Antibody Conjugates

Researchers are aware of the powerful nature of toxins. By modifying their cell binding domains these toxins have been used in clinical trials. The therapeutic usefulness of linking a plant or a bacterial toxin to a tumor-specific MAB has been investigated in both solid tumors and in hematologic malignancies. The toxins most commonly conjugated with MABs include ricin-A chain, diphtheria toxin, and the genetically modified *Pseudomonas* exotoxin (PE40) (LoBuglio and Saleh, 1992).

Toxins are transported to the tumor cell surface by the MAB, which is targeted to a specific antigen. After binding to the antigen, the complex is internalized. At this point, the toxin escapes to the **cytosol**, crossing the cell membrane, and mediates the inhibition of protein synthesis, leading to cell kill (Gould *et al.*, 1989). Because they inhibit protein synthesis, toxins not only kill dividing cells, but resting cells as well (Vitteta and Thorpe, 1991). Figure 7.3 provides a schematic representation of the pathway of immunotoxin entry (Pastan *et al.*, 1986)

Toxins are selected by their ability to perform the function of cell recognition, to internalize to the cytosol, and to initiate the **catalysis** of proteins. The toxins are modified to prevent their binding to their normal cellular receptors so that healthy cells are not damaged (Pastan *et al.*, 1986).

Although diphtheria toxin has been the most widely studied toxin, recent trials using ricin A-chain and anti-B4-blocked ricin are also under investigation. The A chain inhibits protein synthesis and the B chain mediates binding of the toxin to the cells. The B chain also assists in the translocation of the A chain to the cytosol. Blocked ricin has the advantage of blocking the galactose binding site thus preventing nonspecific binding to cells (Grossbard *et al.*, 1992a).

The monoclonal antibody T101 in conjugation with ricin A-toxin has been used to treat patients with chronic lymphocytic leukemia. Although these patients experienced a rapid fall in circulating leukemic cells, no clinical responses were observed (Blakey and Thorpe, 1988; Hertler *et al.*, 1988; Laurent *et al.*, 1986). Metastatic melanoma has been treated with a ricin A-chain toxin conjugated with Xomazyme-mel (antimelanoma associated antigen). Only modest responses were noted. These trials were hampered by capillary leak syndrome and the development of human anti-mouse antibody (HAMA) and antibody to the ricin A-chain (HARA) (Hertler *et al.*, 1987; Spitler *et al.*, 1987).

Twenty-five patients with B-cell lymphoma were treated with anti-CD19 MAB conjugated to ricin. The galactose binding sites were blocked in an effort to reduce toxicity (Grossbard *et al.*, 1992a). Nine patients had partial or mixed responses, and 1 patient had a complete remission. In a second trial of B-cell lymphoma, 15 patients received the monoclonal antibody RFB4, which was conjugated to deglycosylated ricin A-chain. One third of these heavily pretreated patients demonstrated a clinical response (Vitetta *et al.*, 1991). Although the response rates are modestly higher for patients with non-Hodgkin's lymphoma compared to solid tumors, durable remissions are infrequent. Furthermore, the rate of immunogenicity (i.e., HAMA or HARA response) was lower (between 0% and 30%). Interestingly, most of the immune responses were against the toxin molecule rather than the murine antibody (Maloney *et al.*, 1992b).

Trials have been limited by toxicity, immunogenicity of the murine antibody and the immunotoxin, and low response rates with short durations. In a review of 7 immunotoxin-antibody trials for patients with solid tumors (breast, ovarian, melanoma, and colon cancer) the response rates were less than 30% with relapses occurring within 5 months.

In addition, between 50% and 100% of the patients developed antihuman or antitoxin antibody responses (Maloney *et al.,* in press).

ADVERSE EFFECTS

Monoclonal antibody therapy is a desirable approach to the treatment of solid tumors, leukemias, and non-Hodgkin's lymphomas because the antibody directly targets the tumor-associated antigen and, in most cases, preserves the integrity of normal cells. This targeting allows severe, acute, and long-term toxic effects to be avoided. The type and severity of adverse reactions will depend on whether the antibody is administered unconjugated, or conjugated to radioisotopes, chemotherapy or immunotoxins.

In the Stanford University Medical Center experience with anti-idiotype antibodies for the treatment of non-Hodgkin's B-cell lymphomas, infusion-related toxic effects such as fevers ($T > 38°C$), chills, rigors, urticaria, mucosal congestion, nausea, diarrhea, and myalgias/arthralgias have been observed. More severe toxic effects, although rare, have included bronchospasm, increased respiratory secretions, and hypotension (Maloney *et al.,* 1992a; Maloney *et al.,* 1992b; Meeker *et al.,* 1985; Miller *et al.,* 1982). It has been postulated that respiratory symptoms may occur as the result of pulmonary leukostasis which is a consequence of sequestration of antibody-coated tumor cells in the pulmonary vasculature. This leads to wheezing, dyspnea, and in some cases hypotension (Press *et al.,* 1987).

Toxic reactions are typically associated with high levels of circulating tumor cells and high idiotype levels and are observed within the first 1 to 3 treatments. It has been noted that a few patients in whom antibody excess cannot be achieved, toxic effects have been documented throughout the course of treatment. Once the free idiotype protein or idiotype-positive cells have been cleared from the serum and an excess of antibody can be achieved, side effects resolve (Brown *et al.,* 1989b).

Early trials involving treatment of lymphoid malignancies with "nonspecific" antibodies, which recognized not only tumor cell antigens but also the tissues from which they arise, revealed many more cases of allergic reaction and anaphylaxis than are now seen (Dillman *et al.,* 1982). Dillman and colleagues were the first to report significant toxic effects with monoclonal antibody infusions. In their studies of patients with B-cell chronic lymphocytic leukemia they noted anaphylaxis, bronchospasm, and allergic reactions that required cessation of therapy. It should be noted that these early trials administered the antibody by bolus or rapid infusion. It has now been shown that with slower infusion, many of these acute toxic effects can be alleviated (Miller *et al.,* 1982).

Tailoring antibodies to the specific antigenic binding site of the tumor cell, which is different from the host's normal B cells, reduces the frequency of these toxic effects. In a review of 47 non-Hodgkin's lymphoma patients receiving a MAB directed against the tumor immunoglobulin idiotype (Maloney *et al.,* in press) there were no reported cases of anaphylaxis or allergic reactions. Furthermore, the most significant toxic effects developed in patients with prolymphocytic leukemia, chronic lymphocytic lymphoma, or in those with a high level of circulating idiotype.

In the group of patients treated with anti-idiotype antibody, hematologic toxic effects were less common. Thrombocytopenia (platelets $< 50,000/mm^3$) was observed in patients whose baseline counts were less than $100,000/mm^3$. In early trials, transient thrombocytopenia was associated with high levels of circulating idiotype protein (Meeker *et al.,* 1985). The cause of thrombocytopenia remains unclear, however, according to Press *et al.* (1987) the reduction in platelets may be the result of small quantities of antibody being absorbed by the Fc receptors to these cells and removed from the circulation by the reticuloendothelial system. Granulocytopenia has also been documented, again in patients whose baseline counts were less than 1000 cells/mm³ (Maloney *et al.*, 1992b) but this too was a transient phenomenon.

An interesting observation, although probably not a toxic effect, was tumor flare in the anti-idiotype MAB studies. This was characterized by swelling, tenderness, and warmth of lymph nodes. This typically occurred between 7 and 14 days after treatment and resolved within 2 to 7 days. Although the etiology of this effect is not certain, it is believed to have been a result of effector cells penetrating the lymph node. This effect was also noted in the early trials that combined anti-idiotype antibody with interferon. Brown *et al.* (1989a) documented swelling in one or more lymph nodes in several patients within the first week of treatment. All tumor sites that exhibited this reaction had major regressions following treatment.

Patients with solid tumors treated with unconjugated monoclonal antibodies to surface membrane antigens experience similar toxicities. These toxic reactions included allergic symptoms, anaphylaxis, urticaria, nausea, vomiting, diarrhea, and mild constitutional symptoms. Universal to patients with these tumors has been the development of a human anti-mouse antibody (HAMA) response. (Discussion of the HAMA response appears later in the chapter). If a HAMA reaction occurs during infusion of the MAB, the reaction is usually manifested by fever, rigors, rash, and neutropenia (Meeker *et al.*, 1985). Meeker and colleagues noted the onset of symptoms within 1 to 2 hours of receiving treatment, with resolution within several days. Other clinical symptoms associated with a HAMA reaction include serum sickness and hypersensitivity reactions (Tjandra *et al.*, 1990).

Myelosuppression has been a dose-limiting factor when administering radiolabeled antibodies. Goldenberg *et al.* (1991) found grade III or IV marrow toxicity even at low doses that were not considered therapeutic (59 mCi of iodine–131). To overcome this adversity, Press *et al.* (1989) have harvested, purged and reinfused bone marrow to patients in a dose-escalation trial. In this phase I trial doses of iodine–131 ranged from 232 to 608 mCi, with myelosuppression occurring between 3 and 5 weeks following treatment. In their most recent study Press *et al.* (1993) treated 19 patients with escalating doses of iodine–131 up to 777 mCi. Seventy-eight percent of the patients required bone marrow reinfusion between 13 and 31 days following therapy. Bone marrow toxicity is due to prolonged circulating antibody-isotope conjugates or free radiolabel that has been released from the conjugate (Maloney *et al.*, in press).

More recently, however, Kaminiski *et al.* (1993) have reported the opposite effects with low doses of iodine–131 (34 to 66 mCi) conjugated to the anti-B1 MAB. Of 9 patients studied, they reported grade 1 hematologic toxic effects in 5 patients and grade 2 hematologic toxic effects in 2 others. The remaining 2 patients had no myelosuppression. Bone marrow reinfusion was not required in any patient.

Nonhematologic toxic effects of radiolabeled antibodies have been mild and include fever, urticaria, pruritus, malaise, and asymptomatic hypothyroidism. The last was observed 1 year after completion of therapy and reflects the inability to achieve complete blockage of iodine–131 uptake in the thyroid by the administration of the protective agent, potassium iodide (Press *et al.*, 1989). Gastrointestinal toxic effects in the form of nausea are thought to be due to gastric irradiation caused by the excretion of free iodine–131 by the stomach. Recently Press *et al.* (1993), in a study of 19 patients, have noted additional toxicity of alopecia (21%), elevated liver function tests (42%), hyperbilirubinemia (37%), and severe cardiopulmonary toxicity (10%).

When antibody and chemotherapy drugs are conjugated, one can expect the usual toxic effects related to antibody alone, and if circulating free drug is present, all of the usual side effects and complications of the drug given alone. Unusual toxic effects resulting from nonspecific binding of the chemoimmunoconjugate to normal tissues may also occur. Myelosuppression is usually the dose-limiting toxic effect.

The most severe toxic effects have been attributed to immunotoxin-conjugated MABs. These effects, which were reversible, were noted even at doses too low to yield detectable binding of the immunoconjugate to the target antigen. Weiner *et al.* (1989) described vascular leak syndrome as an effect of treatment with a recombinant ricin A-chain linked to MAB. This syndrome is characterized by weight gain, edema, dyspnea, decreased albumin levels, and in some cases, hypotension. They suggest the probability that the immunoconjugate was delivering recombinant ricin A-chain to unintended targets. They also showed that ricin toxin A contains immunotoxins that bind to the human monocyte Fc receptors. Others postulate that monocyte activation or death may lead to the release of mediators that bring about capillary leakage (Gould *et al.*, 1989).

Central nervous system toxic effects have been observed with *Pseudomonas* exotoxin (PE40) and ricin A. Gould *et al.* (1989) described delayed debilitating neuropathy 2 to 3 months following treatment, with residual paresthesias lasting over 6 months. Nerve biopsy revealed axonal loss and segmental demyelination. These investigators were able to show that the epitope was present on either the Schwann or the myelin cell, suggesting that the immunotoxin targeted the neural cells. They observed pulmonary edema, weight gain, dyspnea on exertion, arthralgias, fever, and mild elevations in liver enzymes. Because of these toxic effects, further entry of patients into the study was halted.

Grossbard *et al.* (1992b) reported clinically significant hepatotoxicity associated with treatment with B4 blocked ricin. This has also been documented with diphtheria toxin (Pai *et al.*, 1991). The onset of hepatic toxic effects was noted within 24 to 48 hours after infusion and resolved within 7 to 14 days. Elevated SGOT and SGPT levels rose as high as 10 times the upper limit of normal. They postulate this was due to the clearance of the immunotoxin by the reticuloendothelial system rather than to nonspecific antibody binding or free blocked ricin. Interestingly they did not report capillary leak syndrome or neurotoxicity. Tolerable toxic effects such as fevers, malaise, fatigue, nausea, hypoalbuminemia, and thrombocytopenia were also noted.

Given the historical and current data, one can see that the adverse reactions vary according to the type and specificity of MAB utilized. Most toxic effects are transient and respond to standard interventions.

OBSTACLES TO TREATMENT

Antigenic Modulation

Over the years, researchers have been concerned with how tumor cells escape antibody destruction. One of tumor cells' defense mechanisms is antigenic modulation, in which the antigen is removed from the cells' surface by shedding or internalization (Oldham, 1983). If therapeutic antibody is administered during this modulation there may not be sufficient binding to cell surfaces to effect target cell elimination (Dillman, 1984).

Antigenic modulation can occur within hours after antibody administration. Once the antibody stimulus is removed, the antigen is re-expressed, usually within 24 hours. Miller *et al.* (1981) have shown *in vivo* that leukemic cells undergo antigenic modulation as a result of antibody binding to the cell surface. They noted the onset of modulation 1, 6, and 12 hours after treatment, but no change was observed during treatment or within the first hour after treatment. *In vitro* experiments indicated that modulation was time and dose dependent. That is, the longer the cells are exposed to the antibody, the more susceptible they become to modulation (Miller *et al.*, 1981). Additional *in vitro* studies confirmed that modulation resulted in the loss of both antibody and antigen from the cell surface but was reversible once the antibody disappeared (Ritz *et al.*, 1980). Again, modulation began within 24 hours of treatment.

Interestingly, not all surface antigens modulate. For instance, common acute lymphoblastic leukemia antigen (CALLA) and surface immunoglobulin have a high propensity to modulate, whereas histocompatibility antigens do not (Ritz and Schlossman, 1982). Modulation occurs more often with hematopoietic cells than in solid tumor cells (Levy, 1985).

Careful scheduling of the antibody doses is one method of circumventing the effects of modulation (Miller *et al.*, 1981). Other attempts to control modulation have included the use of biological response modifiers such as interferon-alpha to **upregulate** tumor-associated antigens on the cell surface, which leads to better binding (Schlom, 1991).

Human Antimurine Antibodies

Another limitation associated with murine monoclonal antibodies has been the development of human antimurine antibodies (HAMA response). This is an antibody response against the foreign protein or contaminants in the preparation of the antibody (Ritz and Schlossman, 1982). The development of host antibodies against the protein has a neutralizing effect and inhibits antibody binding (Schroff *et al.*, 1985). Meeker *et al.* (1985) noted that once an immune response had begun, further infusions of antibody were incapable of reaching the tumor. Those patients who had an immune response did not demonstrate a clinical response. Serum assays of antibody levels also indicated that this neutralizing effect occurs. Meeker *et al.* reported decreased serum half-life as well as lower antibody levels with a HAMA response, which correlate with the clearance of administered antibody (Meeker *et al.*, 1985). The onset of a HAMA response in hematologic malignancies has been variable and can occur from 10 to 24 days after treatment (Levy, 1985). As previously discussed, toxic effects related to the HAMA response and characterized by anaphylactic or other immune reactions have been observed and appear related to the formation of immune complexes (Schroff *et al.*, 1985).

Although more prevalent in patients with solid tumors, a HAMA response has been observed in patients with hematologic malignancies. There were higher incidences of a HAMA response in early trials with anti-idiotype antibodies for B-cell lymphomas than in current trials. In 1982, Miller and colleagues reported that during treatment with anti-idiotype antibodies, 5 of 11 patients developed a HAMA response; whereas in the more recent trials reported by Brown *et al.* (1989b) only 2 of 11 patients had positive immune responses. In the most recently published trial there were no detectable HAMA responses in 13 patients (Maloney *et al.*, 1992b). The lack of a HAMA response in these patients may be related to the purity of the antibodies, to higher doses of antibody, to prior immunosuppressive therapy, or to immunosuppression by their disease (Brown *et al.*, 1989b).

Modification of MAB

Human MAB. Researchers are studying ways to overcome the HAMA response. One suggestion has been the use of immunosuppressive therapy prior to antibody treatment. The most prevalent method, however, has been through modification of the antibody. The potential of using a human antibody instead of a mouse antibody is one possible approach. The technique for developing human monoclonal antibodies involves immortalizing immune B-cells with Epstein-Barr virus. The immune B-cell is then fused with a human myeloma cell line or a human lymphoblastoid cell line (Dorfman, 1985). Problems encountered with human monoclonals include the paucity of human myeloma cell lines that are fusion-efficient and no readily available human B cells that have been immunized with tumor cells. To immunize human subjects with tumor cells or products is not a viable option (LoBuglio and Saleh, 1992). The few human antibodies available do not allow for wide-scale clinical trials.

Chimeric MAB. A second method of antibody modification is to try to reduce the amount of mouse protein in the antibody by insertion of the human gene that codes for the constant region. Recent technology has made it possible to produce antibodies with a murine variable region combined with a human constant region through use of genetic engineering techniques. The gene for the human constant region is isolated and amplified by PCR in the same fashion as the mouse variable-region gene. Both genes are inserted into a virus that is allowed to infect *Escherichia coli (E. coli).* The viral DNA is inserted into the cellular DNA of the *E. coli* and the cell produces the desired mouse-human antibody. Growing *E. coli* in cultures is much easier than growing the antibody in the mouse and yields larger volumes of pure antibody (Overmyer, 1990). This type of antibody is called a **chimeric** antibody and is named after a mythical beast, the chimera which had the head of a lion, the body of a goat, and the tail of a dragon (Overmyer, 1990). Potential advantages to this type of antibody include less immunogenicity, longer circulation of the antibody, and better cell killing. Cell killing is enhanced because the chimeric antibody maintains the antigenic specificity of the murine antibody and the effector properties of the human Fc receptor (Hozumi and Sandhu, 1993; LoBuglio and Saleh, 1992). It is believed that these antibodies mediate ADCC with human effector cells causing lysis of the tumor cells.

Of course, there is still a possibility that the patient receiving a chimeric MAB would be at risk for developing a **human antihuman antibody response (HAHA)** or a **human antichimeric antibody response (HACA).** There have been reports of HACA responses in patients treated with chimerized antibodies, and it has been noted these responses were to the murine variable regions rather than the human constant region (Khazaeli *et al.,* 1991). Because studies are ongoing in this area, it remains to be seen if the risk of developing an immune response to the humanized portion will be a salient issue.

Clinical trials are being conducted in patients with solid tumors and hematologic malignancies. To date patients with melanoma, colon cancer, cutaneous T-cell lymphoma, and non-Hodgkin's lymphoma have been treated with chimeric MABs. Transient responses to therapy were noted in the patients with cutaneous T-cell lymphoma, however, no therapeutic responses were documented in either study for patients with melanoma or colon cancer (Maloney *et al.,* 1992b). Clinical trials are now underway throughout the United States to evaluate clinical activity and response rate of chimeric anti-CD20 (C2B8) antibody for patients with relapsed lymphoma. Patients will receive multiple doses once a week for 4 weeks, at a set dose of 375 mg/m^2.

"Humanized" MAB.   A third technique to reduce the immunogenicity of the MAB is to include even more human portions in the engineered antibody. MABs thus adapted are termed "humanized" and are differentiated from chimeric antibodies in that they contain a human constant region and a variable region which consists of both the murine **complementarity-determining regions** and the human V-region framework determinants (LoBuglio and Saleh, 1992). Therefore, only a very small portion of the humanized MAB contains genetic material from the mouse. There is insufficient information thus far to determine whether these MABs decrease the incidence of a HAMA response. Figure 7.4 is a schematic representation of the murine, human, chimeric, and humanized antibodies.

Antigen Blockade

Researchers have battled the occurrence of high levels of circulating antigen, which acts as a blockade and prevents antibody from reaching the tumor cells. Of course, this will depend on the normal secretion of the antigen as well as the type of antibody and its affinity (Dillman, 1984). Black (1980) noted that most tumors have the propensity to shed or secrete antigen into the serum. For instance, Leu 1, T101, and J5 antigens are not shed to an extent

Figure 7.4   Schematic diagram of various types of monoclonal antibodies.

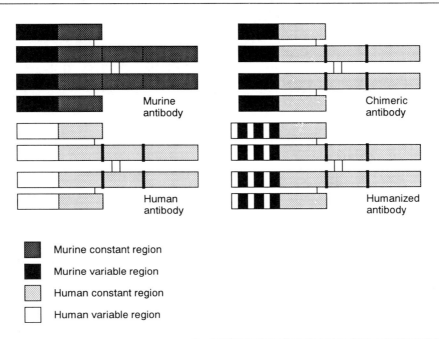

Source: Reprinted with permission from LoBuglio, A., and Saleh, M. 1992. Monoclonal antibody therapy of cancer. *Critical Reviews in Oncology Hematology* 13: p. 273.

that would interfere with therapy (Dillman, 1984), but this has been a concern for patients with B-cell lymphomas treated with anti-idiotype antibody (Meeker *et al.*, 1985). Because serum idiotype can be used as a marker in this disease, it is easier to detect the amount of free antigen. When the circulating antigen is freely secreted, there is a blocking effect on the administered antibody that prevents the antibody from reaching the tumor cell and binding (Brown *et al.*, 1989b). One approach to clearing excess antigen has been the infusion of large quantities of MAB. As already noted, however, this poses a risk of increased toxic effects. Alternatively, Meeker *et al.* (1985) employed the technique of plasmapheresis prior to and during therapy to clear free idiotype from the serum. In this trial, no tumor showed a significant response until excess serum idiotype was depleted and free antibody could

persist. Miller *et al.* (1981) reported an interesting phenomenon in which a patient with T-cell leukemia developed circulating antigen after the first dose of therapy. This suggested that the antigen was released as a result of antibody-induced tumor cell lysis. This has not been a problem in latter trials.

Tumor Heterogeneity

Finally, idiotype-negative variants, or tumor heterogeneity, has also been a difficult problem to overcome when studying and treating hematologic malignancies. In this process, tumor cells secrete mutant forms of surface immunoglobulin that elude the effect of the antibody and allow continued tumor growth. Meeker *et al.* (1985) studied idiotype-negative variants in patients with B-cell lymphoma and found that the change seemed to be related to a somatic mutation in the variable region of the active immunoglobulin genes. This results in amino acid changes in the immunoglobulin molecule and subsequent alteration in the idiotype. Following treatment with anti-idiotype therapy, these variant cells become the prominent population. This is one possible explanation for some of the relapses or progression of disease that is observed (Maloney et al., 1992b). Several trials (discussed earlier) were undertaken to overcome this variance. Unfortunately, the addition of the synergistic agents did not prevent the emergence of idiotype-negative variance (Maloney et al., 1992a; Brown et al., 1989a). Another possible solution would be to treat with multiple antibodies, each recognizing a different portion of the tumor population (Levy, 1985). Tumor heterogeneity is also a problem in the treatment of solid tumors. For example, melanoma tumors can express a variety of melanoma-associated antigens. Administration of a single MAB would not allow for detection of tumors expressing a different melanoma-associated antigen.

Cost

Because of the extensive research and technology needed to develop MABs and antibody conjugates, cost is often identified as an obstacle to treatment. Since most of the antibody trials are still experimental, funding has been provided by grants supported by the National Cancer Institute. At this time patients receiving antibody therapy on these studies do not incur charges, but once the therapy is approved patients would incur treatment-related charges. At Stanford University Medical Center, treatment has been administered on both inpatients and outpatients. The cost per treated patient has been approximately $33,000 for inpatients and $15,000 for outpatients. This does not take into account that the antibody has been supplied gratis by the manufacturing pharmaceutical company.

OTHER USES OF MONOCLONAL ANTIBODIES

The MAB Orthoclone OKT 3 (muromonab-CD3) has been used in the treatment of acute cell-mediated rejection in organ transplants. The antibody reacts with the surface antigen T3 of human T cells and removes the antigen-bearing T cells from circulation, rendering them ineffective in mounting an immune response (Goldstein, 1987). Side effects seen in this setting are similar to those observed with patients being treated for malignancies. Fever, chills, nausea, vomiting, and diarrhea are not uncommon (Moir, 1989; Farrell, 1987). Adverse reactions are more typical during the first hour of infusion and less frequent with the second and third doses. As with the early antibody trials in malignancy, pulmonary edema was observed in these early trials. Assuring that the patient was not in fluid overload prior to treatment helped lessen this side effect (Moir, 1989). Generalized aches and malaise are also common symptoms. Because this MAB suppresses the immune system, patients receiving this form of treatment are at risk for bacterial, fungal, and viral infections. Fevers may not always be a reaction to the antibody but may herald an infection (Moir, 1989).

Resistance of malignant tumors to chemotherapy drugs has been attributed to a multigene family designated mdr^1. These genes encode the membrane proteins called P-glycoproteins 1–5 (Arceci et al., 1993). Murine monoclonal antibody 4E3, which is directed to the human mdr^1-encoded P-glycoprotein, has been used to identify cells that produce this protein. The MAB is thus useful in studying the phenomenon of multidrug resistance in normal and malignant cells (Arceci et al., 1993). Future applications of this antibody may include conjugation to biological toxins or cytotoxic drugs.

Monoclonal antibodies have also been used to treat gram-negative sepsis. A murine IgM MAB, HA–1A, has been targeted to bacterial endotoxin, a causative agent of gram-negative sepsis and other MABs have targeted tumor necrosis factor, one of the prime mediators of septic shock (Greenberg *et al.*, 1992; Klein and Witek-Janusek, 1992). Early results are encouraging that this antibody may have the potential to reduce the early morbidity and mortality in seriously ill patients with gram-negative sepsis (Greenberg *et al.*, 1992). Larger phase III trials are being conducted, but the antibody has not yet been released for commercial use.

Several monoclonal antibodies have greatly enhanced the pathologist's ability to diagnose tumors and to differentiate among subsets of tumors. By utilizing antibodies to surface proteins, predominantly differentiation antigens, the pathologist is able to stain the cells and distinguish cell types and thus the origin of tumors. For example, lymphocytes look the same under the microscope, but when stained with antibodies that have affinity to the surface markers it is easy to identify the subsets of T and B cells.

One can expect an ever expanding use of MABs in the diagnostic arena. For example, research with indium–111 antimyosin antibodies has proven that they are useful in the diagnosis of myocardial infarction. The antibody is specific for acute myocardial necrosis and can thus differentiate between ischemia and chronic infarction (Cimini, 1992).

REGULATORY APPROVAL

As a form of biological therapy, MABs are subject to the same approval process mandated by the FDA (Middleton, 1992) as other biological agents. In addition, biological agents must receive an establishment license application for the product. The law regulating biological agents was actually enacted in July of 1902 as the Virus-Toxin Law. The law specifies manufacturing, inspection, licensing, and labeling requirements. The National Institutes of Health maintained regulatory control of biological agents until 1972, when control

was transferred to the FDA. Most of the MABs currently in testing fall under the category of orphan drugs. On January 4, 1983 the Orphan Drug Act was signed into law and is designed to provide financial incentives for companies to develop new products that might be used in the treatment, diagnosis, or prevention of a rare disease. It was also designed to reduce regulatory barriers. Two examples of monoclonal antibody orphan drugs are murine or human monoclonal antibodies against B-cell lymphoma (Idec Pharmaceutics Corporation, San Diego, CA) and monoclonal antibody 17–1A (Centocor, Malvein, PA) (Wandres and Lau, 1992). OncoScint® CR/OV is the only MAB with FDA approval for use in patients with cancer and is indicated for the detection of disease in patients with colorectal or ovarian cancers. The majority of MABs are given by the intravenous route as a short-term infusion.

FUTURE DIRECTIONS

It is clear that the hybridoma technology developed by Köhler and Milstein has wide-ranging applications for the entire medical field. MABs have been derived that can react with proteins, carbohydrates, nucleic acids, or **haptenated** forms of these molecules (Kummer and Staerz, 1993). It is easy to envision MABs in use in a variety of diagnostic and therapeutic ways. To name a few examples, antibodies are being developed for imaging antifibrin for the diagnosis of deep venous or arterial thromboses, for the targeting of infection and inflammation, and for treating rhesus hemolytic disease. Conjugate technology is being used to develop antibody-enzyme conjugates to target blood clots. Antiplatelet antibodies are conceived for the prevention of intravascular thrombosis (Russell *et al.*, 1992).

Continued development of MABs in the treatment of malignancies will probably focus on diminishing obstacles to treatment. For example, further development and refinement of chimeric or humanized antibodies that have higher affinity for the tumor cells and a reduced risk of causing an immune response represent two possibilities. Human antibodies could be developed using severe combined immunodeficient mice that have been reconstituted with human lymphocytes. These mice could then serve as factories for the development of human antitumor antibodies. Recombinant DNA technology could be used to produce modified toxins that retain the tumoricidal potential but have reduced nonspecific binding. Antibody-drug conjugates more stable than those now available would allow drug release at the tumor site and spare the surrounding healthy tissue. A second type of antibody-drug conjugate, if developed, would allow the antibody to carry multiple non-cross-reacting drugs (LoBuglio and Saleh, 1992; Russell, et al., 1992).

Studies will soon be underway evaluating the use of MABs in the adjuvant treatment of lymphoma. Much like adjuvant chemotherapy, MABs will be administered at a time when patients are in a complete remission following initial chemotherapy. The goal would be to "mop-up" residual cancer cells.

Research has concentrated on the passive administration of antibody therapy, but ideally, active immunotherapy is a more desirable approach. Vaccines have been employed for patients with melanoma, colon cancer, and non-Hodgkin's lymphoma. The most specific vaccine, the idiotype vaccine, has been developed by Kwak and colleagues (Kwak et al., 1992) for patients with B-cell lymphoma. Vaccines for melanoma have used cell surface markers to generate antibodies against the antigen. These antibodies are then reinjected into patients as an immunogen to induce a polyclonal antibody response (Dalgleish and Kennedy, 1988).

As discussed previously, the unique nature of B-cell lymphoma with the presence of the idiotype protein lends itself to tumor-specific therapy. The tumor antigen is used as a vaccine to induce the host to reject cells bearing that antigen. The vaccine is produced by fusing the patient's lymphoma cells with a heterohybridoma with the resulting hybridoma secreting the desired idiotype. The volume of secreted protein is purified by affinity chromatography. Once purified, the idiotype is conjugated with a potent immunogenic protein, keyhole limpet hemocyanin (KLH). This conjugate is then reinjected into the patient for whom it was produced during complete remission. In a study of 9 patients, Kwak et al. (1992) were able to induce specific antibody and/or cellular responses in 7 patients. Although it is too early to make conclusions, one could theorize that tumor recurrence could be prevented if antibodies that recognize the tumor-specific idiotype were produced by the body.

MABs have been used in cancer treatment and detection for over a decade. Although there has been limited success, Goldenberg (1994) points out that MABs have not yet gained a role in standard therapy. They have, however, provided a common tool to the many disciplines involved in the diagnosis and treatment of malignancies.

References

Abbas, A., Lichtman, M., and Prober, J. 1991. Antibodies and antigens. In *Cellular and Molecular immunology*. Philadelphia: W.B. Saunders, pp. 38–68.

Arceci, R., Stieglitz, K., Bras, J., et al. 1993. Monoclonal antibody to an external epitope of the human mdr^1 P-glycoprotein. *Cancer Research* 53: 310–317.

Bajorin, D., Chapman, P., Wong, G., et al. 1992. Treatment with high dose mouse monoclonal (anti-G03) antibody R24 in patients with metastatic melanoma. *Melanoma Research* 2(5–6): 355–362.

Ball, E., Mills, L., and Cornwell, C. 1990. Autologous bone marrow transplantation for acute myeloid leukemia using monoclonal antibody-purged bone marrow. *Blood* 75: 1199–1206.

Basham, T., Kaminski, M., Kitamura, K., et al. 1986. Synergistic antitumor effect of interferon and anti-idiotype monoclonal antibody in murine lymphoma. *Journal of Immunology* 137: 3019–3024.

Benjamini, E., and Leskowitz, S. 1988. *Immunology: A Short Course*. New York: Alan R. Liss, Inc.

Berinstein, N., Starnes, C., and Levy, R. 1988. Enhancement of the therapeutic effect of anti-idiotype antibodies on a murine B-cell lymphoma by IL–2. *Journal of Immunology* 140: 2839–2845.

Berinstein, T., and Levy, R. 1987. Treatment of a murine B-cell lymphoma with monoclonal antibodies and IL–2. *Journal of Immunology* 139: 971–976.

Black, P. 1980. Shedding from normal and cancer cell surfaces. *New England Journal of Medicine* 303: 1415–1416.

Blakey, D., and Thorpe, P. 1988. An overview of therapy with immunotoxins containing ricin or its A chain. *Antibody Immunoconjugate Radiopharmacology* 1: 1–16.

Brown, S., Miller, R., Horning, S., et al. 1989a. Treatment of B-cell lymphoma alone and in combination with alpha interferon. *Blood* 73(3): 651–661.

Brown, S., Miller, R., and Levy, R. 1989b. Anti-idiotype antibody therapy of B-cell lymphoma. *Seminars in Oncology* 16(3): 199–210.

Cheung, N., Laxarus, H., Miraldi, F., et al. 1987. Ganglioside GD2 specific monoclonal antibody 3F8: A phase I study in patients with neuroblastoma and malignant melanoma. *Journal of Clinical Oncology* 5: 1430–1440.

Cimini, D. 1992. Indium–111 antimyosin antibody imaging: A promising new technique in the diagnosis of M.I. *Critical Care Nursing* 12(6): 50–51.

Cooper, E., and Flaum, M. 1988. The use of monoclonal antibodies in blood testing and typing. *Modern Medicine* 56(5): 46–52.

Dalgleish, H., and Kennedy, R. 1988. Anti-idiotype antibodies as immunogens: Idiotype basic vaccines. *Vaccine* 6:215–220.

DeJager, R., Abdel-Nabi, H., Serafini, A., et al. 1993. Current status of cancer immunodetection with radiolabeled human monoclonal antibodies. *Seminars in Nuclear Medicine* 23(2): 165–179.

DeNardo, S., DeNardo, G., O'Grady, L., et al. 1987. Treatment of a patient with a B-cell lymphoma using I–131 Lym–1 monoclonal antibodies. *International Journal of Biological Markers* 2(1): 49–53.

DiJulio, J. 1988. Treatment of B cell and T cell lymphomas with monoclonal antibodies. *Seminars in Oncology Nursing* 4: 102–106.

Dillman, R., Shawler, D., Dillman, J., et al. 1985. Monoclonal antibodies in patients with CLL and CTCL. *Journal of Cellular Biochemistry* 9A: 48 (abstract).

Dillman, R. 1984. Monoclonal antibodies in the treatment of cancer. *Critical Reviews in Oncology/Hematology* 1(4): 357–385.

Dillman, R., Shawler, D., Sobol, R., et al. 1982. Murine monoclonal antibody therapy in two patients with chronic lymphocytic leukemia. *Blood* 59: 1036–1045.

Dorfman, N. 1985. The optimal technological approach to the development of human hybridomas. *Journal of Biologic Response Modifiers* 4: 213–239.

Eary, J., Press, O., Badger, C., et al. 1990. Imaging and treatment of B-cell lymphoma. *Journal of Nuclear Medicine* 31: 1257–1268.

Elias, D., Hirshowitz, L., Kline, L., et al. 1990. Phase I clinical comparison study of monoclonal antibody KS1/4 and KS1/4-methotrexate immunoconjugate in patients with non-small-cell lung cancer. *Cancer Research* 50: 4154–4159.

Epenetos, A., Munro, A., Stewart, S., et al. 1987. Antibody-guided irradiation of advanced ovarian cancer with intraperitoneally administered radiolabeled monoclonal antibodies. *Journal of Clinical Oncology* 5: 1890–1899.

Epenetos, A., 1985. Clinical results with regional antibody-guided irradiation. *Cancer Drug Delivery* 2: 233.

Farrell, M. 1987. Orthoclone OKT 3: A treatment for acute renal allograft rejection. *ANNA Journal* 14: 373–376.

Foon, K., Schroff, R., Mayer, D., et al. 1983. Monoclonal antibody therapy of chronic lymphocytic leukemia and cutaneous T-cell lymphoma: Preliminary observations. In Boss, B., Langman, R., Trowbridge, I. and Dulbecco, R. (eds). *Monoclonal Antibodies and Cancer*. Orlando, FL: Academic Press, pp. 32–39.

Foon, K., Schroff, R., and Gale, R. 1982. Surface markers on leukemia and lymphoma cells: Recent advances. *Blood* 60: 1–19.

Freedman, A., Takvorian, T., Anderson, K., et al. 1990. Autologous bone marrow transplantation in B-cell non-Hodgkin's lymphoma: Very low treatment related mortality in 100 patients in sensitive relapse. *Journal of Clinical Oncology* 7: 1821–1829.

Gold, P., and Freedman, S. 1965. Specific carcinoembryonic antigens of the human digestive system. *Journal of Experimental Medicine* 122: 467–481.

Goldenberg, D. 1994. New developments in monoclonal antibodies for cancer detection and therapy. *CA: A Journal for Clinicians.* 44(1): 43–64.

Goldenberg, D., and Larson, S. 1992. Radioimmunodetection in cancer identification. *Journal of Nuclear Medicine* 33: 803–814.

Goldenberg, D., Horowitz, J., Sharkey, R., et al. 1991. Targeting dosimetry and radioimmunotherapy of B-cell lymphomas with iodine–131-labeled LL2 monoclonal antibody. *Journal of Clinical Oncology* 9: 548–564.

Goldenberg, D., Goldenberg, H., Higginbotham-Ford, E., et al. 1987. Imaging of primary and metastatic liver cancer with I-131 monoclonal and polyclonal antibodies against alpha fetoprotein. *Journal of Clinical Oncology* 5: 1827–1835.

Goldenberg, D., Kim, E., and DeLand, F. 1981. Human chorionic gonadotropin radio-antibodies in the radioimmunodetection of cancer and for disclosure of occult metastases. *Proceedings of the National Academy of Sciences of the USA* 78: 754–758.

Goldenberg, D., Kim, E., DeLand, F., et al. 1980a. Clinical studies of the radioimmunodetection of tumors containing alpha-fetoprotein. *Cancer Research* 40: 984–992.

Goldenberg, D., Kim, E., DeLand, F., et al. 1980b. Radioimmunodetection of cancer using radioactive antibodies to human chorionic gonadotropin. *Science* 208: 1284–1286.

Goldenberg, D. 1978. Immunodiagnosis and immunodetection of colorectal cancer. *Cancer Bulletin* 30: 213–218.

Goldenberg, D., DeLand, F., Kim, E., *et al.* 1978. Use of radiolabeled antibodies to carcinoembryonic antigen for the detection and localization of diverse cancers by external photoscanning. *New England Journal of Medicine* 298: 1384–1388.

Goldstein, G. 1987. Monoclonal antibody specificity: Orthoclone OKT 3 T-cell blocker. *Nephron* 46(Suppl. 1): 5–11.

Gould, B., Borowitz, M., Groves, E., *et al.* 1989. Phase I study of an anti–breast cancer immunotoxin by continuous infusion: Report of a targeted toxic effect not predicted by animal studies. *Journal of Clinical Investigation* 81(10): 775–781.

Greenberg, R., Wilson, K., Kunz, A., *et al.* 1992. Observations using antiendotoxin antibody (E5) as adjuvant therapy in humans with suspected, serious, gram-negative sepsis. *Critical Care Medicine* 20(6): 730–735.

Gribben, J., Freedman, A., Neuberg, D., *et al.* 1991. Immunologic purging of marrow assessed by PCR before autologous bone marrow transplant. *New England Journal of Medicine* 22: 1525–1533.

Grossbard, M., Freedman, A., Ritz, J., *et al.* 1992a. Serotherapy of B-cell neoplasms with anti-B4 blocked ricin: A phase I trial of daily bolus infusion. *Blood* 79: 576–585.

Grossbard, M., Lambert, J., Goldmacher, V., *et al.* 1992b. Correlation between *in vivo* toxicity and preclinical *in vitro* parameters for the immunotoxin anti-B4-blocked ricin. *Cancer Research* 52: 4200–4207.

Hertler, A., Schlossman, D., Borowitz, M., *et al.* 1988. A phase I study of T101-ricin A chain immunotoxin in refractory chronic lymphocytic leukemia. *Journal of Biological Response Modifiers* 7: 97–113.

Hertler, A., Spitler, L., and Frankel, A. 1987. Humoral immune response to a ricin A chain immunotoxin in patients with metastatic melanoma. *Cancer Drug Delivery* 4: 245–253.

Hoppszallern, S. 1993. Radioimmunoimaging : New frontiers in cancer diagnosis and treatment. *Hospital Technology Scanner* 9: 8–11.

Houghton, A., Chapman, P., and Bajorin, D. 1991. Antibodies in cancer therapy. Section 22.3. Melanoma. In DeVita, V., Hellman, S., Rosenberg, S. (eds). *Biologic Therapy of Cancer.* Philadelphia: J.B. Lippincott, pp. 533–550.

Houston, L., and Nowinski, R. 1981. Cell-specific cytotoxicity expressed by a conjugate of ricin and murine monoclonal antibody directed against the Thy 1.1 antigen. *Cancer Research* 41: 3913–3917.

Hozumi, N., and Sandhu, J. 1993. Recombinant antibody technology: Its advent and advances. *Cancer Investigation* 11(6): 714–723.

Irie, R., and Morton, D. 1986. Regression of cutaneous metastatic melanoma by intralesional injection with human monoclonal antibody to ganglioside GD2. *Proceedings of National Academy of Science* 83: 8694–8698.

Kaminski, M., Zasadny, K., Francis, I., *et al.* 1993. Radioimmunotherapy of B-cell lymphoma with [131] anti-B1 (Anti-CD20) antibody. *New England Journal of Medicine* 329(7): 459–465.

Khazaeli, M., Saleh, M., Liu, T., *et al.* 1991. Pharmacokinetic immune response of ^{131}I-chimeric mouse/human B 72.3 (human gamma 4) monoclonal antibody in humans. *Cancer Research* 51(20): 5461–5466.

Khazaeli, M., Saleh, M., Wheeler, R., *et al.* 1988. Phase I trial of multiple large doses of murine monoclonal antibody CO17–1A.II: Pharmacokinetics and immune response. *Journal of National Cancer Institute* 80: 937–942.

Klein, D., and Witek-Janusek, L. 1992. Advances in immunotherapy of sepsis. *Dimensions of Critical Care Nursing* 11(2): 75–89.

Köhler, G., and Milstein, C. 1975. Continuous cultures of fused cells secreting antibody of predefined specificity. *Nature* 256: 495–496.

Kummer, U., and Staerz, M. 1993. Concepts of antibody-mediated cancer therapy. *Cancer Investigation* 11(2): 174–184.

Kwak, L., Campbell, M., Czerwinski, D., *et al.* 1992. Induction of immune responses in patients with B-cell lymphoma against the surface immunoglobulin idiotype expressed by their tumors. *New England Journal of Medicine* 327(17): 1209–1215.

Larson, S., Cheung, N., and Leibel, S. 1991. Radioisotope conjugates. In DeVita, V., Hellman, S., Rosenberg, S. (eds). *Biologic Therapy of Cancer.* Philadelphia: J.B. Lippincott, pp. 563–588.

Larson, S., Carrasquillo, J., Krohn, K., *et al.* 1983. Localization of ^{131}I-labeled p97 specific Fab fragments in human melanoma as a basis for radiotherapy. *Journal of Clinical Investigation* 72: 2101–2114.

Laurent, G., Pris, J., and Farcet, J. 1986. Effects of therapy with T101-ricin A-chain immunotoxin in two leukemia patients. *Blood* 67: 1680–1687.

Levy, R., and Miller, R. 1991. Antibodies in cancer therapy. Section 22.1. B-cell lymphomas. In DeVita, V., Hellman, S., Rosenberg, S. (eds). *Biologic Therapy of Cancer.* Philadelphia: J.B. Lippincott, pp. 512–522.

Levy, R. 1985. Biologicals for cancer treatment: Monoclonal antibodies. *Hospital Practice* 20(11): 67–74, 77, 80–84.

Lictin, A., Iliopoulous, D., Guerry, D., *et al.* 1988. Therapy of melanoma with an anti-melanoma ganglioside monoclonal antibody: A possible mechanism of a complete response (abstract). *Proceedings of the American Society of Clinical Oncology* 7: 247 (Abstract).

LoBuglio, A., and Saleh, M. 1992. Monoclonal antibody therapy of cancer. *Critical Reviews in Oncology/Hematology* 13: 271–282.

LoBuglio, A., Saleh, M., Lee, J., *et al.* 1988. Phase I trial of multiple large doses of murine monoclonal antibody CO17–1A. Clinical aspects. *Journal of the National Cancer Institute* 80: 932–936.

Lowder, J., Meeker, T., and Levy, R. 1985. Monoclonal antibody therapy of lymphoid malignancy. *Cancer Surveys* 4(2): 360–375.

Lotze, M., and Rosenberg, S. 1988. The immunologic treatment of cancer. *CA-A Cancer Journal for Clinicians* 38(2): 68–95.

Maloney, D., Levy, R., and Campbell, M. (in press). The molecular basis of cancer. In Mendelson, E. (ed). *Monoclonal Antibody Therapy*. Philadelphia: W.B. Saunders.

Maloney, D., Brown, S., Czerwinski, D., et al. 1992a. Monoclonal anti-idiotype antibody therapy of B-cell lymphoma: The addition of a short course of chemotherapy does not interfere with the antitumor effect nor prevent the emergence of idiotype negative variant cells. *Blood* 80(6): 1502–1510.

Maloney, D., Levy, R., and Miller, R. 1992b. Monoclonal anti-idiotype therapy of B-cell lymphoma. *Biologic Therapy of Cancer Updates*. Philadelphia: J.B. Lippincott, 2(6): 1–10.

Meeker, T., Lowder, R., Maloney, D., et al. 1985. A clinical trial of anti-idiotype therapy for B cell malignancy. *Blood* 65: 1349–1353.

Middleton, R. 1992. The drug approval process: An introduction. *California Journal of Hospital Pharmacy* 4: 5–11.

Miller, R., Hart, S., Samoszuk, M., et al. 1989. Shared idiotypes expressed by the human B-cell lymphomas. *New England Journal of Medicine* 321: 851–857.

Miller, R., Maloney, D., Warnke, R., et al. 1982. Treatment of B-cell lymphoma with monoclonal anti-idiotype antibody. *New England Journal of Medicine* 306: 517–522.

Miller, R., Maloney, D., McKillop, J., et al. 1981. *In vivo* effects of murine hybridoma monoclonal antibody in patients with T-cell leukemia. *Blood* 58(1): 78–86.

Miller, R., Oseroff, A., Stratte, P., et al. 1983. Monoclonal antibody therapeutic trials in seven patients with T-cell lymphoma. *Blood* 62: 988–995.

Moir, E. 1989. Nursing care of patients receiving Orthoclone OKT 3. *ANNA Journal* 16(5): 327–328, 366.

Mulshine, J., Magnani, J., and Linnoila, R. 1991. Antibodies in cancer therapy. Section 22.5. Applications of monoclonal antibodies in the treatment of solid tumors. In DeVita, V., Hellman, S., Rosenberg, S. (eds). *Biologic Therapy of Cancer*. Philadelphia: J.B. Lippincott, pp. 563–588.

Murray, J. In press. Radioimmunotherapy of colorectal cancer. In Goldenberg, D. (ed.). *Cancer Therapy with Radiolabeled Antibodies*. Boca Raton, FL: CRC Press.

Murray, J., Macey, D., Kasi, L., et al. 1994. Phase II radioimmunotherapy trial with ^{131}I-CC49 in colorectal cancer. *Cancer* 73: 1057–1066.

Murray, J., Cunningham, J., Brewer, H., et al. 1994. Phase I trial of murine monoclonal antibody 14G2a administered by prolonged intravenous infusion in patients with neuroectodermal tumors. *Journal of Clinical Oncology* 12(1): 184–193.

Negrin, R., Kiem, H., Schmidt-Wolf, H., et al. 1991. Use of polymerase chain reaction to monitor the effectiveness of *ex vivo* tumor cell purging. *Blood* 77(3): 654–660.

Oldham, R. 1991. Custom-tailored drug immunoconjugates in cancer therapy. *Molecular Biotherapy* 3: 148–162.

Oldham, R. 1983. Monoclonal antibody in cancer therapy. *Journal of Clinical Oncology* 1(9): 582–590.

Overmyer, R. 1990. Genetically engineered antibodies improve the therapeutic efficacy of drugs. *Modern Medicine* 58: 38–45.

Pai, L., Bookmen, M., and Ozols, R. 1991. Clinical evaluation of intraperitoneal pseudomonas exotoxin immunoconjugate OVB–3PE in patients with ovarian cancer. *Journal of Clinical Oncology* 9: 2095–2103.

Pastan, D., Willingham, M., and Fitzgerald, D. 1986. Immunotoxins. *Cell* 47: 641–648.

Pimm, M., Jones, J., Price, M., et al. 1982. Tumor localization of monoclonal antibody against a rat mammary carcinoma and suppression of tumor growth with adriamycin-antibody conjugates. *Cancer Immunology Immunotherapy* 12: 125–134.

Press, O., Eary, J., Appelbaum, F., et al. 1993. Radiolabeled antibody therapy of B-cell lymphoma with autologous bone marrow support. *New England Journal of Medicine* 329(12): 1219–1224.

Press, O., Eary, J., Badger, C., et al. 1989. Treatment of refractory non-Hodgkin's lymphoma with radiolabeled MB–1 (Anti-CD37) antibody. *Journal of Clinical Oncology* 7: 1027–1038.

Press, O., Appelbaum, F., Ledbetter, J., et al. 1987. Monoclonal antibody 1F5 (anti-CD20) serotherapy of human B cell lymphomas. *Blood* 69: 584–591.

Redwood, W., Tom, T., and Strand, M. 1984. Specificity, efficacy, and toxicity of radioimmunotherapy in erythroleukemic mice. *Cancer Research* 44: 5681–5687.

Ritz, J., and Schlossman, S. 1982. Utilization of monoclonal antibodies in the treatment of leukemia and lymphoma. *Blood* 59(1): 1–11.

Ritz, J., Pesando, J., Notis-McConarty, J., et al. 1980. Modulation of human acute lymphoblastic leukemia antigen induced by monoclonal antibody *in vitro*. *Journal of Immunology* 125(4): 1506–1514.

Rosen, S., Zimmer, A., Goldman-Leiken, R., et al. 1987. Radioimmunodetection and radioimmunotherapy of cutaneous T-cell lymphomas using ^{131}I-labeled monoclonal antibody: An Illinois Cancer Council Study. *Journal of Clinical Oncology* 5: 562–573.

Rosenberg, S., and Terry, W. 1977. Passive immunotherapy of cancer in animals and man. *Advances in Cancer Research* 25: 323–388.

Russell, S., Llewelyn, M., and Hawkins, R. 1992. Principles of antibody therapy. *British Medical Journal* 305: 1424–1429.

Saleh, M., LoBuglio, A., Plott, W., et al. 1990. A phase II trial of murine monoclonal antibody 17–1A and interferon-gamma: Clinical and immunologic data. *Cancer Immunology and Immunotherapy* 32: 185–190.

Schlom, J. 1991. Antibodies in cancer therapy: Basic principles of monoclonal antibodies. In DeVita, V., Hellman, S., Rosenberg, S. (eds). *Biologic Therapy of Cancer.* Philadelphia: J.B. Lippincott, pp. 464–482.

Schroff, R., Foon, K., Beatty, S., *et al.* 1985. Human anti-murine immunoglobulin responses in patients receiving monoclonal antibody therapy. *Cancer Research Update* 45: 879–885.

Sears, H., Atkinson, B., Mattis, J., *et al.* 1982. Phase I clinical trial of monoclonal antibody in treatment of gastrointestinal tumors. *Lancet* 1: 762–765.

Spitler, L., del Rio, M., Khentigan, A., *et al.* 1987. Therapy of patients with malignant melanoma using a monoclonal antimelanoma antibody-ricin A chain immunotoxin. *Cancer Research* 47: 1717–1723.

Thorpe, P., and Ross, W. 1982. The preparation and cytotoxic properties of antibody-toxin conjugates. *Immunology Review* 62: 119–158.

Tjandra, J., Ramidi, L., and McKenzie, I. 1990. Development of human anti-murine antibody (HAMA) response in patients. *Immunology Cell Biology* 68: 367–376.

Vadhan-Raj, S., Cordon-Cardo, C., Carswell, E., *et al.* 1988. Phase I trial of a mouse monoclonal antibody against GD3 ganglioside in patients with melanoma: Induction of inflammatory responses at tumor sites. *Journal of Clinical Oncology* 6: 1636–1648.

Vitetta, E., and Thorpe, P. 1991. Immunotoxins. In DeVita, V., Hellman, S., Rosenberg, S. (eds). *Biologic Therapy of Cancer.* Philadelphia: J.B. Lippincott, pp. 482–511.

Vitetta, E., Stone, M., Amlot, P., *et al.* 1991. Phase I immunotoxin trial in patients with B-cell lymphoma. *Cancer Research* 51: 4052–4058.

Vitetta, E., Frolick, K., Uhr, J. 1982. Neoplastic B cells as targets for antibody-ricin A chain immunotoxins. *Immunology Review* 62: 9–183.

Vriesendorp, H., Herpst, J., Germack, M., *et al.* 1991. Phase I/II studies of yttrium-labeled antiferritin treatment for end-stage Hodgkin's disease, including Radiation Therapy Oncology Group 87–01. *Journal of Clinical Oncology* 9: 918–928.

Waldman, T. 1991. Antibodies in cancer therapy. Section 22.2. T-cell leukemia/lymphoma. In DeVita, V., Hellman, S., Rosenberg, S. (eds). *Biologic Therapy of Cancer.* Philadelphia: J.B. Lippincott, pp. 523–532.

Wandres, D., and Lau, J. 1992. An overview of orphan drugs. *California Journal of Hospital Pharmacy* 4: 12–13.

Weiner, L., O'Dwyer, J., Kitson, J., *et al.* 1989. Phase I evaluation of an anti-breast carcinoma monoclonal antibody 260F-6 recombinant ricin A chain immunoconjugate. *Cancer Research* 49: 4062–4067.

CHAPTER 8 | Tumor Necrosis Factor

Lynne Brophy, RN, MSN, OCN

For centuries, spontaneous regression and even complete eradication of some tumors have been noticed in patients who have had fever or inflammation (Westphal, 1987; Westphal *et al.*, 1985; Nauts *et al.*, 1953). These findings encouraged physicians in the 19th century to inject cancer patients with pus from patients with erysipelas to see if their tumors would regress. In the late 19th century, Dr. William Coley, a surgeon practicing in New York City, recognized that people often died of sepsis after such treatment. He administered a mixture of gram positive and gram negative bacteria to patients with cutaneous, easily measurable primary or metastatic tumors. Administration of his "Coley's toxins" often elicited a tumor response, including some complete clinical responses (Coley, 1893).

A half-century later, Hartwell and others (1943) discovered that the active ingredient in Coley's toxins was **endotoxin** or lipopolysac-charide, a component of the bacterial cell wall (Westphal *et al.* 1985; Hartwell *et al.*, 1943). Old and others isolated a substance that was produced by activated macrophages, monocytes, and lymphocytes after exposure to endotoxin and called it tumor necrosis factor, or TNF (Carswell *et al.*, 1975). TNF appeared to be responsible for the biological effects seen after a patient was exposed to endotoxin. The gene for TNF was cloned in 1984, making it possible to produce recombinant TNF in large quantities (Old, 1988). With an available supply of TNF, further delineation of its biological activities and clinical trials evaluating its efficacy in cancer patients began.

Two types of TNF exist, and are nearly identical in molecular structure. The first, TNF-alpha (TNF-α), or cachectin, is the cytokine produced by activated macrophages, monocytes, and lymphocytes that was already mentioned (Tracey and Cerami, 1992). It plays a role in tumor necrosis and cell-mediated killing of bacteria, parasites, and neoplastic cells (Spriggs, 1991). The second, TNF-beta (TNF-β), or lymphotoxin, is a cytokine produced by lymphocytes and also has the ability to lyse tumor cells (Spriggs, 1991). Lymphotoxin has some of the same antiproliferative properties as TNF-α and both have multiple effects on normal and tumor cells. Both are induced by other cytokines such as interferon-gamma (IFN-γ) and interleukin–1 (IL–1) and play roles in hemostasis, tissue necrosis, tumor cell destruction, differentiation of leukocytes, septic shock and, cachexia. The focus of this chapter is the biological and therapeutic effects of TNF-α, which will be referred to simply as TNF.

BIOLOGICAL ACTIONS

Vascular Changes

TNF is named for its ability to cause necrosis in tumors and healthy tissue by reducing or stopping the flow of blood to these tissues. This agent acts by damaging the endothelial or inner lining of blood vessels, causing a narrowing or blockage of the lumen of the vessel, or by triggering intravascular coagulation. When normal endothelial cells lining blood vessel walls are exposed to TNF, procoagulant activity is increased: TNF augments secretion of inhibitors of tissue plasminogen activator (a substance capable of initiating fibrinolysis) and stimulates release of platelet-activating factor, resulting in an increased risk of disseminated intravascular coagulation (Medcalf *et al.*, 1988; Schleef and Loskutoff, 1988; Van *et al.*, 1988). Platelet-activing factor increases platelet aggregation, causes bronchoconstriction, activates leukocytes, increases capillary permeability, and decreases cardiac output resulting in hypotension (Stroud, 1990; Littleton, 1988).

When blood begins to clot, inflammatory mediators are released, antigen expression increases, and the functioning of the blood vessel wall changes. These changes result in leakage of fluid into the extravascular space, or swelling. When TNF levels are very high, as in the case of septic shock, the fluid leakage increases incrementally. This phenomenon is known as capillary leak syndrome, and results in hypotension due to decreased intravascular volume.

Effects on Hematopoietic Cells

The activities of TNF in the body increase the number of white blood cells and augment the functioning of the immune system. Tumor necrosis factor affects leukocytes, or white blood cells, in various ways. It induces monocyte differentiation such that a portion of monocytes produced become macrophages, activates monocytes, and mediates monocyte cytotoxicity (Spriggs, 1991). When monocytes are exposed to TNF, their maturation and metabolic rate increases. After this exposure, monocytes secrete cytokines that increase antibody expression and cytokine secretion by other white blood cells. When the production of more lymphocytes is needed, TNF inhibits the proliferation of myeloid cells by decreasing production of white blood cell precursors (Murase *et al.*, 1987; Broxmeyer *et al.*, 1986).

Activation of Immune Mechanisms

Tumor necrosis factor has an indirect role in the production of antibodies and cells needed for cell-mediated immunity through induction of interleukin–6 (IL–6). The changes in antibody expression begin when TNF stimulates production of IL–6 by lymphocytes. Interleukin–6 then stimulates proliferation of B cells and has been shown to inhibit the growth of breast cancer and leukemia-lymphoma cells in animal studies (Spriggs, 1991; Chen *et al.*, 1988). T cells exposed to TNF express more receptors for IL–2, resulting in greater proliferation of T cells (Scheurich *et al.*, 1987), and they also produce more granulocyte colony-stimulating factor and granulocyte macrophage colony-stimulating factor (Lu *et al.*, 1988). (Lymphotoxin (TNF-β) can inhibit these activities of TNF, however). One specific example of an immune system function enhanced by TNF is destruction of foreign or abnormal cells: natural killer and lymphokine-activated T cells triggered by TNF play leading roles in the destruction of tumor cells and pathogens.

Inflammation

As a cytokine, TNF assists in the process of destroying abnormal cells other than tumor cells, such as pathogens. It indirectly destroys pathogens by serving as a mediator in the process of inflammation. Inflammation begins when bacteria invade the tissues of the body. When bacteria that have lipoprotein lipase in their cell walls enter the bloodstream, TNF levels in the serum rise and peak within 90 minutes (Spriggs, 1991). Tumor necrosis factor and lymphotoxin levels are also increased by other cytokines activated (e.g., increased IFN-γ levels) after bacterial invasion. As TNF levels rise, cytokines active in the inflammatory process, such as platelet-activating factor, colony-stimulating factors, neutrophil chemotactic factor, and IL–6 are also produced in increased quantities (Bussolino, et al., 1988; Lapierre et al., 1988; Broudy et al., 1987; Hajjar et al., 1987; Seelentag et al., 1987). After endothelial cells are exposed to increased levels of TNF, they express antigens and leukocyte adhesion molecules that sit on endothelial cell surfaces and increase cellular adhesiveness to leukocytes (Spriggs, 1991; Vadas and Prudzanski, 1990). This makes it easier for white blood cells to stick to the endothelial lining of blood vessels, searching for pathogens to destroy. The effectiveness of this response seems to be dependent on the endothelial cells' receptiveness to TNF (Spriggs, 1991). As the white blood cells flood the intravascular and extravascular sites of invasion by a pathogen, swelling increases and the site becomes inflamed.

After this process, which is called **margination,** has begun, TNF has the ability to directly and indirectly increase the effectiveness of white blood cells involved in humoral and cell-mediated immunity. Tumor necrosis factor indirectly stimulates chemotaxis of polymorphonuclear neutrophils (PMNs) by increasing monocytes' release of monocyte-derived neutrophil chemotactic factor (Spriggs, 1991). This factor aids PMNs in attracting other PMNs to sites where activated monocytes are found, thereby increasing phagocytosis in the area. Exposure to TNF also increases the ability of PMNs to kill pathogens and tumor cells (Djeu, et al., 1988; Shau, 1988; Djeu and Blanchard, 1987; Djeu et al., 1986). Interleukin–1 and TNF activate natural killer cells, T cells, PMNs, and monocytes during the inflammatory process, and TNF amplifies and mediates antibody-dependent cell-mediated cytotoxicity by natural killer and lymphokine-activated killer T cells (Lattime et al. 1988; Ortaldo, 1986). Newly produced antibodies then travel to the site of infection and inflammation and detect and destroy antigens. The increased production of these various cytokines is thought to contribute to the progression from localized inflammation to a systemic inflammatory response.

Systemic inflammatory responses occur in a progressive series of stages called the systemic inflammatory response syndrome (SIRS); septic shock is a late stage of this syndrome. When infection occurs, early inflammatory changes are characterized by increased temperature, tachycardia, tachypnea, hypoxia, and leukopenia or leukocytosis (Stroud, 1990; Littleton, 1988). Interleukin–1, or endogenous pyrogen, is one of the cytokines stimulated by TNF during SIRS. (Table 8.1 compares the biological actions of TNF and IL–1, highlighting their many similarities). After an infectious agent, such as a gram negative bacteria, enters the bloodstream, macrophages are stimulated by toxins produced by this agent. These macrophages produce TNF, the level of which peaks in the blood stream within 2 hours (Fraker et al., 1992; Hesse et al., 1988). Tumor necrosis factor induces fever by stimulating IL–1 production (fever is discussed in detail in Chapter 12), but this stimulation can be inhibited by the administration of dexame-

Table 8.1 Similarities between TNF and Il-1

	TNF	IL-1
Pyrogen	x	x
Bone resorption	x	x
Lipoprotein lipase inhibition	x	x
Procoagulant release	x	x
Endothelial-cell adhesion molecules expression	x	x
Induce colony-stimulating factors	x	x
Induce IL-1, IL-6, and TNF	x	x
Radioprotective effects	x	x
Induce myeloid differentiation	x	x
Leukocyte chemotaxis	x/0	x
Neutrophil activation	x	x
Monocyte activation	x	x
T-cell activation	x	x
Direct tumor cell cytotoxicity	x	0
Fibroblast proliferation	x	x
Thymocyte proliferation	0	x

Source: Reprinted with permission from: Spriggs, D. 1991. Tumor necrosis factor: Basic principles and preclinical studies. In DeVita, V., Hellman, S., Rosenberg, S. (eds). *Biologic Therapy of Cancer.* Philadelphia: J.B. Lippincott, pp. 365 Table 16–11.

thasone (Spriggs, 1991). The activation of cytokine and humoral cascades (complement, coagulation, and kinin) are manifested by the symptoms of late SIRS: fever, hypotension, intravascular coagulation, inflammation, and multisystem organ failure. Efforts to blunt the negative effects of TNF during SIRS are described later in this chapter.

Immunologic Surveillance

Tumor necrosis factor clearly plays an important role in the body's defense against tumor development and infection, but it also has a role in destroying tumors that already are in place. The exact mechanisms of TNF's cytotoxic actions against tumor cells are not yet known, but two clues have been discovered. First, it is known that TNF and IFN-γ act synergistically to destroy tumor cells (Old, 1988): more tumor cells are killed when levels of these cytokines are increased. Second, TNF, along with IL–2 and IL–1, indirectly plays a

role in tumor cell killing by activating natural killer cells (Spriggs, 1991). Proposed antitumor mechanisms include direct action by killing tumor cells or indirect activity through blocking tumor blood vessels, promotion of the inflammatory response, stimulation of macrophage cytotoxicity and tumor-specific cytotoxic antibodies (Balkwill, 1989).

Lipid Metabolism

Another effect of TNF on the body is **cachexia**, or wasting of body fat and protein, which is caused by accelerated lipid metabolism. Cachexia results in weight loss and is accompanied by anorexia and wasting of the body tissues. Both TNF and lymphotoxin contribute to cachexia by reversing the growth of adipocytes (fat cells), resulting in impaired lipogenesis and a catabolic state (Torti *et al.,* 1989). Tumor necrosis factor also influences the activity of lipase, the enzyme that assists with fat processing and storage in the body, in two ways. It increases lipase activity, thereby increasing the rate at which fats are used, and inhibits the activity of enzymes that lyse lipids (Zechner *et al.,* 1988; Min and Spiegelman, 1986; Pekala *et al.,* 1983). It also changes the basal metabolic rate by stimulating hepatic cells to synthesize more lipids, DNA, albumin, transferrin, and acute phase proteins, including some forms of complement (Feingold *et al.,* 1988; Grunfeld *et al.,* 1988; Feingold and Grunfeld, 1987). It has been hypothesized that TNF acts as an endogenous antineoplastic agent by preventing the provision of energy (fat) to tumor cells in the body while they grow (Urban *et al.,* 1986).

For these and many other reasons, recombinant TNF has been given as an antineoplastic agent in many clinical studies during the past decade. The rationale for its clinical use is that the biological effects seen in preclinical studies, including its ability to survey and destroy tumor cells, block the blood supply to tumors, and indirectly induce fever, and its indirect role in antibody production would translate to tumor destruction in humans.

CLINICAL STUDIES

Recombinant TNF has been given as therapy for melanoma, colorectal carcinoma, AIDS-related Kaposi's sarcoma, B-cell lymphoma, non-small-cell lung cancer, ovarian cancer, and glioma (Lienard *et al.*, 1992a; Lienard *et al.*, 1992b; Yoshida *et al.*, 1992; del Giglio *et al.*, 1991; Heim *et al.*, 1990; Kauffmann *et al.*, 1990; Schaadt *et al.*, 1990; Yang *et al.*, 1990; Kahn *et al.*, 1989; Chapman *et al.*, 1987). To date, TNF has not provided significant effective palliative or curative therapy for any type of cancer. Important clinical trials with recombinant human TNF are summarized in Tables 8.2–8.4. Occasional partial responses and rare complete responses have been seen. Toxicity, maximum tolerated doses, and responses in these clinical trials may vary because of differences in preparation of TNF, patient populations, treatment schedules, and side effect interventions (Alexander and Rosenberg, 1991). Patients who have received TNF in phase I clinical trials have often been heavily treated before and for this reason may not have responded well to the therapy.

Dosing

Recombinant TNF can be administered intravenously, intra-arterially, intratumorally, intramuscularly, or subcutaneously. Intravenous therapy can be given as a bolus or by continuous infusion. When given intravenously, recombinant TNF has a half-life of 16 minutes, which accounts for the typical transience of its side effects (Blick *et al.*, 1987). No one route or schedule for administering TNF has proven to be most successful. Long continuous intravenous infusions may provide the highest blood levels and longest exposure to TNF. The maximum tolerated doses of TNF in various clinical trials are highlighted in Tables 8.2–8.4.

COMBINATION THERAPY

With the goal of increasing its efficacy as an antineoplastic agent, TNF has been given in clinical trials in combination with other agents with which it is known to be synergistic. The cytotoxic abilities of TNF were enhanced *in vitro* when TNF was combined with the IFNs, mitotic inhibiting agents, actinomycin-D, 5-fluorouracil, cyclophosphamide, cisplatin, doxorubicin, or etopside, or with ionizing radiation or induced hyperthermia (Spriggs, 1991; Demetri *et al.*, 1989; Williamson *et al.*, 1983). Clinical trials of some of these combinations are in progress and have not been widely reported in the literature. One of the difficulties in administering TNF in combination with other antineoplastic agents is the additive toxicities and, in some cases, a side-effect pattern very different from that seen with single-agent TNF therapy.

Human studies of TNF in combination with other cytokines have revealed some differences in side-effect patterns (Negrier *et al.*, 1992; Yang *et al.*, 1990; Kurzrock *et al.*, 1989). Some of this activity may be due to the ability of IFN-γ to increase the expression of TNF receptors on cell surfaces, thereby enhancing the effect of TNF on human cells (Aggarwal *et al.*, 1985). Interferon-gamma has the ability to make TNF-resistant cells sensitive to TNF's antiproliferative effects (Fransen *et al.*, 1986; Sugarman *et al.*, 1985). Abbruzzese and others (1989) administered intramuscular IFN-γ every day and recombinant TNF by intravenous bolus every 8 hours for five days to patients with advanced gastrointestinal cancer. Because of hyperbilirubinemia, the maximum tolerated dose was established at 150 µg/m^2/day for both agents. Demetri and colleagues (1989) administered subcutaneous interferon-gamma daily and recombinant TNF by intravenous bolus. They found the dose limiting toxicity was hypotension at a dose of 136 µg/m^2 of rTNF and 200 µg/m^2 of IFN-γ.

The rationale for administering TNF and IL–2 together stems from preclinical studies.

Table 8.2 Phase I studies of recombinant TNF in patients with advanced malignancy–intravenous (IV) bolus administration

Author	Manufacturer	N	Histologic Type and Site*	Administration	MTD †	Dose-Limiting Toxicity
Kimura et al.	Asahi	33	Lung Gastric Colon	Single IV bolus	227µg/m²	Hypotension
Moritz et al.	Knoll	19	Colon CML‡ Renal	Daily IV bolus x 5 every 3 weeks	200µg/m²	Hypotension
Feinberg et al.	Genentech	39	Colon Melanoma Lung	Daily IV bolus x 5 every 2 weeks	200µg/m²	Constitutional symptoms, hypotension
Creagan et al.	Genentech	27	Colon Melanoma Pancreas	Daily IV bolus x 5 every 2–3 weeks	150µg/m²	Hypotension, phlebitis
Taguchi	Dainippon	43	Gastric Colorectal Hepatoma	Daily IV bolus x 3 every week§	333µg/pt‖	Hypotension
Lenk et al.	Asahi	15	Not given	Single IV bolus	782µg/m²	Hypotension
Bollon et al.	Wadley Institutes	18	Colon Lung Breast	IV bolus every other day	15 mg/kg¶	Constitutional symptoms, nausea and vomiting, diarrhea
Creaven et al.	Asahi	29	Renal Colon Lung	Single IV bolus	218µg/m²	Hypotension
Creaven et al.	Asahi	33	Renal Lung Head and neck	Daily IV bolus x 5	272µg/m²	Hepatotoxicity, hypotension
Walsh et al.	Knoll	16	Colon Melanoma Sarcoma	IV bolus 3 times weekly	> 200# µg/m²	NA**
Selby et al.	Asahi	18	Melanoma Lymphoma	Single IV bolus every 2 weeks x 3	363µg/m²	Hypotension, hepatotoxicity, leukopenia
Rosenberg et al.	Cetus	39	Melanoma Renal Colorectal Breast	Daily IV bolus x 3	300µg/m²	Hypotension

* Histologic type and site shown are the most frequent for each series.
† Maximum tolerated dose calculated from manufacturer's specific activity.
‡ Chronic myelogenous leukemia.
§ Study also describes ten patients given intratumoral injection not included here.
‖ Dose given in micrograms per patient, body-surface area not stated.
¶ Dose not administered per body-surface area.
# MTD not yet reached.
** Not yet applicable.

Source: Alexander: *Biologic Therapy of Cancer* © 1991 J.B. Lippincott. Reprinted by permission of the current copyright holder Boston Jones and Bartlett Publishers.

Table 8.3   Phase I stuies of recombinant TNF in patients with advanced malignancy–intramuscular (IM) and mixed administration

Author	Manufacturer	N	Histologic Type and Site*	Administration	MTD	Dose-Limiting Toxicity
Bartsch et al.	Genentech	30	Colorectal Renal Lung	IM thrice weekly for 8 weeks	150μg/m²	Hypotension, constitutional symptoms, local reaction at injection site
Jakubowski et al.	Genentech	19	Gastrointestinal Melanoma Breast	IM daily for 5 days every other week	150μg/m²	Local reaction at injection site, hepatotoxicity, leukopenia, thrombocytopenia
Blick et al.	Genentech	20	Colon Renal Multiple myeloma	Alternating IM and IV bolus twice weekly for 4 weeks	ND‡	NA§
Chapman et al	Genentech	26	Melanoma Renal Sarcoma Breast Colon	Alternating SQ and IV bolus twice weekly for 4 weeks‖	ND	NA

* Histologic type and site shown are the most frequent for each series.
† Maximum tolerated dose calculated from manufacturer's specific activity.
‡ Not determined.
§ Not applicable.
‖ SQ, subcutaneous.

Source: Alexander: *Biologic Therapy of Cancer* © 1991 J.B. Lippincott. Reprinted by permission of the current copyright holder Boston Jones and Bartlett Publishers.

The need for participation of activated lymphocytes in the destruction of murine tumors (Asher *et al.*, 1989) during treatment with TNF suggested strategies to augment antitumor effects of lymphocytes might increase the therapeutic response to TNF. Interleukin–2 is known to play a pivotal role in stimulation of cytotoxic lymphocytes. Negrier and others (1992) conducted a clinical trial of continuous intravenous infusion of IL–2 (18 MIU/m²/day) for six days followed by single bolus infusions of TNF daily for three days. Patients on this trial had a variety of refractory malignancies. The side-effect profile of the combination of TNF and IL–2 is different from that of single-agent TNF therapy. The dose-limiting side effect on this trial was hypotension, and

the maximum tolerated dose of TNF was judged to be 120 μg/m²/day. Despite the fact that all patients received an intravenous infusion of indomethacin during the entire length of therapy, they experienced all the side effects seen with TNF and IL–2 when given as single agents. However, patients who received the combination regimen developed hypotension requiring dopamine therapy earlier in the treatment cycles and at lower doses of TNF (60 to 80 μg/m²/day). One third of the patients treated on this study also experienced life-threatening pulmonary toxic effects in the form of adult respiratory distress syndrome, anaphylaxis, or bronchospasm. Pulmonary toxic effects were more common and severe in the group

Table 8.4 Phase I studies of recombinant TNF in patients with advanced malignancy—continuous intravenous (IV) administration

Author	Manufacturer	N	Histologic Type and Site	Administration	MTD † μg/m²/ day	Dose-Limiting Toxicity
Spriggs et al.	Asahi	50	Lung Colon Breast	24 hours continuous IV infusion every 3 weeks	545	Hypotension
Steinmetz et al.	Asahi	16	Not given	24 hours continuous IV infusion	261‡	Hypotension, fever, fluid retention, altered sensorium
Sherman et al.	Asahi	19	Colorectal Breast Lung	5 days continuous IV infusion every 28 days	136	Thrombocytopenia, leukopenia
Wiedenmann et al.	Knoll	15	Colorectal Renal	24 hours continuous IV infusion once or twice weekly	200	Fever, chills, myalgias, fatigue, thrombocytopenia
Schwartz et al.	Cetus	18	Colon Renal	5 days continuous IV infusion every 2 weeks	30–40§	Fatigue, confusion, thrombocytopenia, seizures, arrhythmia, hypotension

* Histologic type and site shown are the most frequent for each series.
† Maximum tolerated dose calculated from manufacturer's specific activity.
‡ Without cyclooxygenase inhibitors to ameliorate toxicity.
§ Study included intrapatient dose escalation.

Source: Alexander: Biologic Therapy of Cancer © 1991 J.B. Lippincott. Reprinted by permission of the current copyright holder Boston Jones and Bartlett Publishers.

that received the combination than in patients who received TNF or IL–2 alone. Only two partial remissions were seen in this study, one in a person with breast cancer and the other in a person with renal cell carcinoma. The authors reported they have started a phase II trial of the combination of TNF and IL–2 for women with advanced breast cancer (Negrier et al., 1992).

Researchers have begun to combine TNF with chemotherapeutic agents in attempts to achieve synergistic toxicity. TNF has been given with etoposide, melphalan, and as an accompaniment to induced hyperthermia. Published reports have focused on the side effects seen with these combinations, not the responses. In two different studies of combinations of TNF and etoposide, it was found

that patients experienced not only the side effects seen with single-agent TNF and etoposide therapy, but also a profound myelosuppression (Sherman et al., 1992; Orr et al., 1989). Only Lienard and others (1992) have achieved one of the few exciting results with combination therapy: they administered TNF via isolated limb perfusion with IFN-gamma, melphalan, or as an accompaniment to hyperthermia to patients with refractory melanoma or sarcoma. Eighty-nine percent of patients in this trial responded to therapy. This study, which indicates an exciting new direction for TNF therapy, will be discussed in Chapter 16. Other human studies have investigated ways of stopping the actions of TNF in the body, for example, during SIRS, in order to decrease tissue damage (Exley, 1990).

REGULATORY APPROVAL

Tumor necrosis factor has not yet been approved by the Food and Drug Administration (FDA) for open-label use as an antineoplastic agent.

ADVERSE EFFECTS

The multiple side effects associated with therapeutic administration of TNF reflect the protein's many physiological effects. The side-effect profile associated with TNF therapy is very much dependent on the dose and route used. For example, patients receiving high-dose intravenous therapy are more likely to have hypotension, fever, severe rigors, and focal neurological deficits such as aphasia. Individuals receiving low-dose subcutaneous therapy may experience local skin reaction at the injection site and mild flu-like symptoms. It is very important for the clinician to be aware of the self-limiting transitory nature of the side effects associated with TNF therapy.

A transient but significant side effect of TNF therapy is chills, which can progress to severe rigors and are usually followed by fever. Flu-like symptoms accompany the development of fever during and after TNF therapy and may include fatigue, anorexia, nausea, vomiting, diarrhea, malaise, and headaches (Alexander and Rosenberg, 1991). Chills related to TNF are a part of the physiological stage of fever. Fever begins with TNF stimulating the production of IL–1; IL–1 then stimulates the hypothalamus to produce fever. Moldawer and Figlin (1988) reported TNF-associated headaches as being dull, aching, frontal in location, and decreasing in severity and frequency as therapy progresses. Vasoconstriction and **piloerection** of the skin are followed by shivering or chilling. The chilling phase can be, but is not always, followed by rigoring, a generalized, involuntary shaking of the body. The rigor or chill increases the body temperature, after which the chilling or rigoring stops and a sensation of warmth returns.

Fever and chills may appear at all dose levels of TNF therapy. Severe chills or rigors are one of the hallmarks of high-dose TNF therapy and are quite frightening to the patient and his/her significant other. Chills can begin as soon as an hour after beginning TNF therapy and are followed by fever. The pattern of fever onset, duration, and curve associated with TNF therapy varies according to dose and schedule of therapy (Creaven *et al.,* 1989; Blick *et al.,* 1987; Feinberg *et al.,* 1987). Mild chills associated with low-dose TNF therapy will last for only a short time and usually cause only minor discomfort. Severe rigoring, lasting longer than a few minutes and causing the patient and the bed to shake, is quite uncomfortable and frightening. Refer to Chapter 12 for guidance on how to handle chills and rigors.

Flu-like symptoms can be accompanied by hypotension and capillary leak syndrome. Hypotension occurs at different time points during therapy, depending on the route of administration and the dose of TNF, and has been the dose-limiting side effect in many clinical trials (Alexander and Rosenberg, 1991; Taguchi, 1987; Feinberg *et al.,* 1987). Any patient who receives TNF may experience hypotension, but those with a history of cardiac disease are more susceptible. Hypotension is most common in persons receiving intravenous therapy in doses equal to or greater than 100 $\mu g/m^2$ and almost always occurs in patients who receive 200 $\mu g/m^2$ or more of TNF intravenously. Because of this, 200 $\mu g/m^2$ has often been considered the maximum tolerated dose in clinical trials. The hypotension experienced by persons receiving TNF may be a result of capillary leak syndrome (Tracey and Cerami, 1992). When doses are higher than 100 $\mu g/m^2$, patients are often prehydrated with a bolus of normal saline.

Although TNF is not a vesicant, it can cause irritation of the skin characterized by erythema with or without induration and tenderness (Moldawer and Figlin, 1988). Injection site reactions are most common with intramuscular and subcutaneous TNF therapy. Reactions to TNF doses of less than 150 $\mu g/m^2$

usually occur 24 to 48 hours after the injection, resolve within two to three days, and are self-limiting (Jakubowski *et al.*, 1989; Moldawer and Figlin, 1988). No therapy is needed for these minor reactions. Patients who receive TNF doses equal to or more than 150 μg/m² intramuscularly or 100 μg/m² subcutaneously are at risk for more severe skin reactions, which may include bulla formation at the injection site followed by ulceration and ensuing necrosis. Bulla formation can be prevented by dividing the dose and administering it into two sites, preferably the deltoid areas (Zamkoff *et al.*, 1989). The cause of this skin reaction is not known.

Other transitory acute reactions to TNF, such as changes in laboratory values, are like skin reactions in that they usually prove to be harmless. Multiple transitory changes in laboratory parameters may be seen at some dose levels. Changes in the complete blood count may include leukopenia, thrombocytopenia, and transient leukocytosis, especially elevations in monocyte counts. Increases in white blood cell counts during and after administration of TNF have stimulated the production of colony-stimulating factors, which increase production of white blood cells. Leukocytosis is transient: the leukocyte count usually does not exceed 20,000/mm³ for more than a day and the elevated leukocyte count resolves completely within a few days after therapy has ended. Thrombocytopenia is most common in patients who receive continuous intravenous or lengthy intramuscular therapy and is a result of platelets being used during the process of capillary thrombosis and hemorrhagic necrosis (Moldawer and Figlin, 1988). Thrombocytopenia can be accompanied by elevated levels of fibrin degradation products and reduced levels of fibrinogen, both of which resolve within a few days (Creaven *et al.*, 1987; Kimura *et al.*, 1987). Brown and others (1991) discovered laboratory evidence of disseminated intravascular coagulopathy in 11 of 22 patients treated with intravenous bolus infusions of TNF (30 minutes daily × five days). In addition, 3 of the 11 patients had clinical signs of coagulopathy, including pulmonary emboli. Tumor necrosis factor stimulates acute phase protein biosynthesis by the liver, resulting in increased hepatic transaminase levels, particularly SGOT, SGPT, and BUN, and severe hypophosphatemia, which may be accompanied by cardiac arrhythmias (Tracey and Cerami, 1992; del Giglio *et al.*, 1991; Taguchi, 1987). Administration of TNF may also affect other tests such as lung diffusion capacity (DLCO).

Some patients who receive TNF therapy, both those with and without previous lung disease, have experienced dyspnea during and after administration of TNF and, when tested during or after therapy, have been found to have decreased DLCO (Kuei *et al.*, 1989; Moldawer and Figlin, 1988; Creaven *et al.*, 1987; Kiura, 1987; Taguchi, 1988). Morice and others (1987) noted dyspnea in patients who received TNF on a phase I clinical trial. Pulmonary function testing on these patients revealed that patients who received moderate to high doses of TNF (> 50 μg/m²), or greater cumulative doses, had acute, reversible changes in respiratory function as evidenced by decreased DLCO values. The DLCO levels returned to near baseline levels in all patients within two weeks after discontinuing therapy. Morice and his colleagues (1987) suggested that changes in respiratory function were due to endothelial changes within the lung and to pulmonary edema. Kuei and colleagues (1989) felt that cytotoxic damage occurred to alveolar capillary endothelium resulting in increased capillary leak. They also found higher rates of decreased pulmonary function in patients receiving intramuscular TNF. The potential for these changes make it advisable to do pulmonary function testing before TNF therapy and to monitor the respiratory status of patients carefully for dyspnea while they are receiving TNF. Further research is needed to determine what level of baseline respiratory dysfunction indicates that a patient is not able to receive TNF therapy.

Patients with baseline neurological deficits may not be good candidates for TNF therapy because of the risk of central nervous system (CNS) toxicity. Toxic effects of the CNS can include focal neurological deficits, such as aphasia, confusion, seizures, and cerebral vascular accidents (Moldawer and Figlin, 1988). Patients who experience these side effects should have therapy discontinued immediately and be carefully evaluated to determine the cause of the symptoms.

Clinicians caring for persons who are receiving TNF must be vigilant in assessing for the toxic effects of TNF therapy. When the treatment dose, route, and schedule have been chosen, patients should be educated about when fever and flu-like symptoms may occur (if known). In general, persons with a history of coagulation, cardiac, pulmonary, hepatic, renal or neurologic disorders may not be good candidates for TNF therapy.

Clinicians administering TNF in combination with other antineoplastic agents must be aware that side effect profiles may change or side effects may worsen when combination therapy is given. For example, side effects in patients who received TNF and IFN-γ included fever and flu-like symptoms, which differed from those in patients who received TNF alone: although hepatic transaminase levels did not increase significantly in patients who received TNF alone, alkaline phosphatase and lactic acid dehydrogenase did increase in the patients who received the combination (DeMulder *et al.,* 1989).

SUMMARY

Tumor necrosis factor has not proven to be the "magic bullet" many people hoped it would be. Of course, TNF, like other biological response modifiers, is very different from chemotherapeutic agents in that it has a wide range of effects on both normal and cancer cells. For this reason, routes and schedules of administration traditionally used with chemotherapy have not been very effective with TNF. Clinical trials with TNF continue, despite disappointing results in the past, in order to find the most effective way to give TNF.

Future clinical trials will need to employ the maximal tolerated dose of TNF, since the success of TNF therapy seems to depend on high concentrations, and responses are more common with higher doses (Frei and Spriggs, 1989). Although TNF therapy in animal experiments has usually resulted in necrosis of the vascular supply to the tumor, this has not always been the case in human trials, giving clinical researchers the clue that higher blood concentrations of TNF may be needed to have this effect. Unfortunately, severe side effects are associated with high blood concentrations of TNF in humans. In the future, dexamethasone and other inhibitors of inflammation may be given to prevent or minimize the side effects associated with SIRS.

The schedule and route of administration of TNF therapy may need to be changed. In the future, TNF will most likely be given intravenously for 12 to 36 hours to keep the concentration of TNF in the blood high, thereby maximizing its effects. More information needs to be gathered about how TNF gets into the tumor's vasculature and which methods assist in this process. Future routes of administration may include intra-arterial or intratumoral therapy as a means to assist TNF in reaching tumor neovasculature. Moreover, other BRMs or chemotherapy may be given before, in conjunction with, or after administration of TNF in an attempt to produce a synergistic effect against tumor cells. The challenge that lies ahead is to find the most effective way of combining these methods to kill tumor cells with the fewest and mildest side effects.

Future clinical trials may attempt to block the adverse effects of TNF during SIRS. The damaging effects of TNF on healthy body tissues have already been discussed. It has been hypothesized that if the systemic effects of TNF could be blunted during SIRS, the syndrome would not progress into septic shock and multisystem organ failure. In one laboratory study, it was discovered that TNF production in the body can be slowed through administration of dexamethasone before the cells are exposed to bacteria (Spriggs, 1991).

When white blood cells that produce TNF are exposed first to lipopolysaccharide, the main component of bacterial cell walls, and then to dexamethasone, TNF production is slowed (Beutler *et al.*, 1986). Although this is helpful information, the key step in this research will be to discover whether small amounts of dexamethasone should be given to patients with sepsis early in the SIRS process to prevent damage.

An alternative method of blunting the effect of TNF during sepsis may be use of a monoclonal antibody that is targeted to attach to TNF. In an attempt to reduce TNF-related morbidity during sepsis, monoclonal antibodies to TNF have been developed and administered to laboratory animals and humans with sepsis in clinical trials. The anti-TNF monoclonal antibody was most successful in animal experiments when it was given 2 hours before endotoxin challenge (Tracey *et al.*, 1987). Naturally, in the clinical setting health care workers are not able to predict pathogenic invasion 2 hours before it occurs. Exley and others (1990) administered an anti-TNF monoclonal antibody to 14 persons with severe sepsis. They found that, despite improvments in mean arterial pressure one day after administration, 11 of 14 patients in the study later died of sepsis. Further studies are needed to determine the role of anti-TNF antibodies in the treatent of sepsis and to discover the optimal time to administer anti-TNF monoclonal antibodies in SIRS.

Future clinical trials may employ TNF-β (lyphotoxin) as an antineoplastic agent; none have yet been reported. It is known that lyphotoxin's cytotoxic activity is increased when doxorubicin, cyclophosphamide, etoposide, or bleoycin is given *in vitro* (Spriggs, 1991). It is interesting to note that despite the fact that the structures of lyphotoxin and TNF are similar, they are synergistic with different chemotherapeutic agents. Perhaps one day we will have the ability to manipulate the effects of TNF-α and TNF-β to patients' therapeutic advantage.

References

Abbruzzesse, J., Levin, B., Ajani, J., *et al.* 1989. Phase I trial of recombinant human gamma interferon and recombinant human tumor necrosis factor in patients with advanced gastrointestinal cancer. *Cancer Research* 49(14): 4057–4061.

Aggarwal, B., Eessalu, E., and Hass, P. 1985. Characterization of receptors for human tumor necrosis factor and their regulation by gamma-interferon. *Nature* 318(6047): 665–667.

Alexander, R., and Rosenberg, S. 1991. Tumor necrosis factor: Clinical applications. In DeVita, V., Hellman, S., Rosenberg, S. (eds). *Biologic Therapy of Cancer.* Philadelphia: J.B. Lippincott, pp. 378–392.

Asher, A., Mulé, J., and Rosenberg, S. 1989. Recombinant human tumor necrosis factor mediates regression of a murine sarcoma in vivo via Lyt–2+ cells. *Cancer Immunology and Immunotherapy* 28(2): 153–156.

Balkwill, F. 1989. Tumor Necrosis Factor. In Balkwill, F. (ed). *Cytokines in Cancer Therapy.* Oxford: Oxford University Press, pp. 54–87.

Bartsch, H., Nagel, G., Mull, R., *et al.* 1988. Phase I study of recombinant human tumor necrosis factor-alpha in patients with advanced malignancies. *Molecular biotherapy* 1: 21–29.

Beutler, B., Krochin, N., Milsark, I., *et al.* 1986. Control of cachectin (tumor necrosis factor) synthesis: mechanisms of endotoxin resistance. *Science* 232(4753): 977–980.

Blick, M., Sherwin, S., and Rosenblum, M. 1987. Phase I study of recombinant tumor necrosis factor in cancer patients. *Cancer Research* 47: 2986–2989.

Bollon, A., Berent, S., Torczynski, R., *et al.* 1988. Human cytokines, tumor necrosis factor, and interferons: Gene cloning, animal studies, and clinical trials. *Journal of Cell Biochemistry* 36: 353–367.

Broudy, V., Harlan, J., and Adamson, J. 1987. Disparate effects of tumor necrosis factor-alpha/cachectin and tumor necrosis factor-beta/lymphotoxin on hematopoietic growth factor production and neutrophil adhesion molecule expression by cultured human endothelial cells. *Journal of Immunology* 138(12): 4298–4302.

Brown, T., Goddman, P., Fleming, T., *et al.* 1991. A phase II trial of recombinant tumor necrosis factor in patients with adenocarcinoma of the pancreas: A southwest oncology group study. *Journal of Immunotherapy* 10(5): 376–378.

Broxeyer, H., Williams, D., Lu, L., *et al.* 1986. The suppressive influences of human tumor necrosis factors on bone marrow hematopoietic progenitor cells from normal donors and patients with leukemia: Synergism of tumor necrosis factor and interferon-gamma. *Journal of Immunology* 136(12): 4487–4495.

Bussolino, F., Cammussi, G., and Baglioni, C. 1988. Synthesis and release of platelet-activating factor by human vascular endothelial cells treated with tumor necrosis factor or interleukin–1 alpha. *Journal of Biological Chemistry* 263(24): 11856–11861.

Carswell, E., Old, L., Kassel, R., et al. 1975. An endotoxin-induced serum factor which causes necrosis of tumors. *Proceedings of the National Academy of Sciences USA* 72: 3666–3670.

Chapman, P., Lester, T., Casper, E., et al. 1987. Clinical pharmacology of recombinant human tumor necrosis factor in patients with advanced cancer. *Journal of Clinical Oncology* 2(12): 1942–1951.

Chen, L., Mory, Y., Zilbertein, A., et al. 1988. Growth inhibition of human breast carcinoma and leukemia/lymphoma cell lines by recombinant interferon-beta 2. *Proceedings of the National Academy of Sciences USA* 85: 8037–8041.

Coley, W. 1893. The treatment of malignant tumors by repeated inoculations of erysipelas, with a report of ten original cases. *American Journal of Medical Science* 105: 487–511.

Creagan, E., Kovach, J., Moertel, C., et al. 1988. A phase I clinical trial of recombinant human tumor necrosis factor. *Cancer* 62: 24676–2471.

Creaven, P., Brenner, D., Cowens, W. 1989. Phase I clinical trial of recombinant human tumor necrosis factor (rH-TNF) given on a daily × 5 schedule. *Cancer Chemotherapy and Pharmacology* 23(3): 186–191.

Creaven, P., Plager, J., Dupere, S., et al. 1987. Phase I clinical trial of recombinant human tumor necrosis factor. *Cancer Chemotherapy and Pharmacology* 20: 137–144.

del Giglio, A., Zukiwski, A., Ali, K., et al. 1991. Severe, symptomatic, dose-limiting hypophosphatemia induced by hepatic arterial infusion of recombinant tumor necrosis factor in patients with liver metastases. *Cancer* 67(10): 2459–2461.

DeMulder, P., Debruyne, F., Rikken, G., et al. 1989. Recombinant tumor necrosis factor alpha and interferon-gamma in the treatent of advanced renal cell carcinoma. *Proceedings of the American Society of Clinical Oncology* 7: 164 (abstract).

Demetri, G., Spriggs, D., Sherman, M., Arthur, K. 1989. A phase I trial of recombinant human tumor necrosis factor and interferon-gamma: effects of combination cytokine administration in vivo. *Journal of Clinical Oncology* 7(10); 1545–1553.

Djeu, J., Blanchard, D., Klein, T., et al. 1988. Protective effects of tumor necrosis factor in experimental *Legionella pneumophilia* infections of mice via activation of PMN function. *Journal of Leukocyte Biology* 43(5): 429–435.

Djeu, J., and Blanchard, D. 1987. Regulation of human polymorphonuclear neutrophil (PMN) activity against *Candida albicans* by large granular lymphocytes via release of a PMN-activating factor. *Journal of Immunology* 139(8): 2761–2767.

Djeu, J., Blanchard, D., Halkias, D., et al. 1986. Growth inhibition of *Candida albicans* by human polymorphonuclear neutrophils: Activation by interferon-gamma and tumor necrosis factor. *Journal of Immunology* 137(9): 2980–2984.

Exley, A., Cohen, J., Buurman, W., et al. 1990. Monoclonal antibody to TNF in severe septic shock. *Lancet* 335: 1275–1277.

Feinberg, B., Kurzrock, R., Talpaz, M., et al. 1988. A phase I trial of intravenously-administered recombinant tumor necrosis factor-alpha in cancer patients. *Journal of Clinical Oncology* 6: 1328–1334.

Feinberg, B., Kurzrock, R., Blick, M., et al. 1987. Phase I study of recombinant tumor necrosis factor in patients with disseminated cancer. *Proceedings of the American Society of Clinical Oncology* 6: 238 (abstract).

Feingold, K., and Grunfeld, C. 1987. Tumor necrosis factor-alpha stimulates hepatic lipogenesis in the rat *in vivo. Journal of Clinical Investigation* 80(1): 184–190.

Feingold, K., Soued, M., and Grunfeld, C. 1988. Tumor necrosis factor stimulates DNA synthesis in the liver of rats. *Biochemical and Biophysical Research Communications* 153(2): 576–582.

Figlin, R., de Kerion, J., and Sarna, G. 1988. Phase II study of recombinant tumor necrosis factor (rTNF) in patients with metastatic renal cell carcinoma (rCCa) and malignant melanoma (MM). *Proceedings of the American Society of Clinical Oncology* 7: 169 (abstract).

Fraker, D., Alexander, H., and Norton, J. 1992. Biologic therapy of sepsis: The role of antibodies to endotoxin and tumor necrosis factor and the interleukin–1 receptor antagonist. In DeVita, V., Hellman, S., & Rosenberg, S. (eds). *Biologic Therapy of Cancer Updates* 2(3) Philadelphia: J.B. Lippincott, pp. 1–12.

Fransen, L., Van, D., Ruysschaert, R., et al. 1986. Recombinant tumor necrosis factor: Its effect and its synergism with interferon-gamma on a variety of normal and transformed human cell lines. *European Journal of Cancer and Clinical Oncology* 22(4): 419–426.

Frei, E., and Spriggs, D. 1989. Tumor necrosis factor: Still a promising agent. *Journal of Clinical Oncology* 7(3): 291–294.

Grunfeld, C., Verdier, J., Neese, R., et al. 1988. Mechanisms by which tumor necrosis factor stimulates hepatic fatty acid synthesis *in vivo. Journal of Lipid Research* 29(10): 1327–1335.

Hajjar, K., Hajjar, D., Silverstein, R., et al. 1987. Tumor necrosis factor-mediated release of platelet-derived growth factor from cultured endothelial cells. *Journal of Experimental Medicine* 166(1): 1235–1245.

Hartwell, J., Shear, M., and Adams, J. 1943. Nature of the hemmorrhage-producing fraction from *Serratia marcescens (B. prodigiosus)* culture filtrates. *Journal of the National Cancer Institute* 4: 107–122.

Heim, M., Siegund, R., Illiger, H., et al. 1990. Tumor necrosis factor in advanced colorectal cancer: A phase II study. A trial of the phase I/II study group of the Association for Medical Oncology of the German Cancer Society. *Onkologie* 13(6): 444–447.

Hesse, D., Tracey, K., Fong, H., et al. 1988. Cytokine appearance in human endotoxemia and primate bacteremia. *Surgery, Gynecology and Obstetrics* 166(2): 147–153.

Jakubowski, A., Casper, E., Gabrilove, J., et al. 1989. Phase I trial of intramuscularly administered tumor necrosis factor in patients with advanced cancer. *Journal of Clinical Oncology* 7(3): 298–303.

Kahn, J., Kaplan, L., Volberding, P., et al. 1989. Intralesional recombinant tumor necrosis factor-alpha for AIDS-associated Kaposi's sarcoma: A randomized, double-blind trial. *Journal of Acquired Immune Deficiency Syndrome* 2(3): 217–223.

Kauffmann, M., Schid, H., Raeth, U., et al. 1990. Therapy of ascites with tumor necrosis factor in ovarian cancer. *Geburtshilfe und Frauenheilkunde* 50(9): 678–682.

Kimura, K., Taguchi, T., Urushizaki, I., et al. 1987. Phase I study of recombinant human tumor necrosis factor. *Cancer Chemotherapy and Pharmacology* 20: 223–229.

Kuei, J., Tashkin, D., and Figlin, R. 1989. Pulmonary toxicity of recombinant human tumor necrosis factor. *Chest* 96(2): 334–338.

Kurzrock, R., Feinberg, B., Talpaz, M., et al. 1989. Phase I study of a combination of recombinant tumor necrosis factor-alpha and recombinant interferon-gamma in cancer patients. *Journal of Interferon Research* 9(4): 435–444.

Lapierre, L., Fiers, W., and Pober, J. 1988. Three distinct classes of regulatory cytokines control endothelial cell MHC antigen expression. Interactions with immune gamma interferon differentiate the effects of tumor necrosis factor and lymphotoxin from those of leukocyte alpha and fibroblast beta interferons. *Journal of Experimental Medicine* 167(3): 794–804.

Lattime, E., Stoppacciaro, A., Khan, A., et al. 1988. Human natural cytotoxic activity mediated by tumor necrosis factor: Regulation by interleukin–2. *Journal of the National Cancer Institute* 80(13): 1035–1038.

Lenk, H., Tanneberger, S., Müller, U., et al. 1988. Human pharmacological investigation of a human recombinant tumor necrosis factor preparation (PAC–4D), a phase-I trial. *Archives Geschwulstforsch* 58: 89–97.

Lienard, D., Ewalenko, P., Delotte, J., et al. 1992a. High-dose recombinant tumor necrosis factor alpha in combination with interferon gamma and melphalan in isolation perfusion of the limbs for melanoma and sarcoma. *Journal of Clinical Oncology* 10: 52–60.

Liernard, D., Lejeune, F., and Ewalenko, P. 1992b. In transit metastases of malignant melanoma treated by high dose rTNF-alpha in combination with interferon-gamma and melphalan in isolation perfusion. *World Journal of Surgery* 16(2): 234–240.

Littleton, M. 1988. Pathophysiology of sepsis and septic shock. *Critical Care Nursing Quarterly* 11: 30–47.

Lu, L., Srour, E., Warren, D., et al. 1988. Enhancement of release of granulocyte and granulocyte-macrophage colony-stimulating factors from phytohemagglutinin-stimulated sorted subsets of human T lymphocytes by recombinant human tumor necrosis factor-alpha. Synergism with recombinant human IFN-gamma. *Journal of Immunology* 141(1): 201–207.

Medcalf, R., Kruithof, E., Schleuning, W. 1988. Plasminogen activator inhibitor 1 and 2 are tumor necrosis factor/cachectin-responsive genes. *Journal of Experimental Medicine* 168(2): 751–759.

Min, H., and Spiegelann, B. 1986. Adipsin, the adipocyte serine protease: Gene structure and control of expression by tumor necrosis factor. *Nucleic Acids Research* 14(22): 8879–8892.

Moldawer, N., and Figlin, R. 1988. Tumor necrosis factor: Current clinical status and implications for nursing management. *Seminars in Oncology Nursing* 4(2): 120–125.

Morice, R., Blick, M., Ali, M., et al. 1987. Pulmonary toxicity of recombinant tumor necrosis factor (rTNF). *Proceedings of American Society for Clinical Oncology* 6: 29 (abstract).

Moritz, T., Niederle, N., Baumann, J., et al. 1989. Phase I study of recombinant human tumor necrosis factor alpha in advanced malignant disease. *Cancer Immunology and Immunotherapy* 29: 144–150.

Murase, T., Hotta, T., Saito, H., et al. 1987. Effect of recombinant human tumor necrosis factor on the colony growth of human leukemia progenitor cells and normal hematopoietic progenitor cells. *Blood* 69(2): 467–472.

Nauts, H., Fowler, G., and Bogatko, F. 1953. A review of the influence of bacterial infection and of bacterial products (Coley's toxins) on malignant tumors in man. *Acta Medica Scandinavica Supplementum* 276: 1–103.

Negrier, M., Pourreau, C., Paler, P., et al. 1992. Phase I trial of recombinant interleukin–2 followed by recombinant tumor necrosis factor in patients with metastatic cancer. *Journal of Immunotherapy* 11: 93–102.

Old, L. 1988. Tumor necrosis factor. *Scientific American* 141: 59–60, 69–75.

Orr, D., Oldham, R., Lewis, M., et al. 1989. Phase I study of the sequenced administration of etoposide (VP–16) and recombinant tumor necrosis factor (rTNF; Cetus) in patients with advanced malignancy. *Proceedings of the American Society of Clinical Oncology* 8: A741 (abstract).

Ortaldo, J. 1986. Comparison of natural killer and natural cytotoxic cells: Characteristics, regulation and mechanism of action. *Pathology and Immunopathology Research* 5(3–5): 203–218.

Pekala, P., Kawakai, M., Angus, C., et al. 1983. Selective inhibition of synthesis enzymes for *de novo* fatty acid biosynthesis by an endotoxin induced mediator from exudate cells. *Proceedings of the National Academy of Science USA* 80: 2743–2747.

Rosenberg, S., Lotze, M., Yang, J., et al. 1989. Experience with the use of high dose interleukin–2 in the treatment of 652 patients with cancer. *Annals of Surgery* 210: 474–485.

Schaadt, M., Pfreundschuh, M., Lorscheidt, G., *et al.* 1990. Phase II study of recombinant human tumor necrosis factor in colorectal carcinoma. *Journal of Biological Response Modifiers* 9: 247–250.

Schleef, R., and Loskutoff, D. 1988. Fibrinolytic system of vascular endothelial cells. Role of plasminogen activator inhibitors. *Haemostasis* 18(4–6): 328–341.

Scheurich, P., Thoa, B., Ucer, U., *et al.* 1987. Immunoregulatory activity of recombinant human tumor necrosis factor (TNF)-alpha: Induction of TNF receptors on human T cells and TNF-alpha-mediated enhancement of T cell responses. *Journal of Immunology* 138(6): 1786–1790.

Schwartz, J., Scuderi, P., Wiggins, C., *et al.* 1989. A phase I trial of recombinant tumor necrosis factor (rTNF) administered by continuous intravenous infusion in patients with disseminated malignancy. *Biotherapy* 1(3): 207–214.

Seelentag, W., Mermod, J., Montesano, R., *et al.* 1987. Additive effects of interleukin–1 and tumor necrosis factor-alpha on the accumulation of the three granulocyte and macrophage colony-stimulating factor mRNAs in human endothelial cells. *EMBO Journal* 6(8): 2261–2265.

Selby, P., Hobbs, S., Viner, C., *et al.* 1987. Tumor necrosis factor in man: Clinical and biological observations. *British Journal of Cancer* 56: 803–808.

Shau, H. 1988. Characteristics and mechanisms of neutrophil-mediated cytostasis induced by tumor necrosis factor. *Journal of Immunology* 141(1): 234–240.

Sherman, M., Spriggs, D., Arthur, K., *et al.* 1992. Enhanced myelosuppression in a phase I trial of recombinant human tumor necrosis factor in combination with etoposide. *Proceedings of the American Association for Cancer Research* 33: A1468 (abstract).

Sherman, M., Spriggs, D., Arthur, K., *et al.* 1988. Recombinant tumor necrosis factor administered as a five day continuous infusion in cancer patients: Phase I toxicity and effects on lipid metabolism. *Journal of Clinical Oncology* 6(2): 344–350.

Spriggs, D. 1991. Tumor necrosis factor: Basic principles and preclinical studies. In DeVita, V., Hellman, S., Rosenberg, S. (eds). *Biologic Therapy of Cancer*. Philadelphia: J.B. Lippincott, pp. 354–377.

Spriggs, D., Sherman, M., Michie, H., *et al.* 1988. Recombinant human tumor necrosis factor administered as a 24-hour intravenous infusion. A phase I and pharmacologic study. *Journal of the National Cancer Institute* 80: 1039–1044.

Steinmetz, T., Schaadt, M., Gähl, R., *et al.* 1988. Phase I study of 24-hour continuous intravenous infusion of recombinant human tumor necrosis factor. *Journal of Biologic Response Modifiers* 7: 417–423.

Stroud, M. 1990. Cellular and hormonal mediators of sepsis syndrome. *Critical Care Nursing Clinics of North America* 2: 151–160.

Sugarman, B., Aggarwal, B., Hass, P., *et al.* 1985. Recombinant human tumor necrosis factor-alpha: Effects on proliferation of normal and transformed cells *in vitro. Science* 230(4728): 943–945.

Taguchi, T. 1988. Phase I study of recombinant human tumor necrosis factor (rHu-TNF:PT–050). *Cancer Detection and Prevention* 12: 561–572.

Taguchi, T. 1987. Recombinant human tumor necrosis factor (rHu-TNF): Phase I and early phase II study. *Proceedings of the American Society for Clinical Oncology* 6: 233 (abstract).

Torti, F., Torti, S., Larrick, J., *et al.* 1989. Modulation of adipocyte differentiation by tumor necrosis factor and tumor necrosis factor beta. *Journal of Cell Biology* 108(3): 1105–1113.

Tracey, K., and Cerami, A. 1992. Tumor necrosis factor in the malnutrition (cachexia) of infection and cancer. *American Journal of Tropical Medicine and Hygiene* 47(Suppl 1): 2–7.

Tracey, K., Fong, Y., Hesse, D., *et al.* 1987. Anti-cachectin/TNF monoclonal antibodies prevent septic shock during lethal bacteremia. *Nature* 330: 662–664.

Urban, J., Shepard, H., Rothstein, J., *et al.* 1986. Tumor necrosis factor: A potent effector molecule for tumor cell killing by activated macrophages. *Proceedings of the National Academy of Sciences USA* 83: 8318.

Vadas, P., and Pruzanski, W. 1990. Phospholipase A2 activation is the pivotal step in the effector pathway of inflammation. *Advances in Experimental Medicine and Biology* 275: 83–101.

Van, dB.E.A., Sprengers, E., Jaye, M., *et al.* 1988. Regulation of plasminogen activator inhibitor–1 mRNA in human endothelial cells. *Thrombosis and Haemostasis* 60(1): 63–67.

Walsh, C., Chachoua, A., Hochster, H., *et al.* 1989. Phase I study of recombinant human tumor necrosis factor, abstracted. *Proceedings of the American Society of Clinical Oncology* 8: 193.

Westphal, O. 1987. Hommage à Valy Menkin. In Bonavida, B., Gifford, G., Kirchner, H., *et al.* (eds). *International Conference on Tumor Necrosis Factor and Related Cytokines.* Basel, Switzerland: Karger, pp. 1–6.

Westphal, O., Luderitz, O., Galanos, C., *et al.* 1985. The story of bacterial endotoxin. In Chedid, L., Hadden, Speafico, *et al.* (eds). *Advances in Immunopharmacology: Third International Conference on Immunopharmacology, Florence, 1985.* Oxford: Pergamon Press, pp. 13–34.

Wiedenmann, B., Reichardt, P., Räth, U., *et al.* 1989. Phase-I trial of intravenous continuous infusion of tumor necrosis factor in advanced metastatic carcinomas. *Journal of Cancer Research and Clinical Oncology* 115: 189–192.

Williamson, B., Carswell, E., Rubin, B., *et al.* 1983. Human tumor necrosis factor produced by human B-cell lines: Synergistic cytotoxic interaction with human interferon. *Proceedings of the National Academy of Sciences* 80: 5397–5401.

Yang, S., Owen-Schaub, L., Mendiguren-Rodriguez, A., *et al.* 1990. Combination immunotherapy for non-small-cell lung cancer. Results with interleukin–2 and tumor necrosis factor-alpha. *Journal of Cardiothoracic Surgery* 99(1): 8–12.

Yoshida, J., Wakabayashi, T., Mizuno, M., *et al.* 1992. Clinical effect of intra-arterial tumor necrosis factor-alpha for malignant glioma. *Journal of Neurosurgery* 77(1): 78–83.

Zamkoff, K., Newman, N., Rudolph, A., *et al.* 1989. A phase I trial of subcutaneously administered recombi-

nant tumor necrosis factor to patients with advanced malignancy. *Journal of Biological Response Modifiers* 8: 539–552.

Zechner, R., Newman, T., Sherry, B., *et al.* 1988. Recombinant human cachectin/tumor necrosis factor but not interleukin–1 alpha down-regulates lipoprotein lipase gene expression at the transcriptional level in mouse 3T3-L1 adipocytes. *Molecular and Cellular Biology* 8(6): 2394–2401.

CHAPTER 9 | Immunomodulators, Differentiation Agents, and Vaccines

Grace E. Dean, RN, MSN

In the last 50 years, various biological agents have come into and gone out of vogue. Each of the therapies reviewed in this chapter, however, has survived the test of time and earned its place in the biotherapy arsenal. Two of the earliest forms of biotherapy, bacillus of Calmette and Guérin (BCG) and tumor vaccines, along with two agents recently utilized in cancer care, retinoids and levamisole, will be presented. A brief historical overview, as well as reviews of significant clinical trials and side effects, and of regulatory status, are included in the discussion of each agent.

BACILLUS OF CALMETTE AND GUÉRIN

In the late 1800s, the major public health problem was tuberculosis. In 1908, two French scientists at the Pasteur Institute, León Calmette and Alphonse Guérin, discovered that the addition of a small aliquot of beef bile to the cultured medium of a highly virulent strain of bovine tubercle bacillus caused it to lose its pathogenic characteristic (Hanna *et al.*, 1992). After 13 years of culturing with 231 serial transplants, the tubercle bacillus was **attenuated** and could be used for vaccination. Finally, in 1921, the first human was vaccinated with bacillus Calmette-Guérin (BCG) as the isolated vaccine was designated (Weill-Hallé, 1980).

Old *et al.* (1959) demonstrated that BCG could prevent or delay the occurrence of sarcomas, carcinomas, and ascitic tumors in mice. This study and the work of others led to the clinical use of BCG in the treatment of cancer. Mathé *et al.* (1969) were the first to use BCG as an adjuvant therapy in childhood acute lymphoblastic leukemia. Their positive results were the impetus for several hundred clinical trials using BCG in the treatment of a variety of cancers; some of these trials are still underway.

Bacillus Calmette-Guérin is a microbial material made from an attenuated strain of a live virus, *Mycobacterium bovis*. It has been used for decades for immunization against tuberculosis and as a nonspecific immunopotentiating agent in cancer treatment. As with other biological agents, it is important to have an immunocompetent host, and a small tumor burden is necessary for this type of treatment to be effective (Zbar *et al.*, 1972).

In the treatment of cancer, BCG acts as a nonspecific immunostimulatory agent. This effect is believed to be initiated not by a single mechanism but as the result of a cascade of immunologic events involving both humoral and cellular immunity. T cells, B cells, macrophages, and natural killer cells are all potentiated by a variety of lymphokines and cytokines induced as a result of BCG administration (Mitchell and Murntz, 1979; Murahata and Mitchell, 1976). The exact mechanism by which BCG causes tumor regression remains a mystery, but the local presence of BCG and development of a granuloma are believed to be important (Snodgrass and Hanna, 1973; Hanna *et al.*, 1972).

Mathé *et al.* (1969) used BCG as an adjuvant in the treatment of acute lymphoblastic leukemia. Intensive weekly multisite scarifications (Figure 9.1) with BCG were administered during both the induction and maintenance phases of chemotherapy. Improved survival over historical controls stimulated much interest in the area. Similar improvement in survival was demonstrated when a similar treatment schedule of BCG was used as therapy for acute myeloid leukemia (Freeman *et al.*, 1973). However, it had little effect on the duration of remission.

Preoperative intralesional injections of BCG were used in a randomized trial of 24 head and neck cancer patients. The control group (12 patients) underwent surgery while the experimental group (12 patients) received intralesional BCG prior to surgery. Three years after treatment, the BCG-treated group had a 73% survival rate, and the control group had a 50% survival rate (Bier *et al.*, 1981).

Morton *et al.* (1970) reported complete regression of cutaneous metastases of malignant melanoma in 5 of 8 patients treated with intralesional administration of BCG. Regression of noninjected adjacent nodules in the lymphatic drainage area of the injected lesions were also noted in 2 out of 8 patients. Minor effects were achieved at distant sites or for visceral disease.

Intracavity or intrapleural administration of BCG prior to surgery in stage I or II lung cancer patients was described by McKneally *et al.* (1977). Two years after surgery, 93% of BCG-treated patients were disease free, compared with 67% of patients not treated with BCG. At the 4-year follow-up evaluation, it was determined that postoperative administration of BCG was effective only in stage I lung cancer. To date, however, no one has been able to reproduce the beneficial effect of intrapleural administration of BCG in the treatment of lung cancer.

A landmark study by Morales *et al.* (1976) involved the intravesical use of BCG for treatment of bladder cancer. Twenty-six patients with superficial bladder tumors were treated with a combination of intravesically and intradermally administered BCG. A dramatic reduction was found in the recurrence rate for up to 3 years after treatment. This study led to prospective randomized trials that demonstrated that intravesical BCG was effective without concomitant intradermal BCG (Lamm *et al.*, 1991).

Positive results from studies employing systemic administration of BCG in combination with other agents have also been published. In a Southwest Oncology Group trial involving 652 previously untreated patients with non-Hodgkin's lymphoma, patients were randomly assigned to 1 of 3 remission induction arms (Jones *et al.*, 1983). The 3 treatment arms were: (1) CHOP-BCG which included cyclophosphamide (C), hydroxydaunorubicin (doxorubicin H), vincristine (O), prednisone (P), and BCG; (2) CHOP-Bleo (5 drugs) which included the same drugs as CHOP-BCG except that bleomycin was substituted for BCG; and (3) COP-Bleo in which

Figure 9.1 Scarification technique of BCG administration. A 5-cm-X-5-cm area is anesthetized, then the skin is cleaned and allowed to dry. The vaccine preparation is then spread over the 5-cm-X-5-cm area of skin. Straight lines (ten vertical and ten horizontal) are scratched through the skin layers.

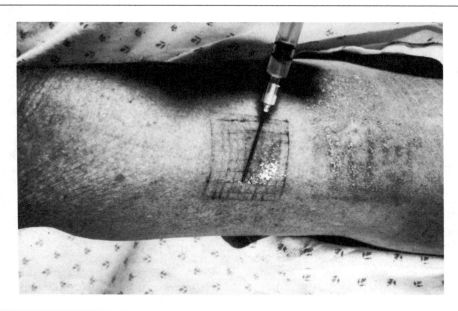

Source: Courtesy of the University of Texas M.D. Anderson Cancer Center, Houston, Texas.

doxorubicin was omitted. Complete response rates in large-cell lymphoma occurred in 68% of patients treated with CHOP-BCG, in 48% of patients treated with CHOP-Bleo, and in 44% of patients treated with COP-Bleo. In a trial of patients with advanced stage IV breast cancer, patients were randomized to receive 5-fluorouracil, doxorubicin (adriamycin), and cyclophosphamide (FAC) with or without BCG (McCulloch *et al.,* 1982). Overall survival was prolonged in the chemoimmunotherapy arm, but the rate and duration of response were only slightly improved. In 121 melanoma patients, a 3-way randomization that involved BCG alone, dacarbazine (DTIC) alone, or DTIC with BCG proved the chemoimmunotherapy arm was superior in delaying recurrence and in significantly increasing the 3-year survival (Wood *et al.,* 1982).

In 1990, the Food and Drug Administration (FDA) approved BCG for intravesical treatment of carcinoma *in situ* of the bladder. Treatment consists of an induction regimen plus maintenance schedule. For the induction phase, 1 ampule of BCG (50 mg; 1 to 8 x 10^7 colony-forming units) is suspended in 50 ml of saline; the solution is administered once per week for a minimum of 6 weeks intravesically and is retained in the bladder for 2 hours. The maintenance schedule consists of this same treatment once a month for up to 12 months. Effectiveness is evaluated every 3 months by cystoscopy and urine cytology tests.

As with other biological response modifiers, side effects depend on the dose, route, schedule, and even the timing of administration (Greenspan, 1986). When BCG is injected into a lesion, a local inflammatory reaction occurs within 4 hours. Within a week, tumor necrosis and ulceration develop that may require a few months to heal. Systemic effects include a flu-like syndrome with fever, fatigue, myalgias, and possibly nausea and vomiting that may last a few days.

Side effects of scarification or intradermal BCG develop more gradually. An erythematous papule forms at the injection site and may heal in a day or two. Pruritis is common and occurs at the site of injection. As patients become sensitized to the treatment, however, the papules will ulcerate. Permanent scarring should be anticipated and patients should be prepared for this.

When BCG is administered intravesically, the toxic effects are often localized, but there may be accompanying systemic symptoms (Hanna *et al.,* 1992). More than half the patients studied reported symptoms of bladder irritability such as dysuria, frequency, and hematuria. In addition, a "flu-like" syndrome consisting of fever, chills, malaise, and myalgias was found in one-third of patients treated. Of those reporting flu-like symptoms, fewer than 10% had severe side effects.

Two major complications may occur when BCG is administered: a hypersensitivity reaction or a disseminated BCG infection. Two cases of immediate hypersensitivity reactions to BCG have been reported that ultimately resulted in deaths (McKhann *et al.,* 1975). Presenting symptoms include fever, chills, hypotension, and oliguria (Groenwald *et al.,* 1987). Thus, emergency equipment should be readily available when initiating therapy. Disseminated BCG infection presents with persistent fever, nausea, vomiting, fatigue, and weight loss. Definitive antimicrobial treatment is needed; many clinicians recommend isoniazid.

Bacillus of Calmette-Guérin has clearly proven to be effective as a vaccine against tuberculosis and as primary treatment for bladder cancer. However, overtreatment (such as regimens that include injections into multiple sites, large doses, and frequently scheduled treatments), is the probable cause for the many studies that have reported negative results when BCG is used alone or in combination with other cancer therapies (Greenspan, 1986). It is well recognized that using smaller doses may be more effective when using biological agents (Hanna *et al.,* 1992).

The most promising future use of BCG is as an adjuvant for a tumor vaccine in the treatment of advanced melanoma and as an adjuvant therapy in treating colon cancer. In the upcoming section on vaccines, the recent work by Berd *et al.* (1990) in using autologous tumor vaccine plus BCG in treating metastatic melanoma will be reviewed along with early work by Hoover *et al.* (1985), which showed encouraging results in the use of postoperative BCG in the treatment of Dukes' stage B and C colorectal cancer.

RETINOIDS

Retinoids have been recognized for more than 50 years for their profound impact on biological functions (Smith *et al.,* 1992). Epidemiologists first realized the importance of retinoids in chemoprevention studies long before clinical oncologists became aware of their usefulness. Dramatic results following treatment of acute promyelocytic leukemia, metastatic squamous cell cancer of the skin and squamous cell carcinoma of the cervix led cancer specialists in early 1990 to obtain an investigational new drug (IND) status for the therapeutic use of retinoids (Smith *et al.,* 1992). This status will allow investigation of the potential use of retinoids in the treatment of a variety of hematopoietic and solid malignancies.

Retinoids are a class of agents consisting of vitamin A (retinol) and other related derivatives (Chomienne *et al.,* 1986). Long known for their effects on a variety of biological functions, retinoids normally perform significant roles in vision, growth, reproduction, epithelial cell differentiation, and immune function (Smith *et al.,* 1992). The dietary sources of retinol are animal products, such as liver, meat, eggs, and milk products, and carotenoids, which are found in fruits and cruciferous vegetables such as cabbage. Following absorption in the small intestine, retinol is transported to the liver, where it is stored. Bound to a retinol-binding protein, retinol is released from the liver at constant rates and transported to the tissues via the bloodstream (DeVet, 1989).

All-*trans*-retinoic acid (tRA) (vitamin A acid, or tretinoin) is a natural retinol metabolite and the photoisomer of 13-*cis*-retinoic acid (cRA) (isotretinoin, or Accutane®), a well-investigated agent used widely in dermatology (Parkinson *et al.*, 1992).

The exact mechanism of action of retinoic acid in cancer treatment and prevention is elusive. A number of preclinical studies have presumed that it exerts a hormone-like action for cell proliferation and/or differentiation (DeVet, 1989). According to this theory, specific binding proteins are believed to be responsible for the transport of retinol into the cell. Once in the cell, retinol acts on the nucleus by binding to nuclear retinoic acid receptors and then mediating gene expression. The potentially beneficial effects of retinoic acid include direct induction of differentiation, direct growth inhibition without differentiation, a paracrine-mediated growth inhibition or differentiation, and induction of apoptosis (programmed cell death) (Smith *et al.*, 1992).

In addition, retinoids have very definite effects on the immune system. They enhance humoral- and cell-mediated immune responses and phagocytosis by macrophages, and according to extensive studies *in vivo* and *in vitro*, they induce prostaglandin synthesis (Dennert *et al.*, 1979; Lotan *et al.*, 1979). Interleukin–2 production by helper T cells which leads to killer T cell proliferation, is also augmented by retinoic acid (Dennert, 1985).

Acute promyelocytic leukemia, an uncommon type of acute myeloid leukemia characterized by the presence of disseminated intravascular coagulation at diagnosis, responds to oral all-*trans*-retinoic acid (tRA) therapy (Stone and Mayer, 1990). In a worldwide series of studies, 90 of 99 patients who had been

previously untreated or were in first relapse achieved a complete remission 1 to 2 months after treatment with tRA (Smith *et al.*, 1992). Thus far, responses last only 2 to 13 months despite continued therapy.

Mycosis fungoides (T-cell lymphoma), a malignancy of the helper-inducer T-cell phenotype, typically involves the skin, with the potential for dissemination to lymph nodes, spleen, liver, and other organs (Kuzel *et al.*, 1991). Patients treated with starting doses of 1–2 mg 13-*cis*-retinoic acid (cRA)/kg/day have shown clinical improvement within 2 to 4 weeks of initiating treatment. Responses have been documented in up to 44% of patients (including 3 complete clinical responses), most of whom had been previously treated (Kessler *et al.*, 1987).

A postoperative chemoprevention trial in patients with squamous cell cancer of the head and neck was conducted by Hong *et al.* (1990). The investigators found that 32 months after cRA therapy ($50–100 \text{ mg}/\text{m}^2/\text{day}$ for 12 months) was initiated, there was a much lower rate of occurrence of second primary tumors (4% in the treated group vs. 24% in the placebo group). However, recurrences from the original tumor were unaffected by cRA (30% recurrence rate in both treated and placebo groups).

The antiproliferative and differentiation effects of retinoids on squamous cell carcinoma cell lines have led investigators to evaluate their use in patients with this tumor. In surgically incurable head and neck squamous cell carcinomas, administration of cRA (3 mg/kg/day) has resulted in partial responses in 3 of 19 patients (Lippman *et al.*, 1987). Another study involving patients with locally advanced or metastatic squamous cell carcinoma of the head and neck had similar results at the same dosage (3 mg/kg/day for at least 6 weeks). Lippman *et al.* (1988) again reported 3 partial responses and 1 complete response of 19 total patients. Both tRA and cRA have been used to treat a variety of skin malignancies including basal cell carcinoma, squamous cell carcinoma, and melanoma. In cutaneous basal cell carcinoma, both topical administration of cRA and tRA have resulted in complete or partial responses in most patients (Sankowski et al., 1987; Epstein, 1986). Lippman and Meyskens (1987) used systemic administration of cRA for locally advanced squamous cell carcinoma of the skin and achieved a 40% to 50% response rate. Topical administration of tRA has been used on subcutaneous metastatic melanoma lesions and resulted in transient local regression of some tumors (Levine and Meyskens, 1980).

Interest in the use of tRA in treatment of sarcomas is growing following a report by Bonhomme et al. (1991). Topically applied tRA (1% gel) was used to treat cutaneous lesions of patients with Kaposi's sarcoma. A 50% reduction in the size of cutaneous lesions was noted in 7 of 8 patients.

Combination trials have also been conducted for treatment of advanced squamous cell carcinoma of the skin and locally advanced squamous cell carcinoma of the cervix. Interferon-alpha (IFN-α) and cRA were used in 28 patients with either locally advanced or metastatic squamous cell carcinoma of the skin (Lippman et al., 1992a). Sixty-eight percent of the patients responded with 7 of 19 responders achieving a complete response. In another study, previously untreated patients with locally advanced squamous cell carcinoma of the cervix received cRA (1 mg/kg/day) and IFN-α (6 MIU subcutaneously daily) (Lippman et al., 1992b). Half of the patients had at least a partial response, and the outpatient regimen was well tolerated.

It is apparent from these small studies that the retinoids have some efficacy in treating a variety of preneoplastic conditions and epithelial tumors. However, this basic work needs to be expanded to understand more fully the mechanism by which reduction of lesions occurs and to understand why some tumors are responsive to retinoids while others are not.

Currently, retinol and tRA are not approved for the prevention or treatment of cancer. Vitamin A capsules (15 mg retinol) have been approved for vitamin A deficiency. Retin A® cream (tretinoin) has been approved for the treatment of acne vulgaris and Accutane® (isotretinoin), an orally administered retinoid, has been approved for treatment of cystic acne.

Acute hypervitaminosis A toxicity exhibits a well-known clinical presentation (Windhorst and Nigra, 1982). Drowsiness, irritability, headache, and vomiting are all symptoms of the toxic effects to the central nervous system (CNS). Dermatologic changes include desquamation; pruritis; alopecia; increased pigmentation; drying and cracking of the lips, mucous membranes, and skin. Fatigue, anorexia, arthralgias, hepatosplenomegaly, and irritation of the eyes are also common. The chronic, low-grade toxic effects seen in the clinical trials of synthetic retinoids are similar to the acute effects just described, but serious CNS effects are rare. Signs and symptoms usually disappear within one to four weeks following discontinuation of treatment.

Smith et al. (1992) found significant differences in the toxic effects of tRA and cRA. Headaches, visual disturbances, dizziness and lethargy were reported more often in patients receiving tRA. There is also a reported relationship between dose and toxic effects in patients treated with tRA. Fewer patients with skin disorders requiring low doses (30 mg/day) of tRA reported headaches than did patients receiving high doses (70–100 mg/day) (4% vs. 50%) (Smith et al., 1992). Therapy had to be discontinued for 11% of patients receiving high doses.

The most significant toxic effect associated with both tRA and cRA is teratogenesis. Both retinoids have the potential to produce a 25-fold increase in the incidence of severe embryopathic changes, including spontaneous abortions and malformations that involve the craniofacial, cardiac, thymic, and CNS structures (Lammer et al., 1985). Women of childbearing potential must be thoroughly counseled concerning the serious risks to the fetus if they should become pregnant while undergoing treatment. In addition, the length of time during which pregnancy must be avoided after treatment has ended has not yet been determined.

A hyperleukocytosis syndrome unique to tRA therapy has been associated with fatal pulmonary complications in several patients with acute promyelocytic leukemia (Frankel *et al.*, 1992). It occurs within the first 2 to 3 weeks of treatment. Symptoms include fever, dyspnea, and pleural effusions; it may be difficult to distinguish the syndrome from a bacterial or fungal infection. This syndrome has been successfully treated with leukapheresis and/or high-dose corticosteroids in some patients.

With the tremendous interest in the use of retinoids in cancer treatment and because the Division of Cancer Treatment at the National Cancer Institute has obtained IND status for retinoic acid, the potential for rational drug development is excellent. Combination trials using retinoic acid with chemotherapy and other biological agents to treat solid tumors and hematologic disorders are already underway.

LEVAMISOLE

In the mid 1960s, a broad-spectrum **anthelmintic** agent was identified and found to have beneficial effects on the immune system (Renoux and Renoux, 1971). These investigators showed that levamisole potentiated the protective effect of a *Brucella* vaccine in mice. Although a tremendous amount of interest and research followed, it was short-lived. The overall conclusion from research conducted in the mid to late 1970s was that levamisole restored depressed or anergic states to normal (DeBrabander *et al.*, 1992).

Levamisole has been effective in treating recurrent and chronic infections, postviral anergy and rheumatic disorders by restoring to normal various functions of T lymphocytes and phagocytes. Only recently have positive results been seen in the treatment of cancer. Three major multicenter clinical trials have revealed that levamisole is an effective adjuvant therapy for melanoma and colon carcinoma (Amery and Bruynseels, 1992). These new findings have stimulated renewed interest and research in the use of levamisole in treating cancer.

A **racemic** compound, tetramisole hydrochloride, was first introduced as an anthelmintic in 1966. It was soon discovered that the anthelmintic activity resided in the levorotatory isomer of levamisole. Today, levamisole is used as a broad-spectrum anthelmintic in the treatment of lungworm and gastrointestinal nematodes in animals and humans. It is administered as a single 5- to 40-mg/kg dose, depending on the parasite involved (Miller, 1980).

The mode of levamisole's action is still not completely understood, but the following effects have been documented in *in vitro* and *ex vivo* experiments: (1) improvement of cell-mediated immune responses, particularly of macrophages and T cells; (2) restoration to normal various functions of T lymphocytes and phagocytes, such as chemotaxis, random migration, adherence, intracellular killing, E rosette formation, and delayed skin hypersensitivity; and (3) synergism with mitogens and antigens in lymphocyte proliferation (Amery and Bruynseels, 1992; Van Wauwe and Janssen, 1991). Levamisole's effect on B lymphocytes remains uncertain at this time, although investigations continue.

Amery *et al.* (1982) reported on the use of levamisole in treating bronchial carcinoma. In a randomized, placebo-controlled study involving 96 patients, levamisole was used as an adjuvant to surgery, oral administration beginning 3 days before the operation. Therapy consisted of 3 consecutive days of treatment every 2 weeks and was to be continued for 3 years if there was no recurrence of disease. Beneficial effects were noted in survival and recurrence rates at doses greater than or equal to 2.5 mg/kg or 80.7 mg/m². After 12 months of treatment, 71% of the levamisole-treated patients were alive, as compared with 41% of the patients in the placebo group.

In melanoma, the most significant levamisole trial reported to date was conducted in Canada (Quirt *et al.*, 1991). In a phase III study involving levamisole therapy for malignant melanoma with poor prognosis, 543 patients were randomly assigned to either a control arm or to a group that received levamisole postoperatively. Levamisole (2.5 mg/kg) was given orally on 2 consecutive days each week for 3 years. The levamisole-treated group demonstrated improved overall survival and a reduced incidence of recurrences as compared with the control group.

Klefstrom *et al.* (1985) used levamisole following irradiation in treating patients with stage II breast carcinoma. In this double-blind trial, 72 patients received either capsules containing levamisole or identical capsules containing placebo on 2 consecutive days each week for up to 1 year. The levamisole dose was 2.5 mg/kg/day. Mean duration of treatment was 6.5 months; several patients discontinued treatment earlier than originally planned because of the toxic effects of the drug (high fever, severe nausea, urticaria, or granulocytopenia). The levamisole group had a slightly better survival rate (p = .059) and a significantly higher disease-free survival rate (p = .042) than did the placebo group.

Two significant trials of the combination of levamisole and 5-fluorouracil (5-FU) in the treatment of colorectal cancer also resulted in renewed interest in the use of levamisole as a biological agent. The first trial, a study by Laurie *et al.* (1989), involved 408 patients with resected Dukes' stage B_2 or C colorectal cancer. The trial consisted of 3 groups: one group received 150 mg levamisole given orally for 3 consecutive days every 2 weeks for 1 year plus 5-FU (450 mg/m²/day IV bolus for 5 days beginning at day 28 and then once/week for one year); the second group received levamisole only for a year; the third group received no further therapy. The combination of levamisole and 5-FU was superior in treating patients with Dukes' stage C disease, with a 5-year survival rate of 49%, to no treatment (5-year survival rate, 37%). There was also a difference in mean disease-free

intervals (23 months with levamisole plus 5-FU and 14 months with no therapy) and tumor recurrences (41% vs. 55%). Treatment with levamisole alone was only marginally beneficial.

A second study by Moertel *et al.* (1990), used a similar treatment scheme, but involved 1296 comparable patients with matched controls. The combination therapy of levamisole plus 5-FU reduced the risk of recurrence by 41% and of overall death by 33% as compared to controls.

Levamisole has been approved by the FDA as an adjuvant treatment in combination with 5-FU following resection of Dukes' stage C colon cancer. Treatment consists of 150 mg (50 mg every 8 hours) of levamisole given orally for 3 consecutive days every 2 weeks for one year. It is recommended that treatment be initiated no earlier than 7 and no later than 30 days following resection.

Levamisole is rapidly absorbed from the gastrointestinal tract. Pharmacokinetic study of a single 50-mg dose revealed that the mean peak plasma level was reached within 1.5 to 2 hours. The drug is metabolized by the liver and excreted mainly by the kidneys (70% over 3 days) (Symoens *et al.*, 1979).

When compared to other biological agents, the side effects of levamisole as a single agent are relatively mild. Gastrointestinal side effects (nausea, vomiting, and diarrhea) are the most common and occur in about 5% to 25% of patients. Flu-like symptoms, fatigue, headache, and dermatitis have also been reported. Granulocytopenia and agranulocytosis have been reported in as many as 10% of patients in some studies (Klefstrom *et al.*, 1985). However, in combination with 5-FU, the side effects are slightly different. Moertel *et al.* (1990) reported toxic effects to the gastrointestinal tract in more than half of the patients (nausea, vomiting, diarrhea, and stomatitis); nearly 25% had dermatitis and alopecia. Up to 14% of the patients had to discontinue combination therapy because of adverse reactions that included life-threatening exfoliative dermatitis, leukopenia, and sepsis.

Three conclusions can be drawn from the results of the different experimental clinical trials: (1) levamisole was more effective on slow-growing tumors than on fast-growing ones; (2) levamisole was more effective in preventing metastases than in shrinking established tumors; and (3) levamisole has been most effective as an adjuvant following resection (DeBrabander *et al.*, 1992).

Much can still be learned through this renewed interest in levamisole. Questions of paramount importance include the effect of levamisole plus 5-FU in treating Dukes' stage B colorectal carcinoma; the relative merits of preoperative and postoperative use of levamisole; the appropriate dosing of levamisole on chemotherapy treatment days; and levamisole's effect on other types of tumors.

TUMOR VACCINES: ACTIVE SPECIFIC IMMUNOTHERAPY

The first use of active specific immunotherapy (ASI) to treat cancer patients was reported by von Leyden and Blumenthal in 1902 (Currie, 1972). An autologous tumor-cell preparation—a vaccine produced from the patient's own tumor—was used on patients with advanced cancer. No objective improvement was found following treatment, although two of the patients reported some improvement in symptoms.

In 1912, Coca, Dorrance, and Lebredo (Currie, 1972) used large quantities of macerated tumor, containing live tumor cells, in preparation of a "tumor vaccine." Both autologous and allogeneic tumor cells were administered subcutaneously repeatedly at 14-day intervals. Seventy-nine patients with an assortment of advanced malignant tumors were treated, and only one patient with breast cancer had a clinical response that lasted four months. Remarkably, only 1 patient developed a tumor at the site of injection. The au-

thors reluctantly concluded that their approach was impractical.

With the evolution of inbred strains of mice came the capability to immunize the mice with small doses of tumor cells. When later challenged with large doses of tumor cells, the immunized mice were protected, whereas nonimmunized mice developed tumors that eventually killed them (Gross, 1943). These results suggested that the immunity of the inbred mice was specific against the tumor used for inoculation. This work, as well as the work of others (Prehn and Maine, 1957; Foley, 1953) established a firm basis for the existence of tumor-specific antigens.

The purpose of ASI is to reintroduce (the host already has the tumor) tumor-associated antigens in a way that will be more **immunogenic** in the host. The goal of this therapy is to achieve rejection of the tumor or at least to enhance the rejection process through augmentation of the host's own potential immunity. Nonspecific active immunotherapy (adjuvants) is used in conjunction with ASI to further augment the immune response.

Our knowledge of tumor-associated antigens is incomplete. There are different types of materials used to obtain the antigens such as whole tumor cells or tumor cell lines. It should be noted that the materials which will be reviewed below are derived from cancer patients who are candidates for immunization.

Whole-cell autologous irradiated tumor used in a vaccine must be obtained from fresh tumor. Many investigators have used this method to treat patients with advanced melanoma, renal cell carcinoma, or microscopic residual colon cancer. With autologous vaccination, treatment is limited to patients with advanced disease in whom sufficient numbers of cells are available to enable preparation of a series of vaccine injections. This process requires surgery to obtain the cells and laboratory support to process and store the material for future use.

Allogeneic vaccines are made from cell lines derived from more than one patient. The cells are irradiated, mechanically disrupted (lysed), or their antigens may be shed into a supernatant fluid. Advantages to this method include the potential for a standard (generic) product, enabling the treatment of large groups of patients, and the ability to prevent recurrence in patients with microscopic residual disease.

Adjuvants

Adjuvants are used in conjunction with ASI to nonspecifically stimulate the immune system. BCG; *Corynebacterium parvum;* DETOX™, a detoxified endotoxin; infecting viruses (Newcastle disease virus and vaccinia vaccine virus); and **Freund's adjuvant** are just a few of the adjuvants that have been used with ASI. Each will be briefly described, except BCG, which was presented earlier.

C. parvum is a gram-positive formalin-killed bacterium that was reportedly first used in humans in the mid 1970s (Scott, 1975). A strong stimulator of the reticuloendothelial system, *C. parvum* also activates macrophages which, in turn, stimulate sensitized B lymphocytes to proliferate and produce antibody (Howard *et al.,*1973).

DETOX™ (Ribi Immunochem Research Inc., Hamilton, MT), a pyrogen-free preparation, is formulated from *Salmonella minnesota* and cell wall skeletons of *Mycobacterium phlei* (Ribi *et al.,* 1984). A nonspecific stimulator, DETOX™ triggers both antibody and cell-mediated immunity.

Vaccinia (smallpox) vaccine virus, has been used as a model for viral oncolysis on the basis of experiments conducted by Cassal *et al.* (1983). In their laboratory, animals treated with viral oncolysates (tumor cells infected with vaccinia virus) were completely resistant to subsequent growth of tumor cells when challenged with uninfected tumor cells, whereas untreated controls developed tumors. Newcastle disease virus is a mouse-adapted neurotropic virus for the immunization of patients with certain cancers and is also used as a viral oncolysate.

Freund's complete adjuvant consists of heat-killed mycobacterial cells suspended in mineral oil (Freund, 1956). It was developed more than 30 years ago and was thought to be the most potent immunoadjuvant for the induction of cell-mediated immunity and humoral antibody formation.

The mechanism of ASI has not been defined. Scientific evidence currently supports multiple theories, including one that helper T lymphocytes (specifically, CD4+) are the keys that unlock the cascade of events critical to rejection of the tumor by the host. Once the tumor-associated antigen is presented to the CD4+ cell, it will activate other helper T cells, as well as macrophages, and both will proliferate and release different cytokines. Ultimately, killer T cells and macrophages, along with other effector cells, will kill the tumor targets.

Clinical Studies

This section is a representation of the clinical work completed in ASI (see Table 9.1). Most of these investigators focused not only on clinical outcomes, but also on laboratory results involving humoral and cell-mediated immune reactions to their particular vaccine preparations. The interested reader is referred to the individual investigator's report for those results.

McCune *et al.* (1981) treated 14 patients with metastatic renal cell carcinoma with a combination of autologous, irradiated tumor cells mixed with *C. parvum.* The vaccine preparation was injected intracutaneously in the shoulder on a weekly basis for 4 to 14 weeks, depending on the amount of available tumor tissue. Tenderness at the injection site, slight chills, and fatigue were the reported side effects. Four patients had complete and/or partial responses of some of their metastatic lesions, whereas other patients' lesions remained stable or progressed. The authors concluded that the most likely cause for the mixed response was the presence of antigen-distinct subpopulations in metastatic cells (McCune *et al.,* 1981).

Table 9.1   Summary of clinical trials

Author (Year)	Tumor Type	Vaccine Type	CY*	N†	Responders (Complete or partial)
McCune et al. (1981)	Renal	Autologous + C. parvum	No	14	4
Sahasrabudhe et al. (1986)	Renal	Autologous + C. parvum	Yes	20	5
Hoover et al. (1985)	Colorectal	Autologous + BCG	No	20	improved survival
Hollinshead et al. (1988)	Lung	Allogeneic + Freund's	MTXF	34	improved survival
Berd et al. (1990)	Melanoma	Autologous + BCG	Yes	40	5
Mitchell et al. (1990)	Melanoma	Allogeneic + DETOX™	Yes	25	4
Scoggin et al. (1992)	Melanoma	Allogeneic Vaccinia	No	48	improved survival

*CY = cyclophosphamide used; †N = number of patients in the study.
FMTX = methotrexate

Another small, multicenter trial was conducted in patients with metastatic renal cell cancer by Sahasrabudhe et al. (1986). Again, autologous irradiated tumor cells mixed with C. parvum were administered intracutaneously to 20 evaluable patients. The patients also received 1 of 3 different dose levels (100, 500, or 1000 mg/m^2) of cyclophosphamide. The drug, which was given intravenously 24 hours before the first vaccine injection, augments the immune response by inhibiting suppressor T-lymphocyte function (Askenase et al. 1975). Side effects were reportedly infrequent and mild. One of the 20 patients had a complete response, and 4 had partial responses.

In an effort to improve the rate of long-term disease-free survival in postsurgical patients with colorectal cancer, Hoover et al. (1985) conducted a randomized two-armed clinical trial of ASI with a total of 40 patients, 20 in each arm. In the group who received treatment, autologous irradiated tumor cells plus BCG were administered intradermally once a week for 3 weeks (4 to 5 weeks after surgery). Treatment with ASI consisted of 3 weekly intradermal injections at the following sites: upper left anterior thigh, upper right anterior thigh, and right deltoid. Patients in the control arm received surgery only. All ASI-treated patients developed ulcerations where BCG had been administered. This side effect began 3 weeks after the injection and resolved within 3 months. Sixty percent of the ASI-treated patients also developed palpable

ipsilateral inguinal adenopathy that resolved within 3 months. At a mean follow-up period of 28 months, 9 recurrences and 4 deaths were noted in the control arm, while the ASI arm had 3 recurrences and no deaths. In this small trial, ASI significantly improved survival rates and reduced recurrence rates.

Use of ASI in treating stage I or II lung cancer was reported by Hollinshead et al. (1988). They treated 34 patients with an allogeneic tumor vaccine and Freund's adjuvant, both given intradermally in the deltoid and thigh, once per month for 3 months. Half of the patients who received ASI were also treated with 1000 mg of methotrexate a week before the first vaccine. Ulcers developed slowly at the injection sites, lasted 7 to 10 days, and usually resolved within 7 months. The 2 treatment groups (ASI alone or ASI plus chemotherapy) were compared to matched controls (30 patients) and, after 5 years, 63% of the ASI treated patients were alive whereas only 33% of the control group had survived.

Berd et al. (1990) reported their experience using ASI in treating melanoma. An autologous irradiated tumor vaccine mixed with BCG was administered intradermally in the upper arms or legs 3 days after intravenous administration of cyclophosphamide 300 mg/m^2. This treatment sequence was repeated every 28 days. Fifty percent of the patients experienced nausea and vomiting after receiving the drug. All patients had local inflammatory reactions that developed into ulcers and drained clear fluid for 3 to 4 weeks after treatment. The number of treatments administered ranged from 2 to 16, with a median number of 5. Of 40 evaluable patients, there were 4 complete responses and 1 partial response. The median duration of response was 10 months. The investigators also reported that 6 of the nonresponders had delayed tumor regressions several months after ASI began. This phenomenon is similar to that reported by McCune *et al.* (1981) with their mixed responders (i.e., some lesions regressed whereas others were stable or progressed). The authors postulated a delayed immune reaction or the presence of shared antigens between the metastatic lesions and the vaccine. Non response may occur when metastatic clones lack shared antigens with the vaccine.

An allogeneic melanoma lysate treated with DETOX™ was used in 25 patients with measureable malignant melanoma (Mitchell *et al.*, 1990). Patients were treated with a low intravenous dose of cyclophosphamide (300 mg/m^2) given 5 to 7 days before the first vaccine. Five injections of the vaccine were administered once a week for 6 weeks. Each vaccine was administered subcutaneously in 2 sites, deep in the deltoid or upper buttocks. Fatigue was reported in about one third of the patients. One patient reported flu-like symptoms lasting 4 to 5 days. Granulomas developed at the injection site in 5 patients, 1 of whom developed a local abscess at the site. There was 1 complete response, 3 partial responses, and 1 case of long-term disease stability that lasted 17 months. The median duration of response was 16 months.

Scoggin and colleagues (1992) treated high-risk stage I or II melanoma patients with vaccinia melanoma oncolysate, a preparation of allogeneic melanoma cell membranes infected with the smallpox virus. Each dose was administered intradermally near major lymph node drainage areas. Forty-eight patients were treated and 24 remained disease-free. The mean disease-free interval was 22 months (range, 17 to 28 months).

A few observations may be drawn from this review of clinical trials involving treatment with ASI. There have been no reports of major large-scale controlled clinical trials testing the ASI theory, although the literature is filled with small studies using different cell preparations, adjuvants, schedules, and routes of administration. Most ASI regimens seem to be less toxic and better tolerated than conventional treatments for cancer. It is difficult to draw any conclusions, however, except to say that a small cohort of patients respond to therapy while the vast majority do not. The heterogeneity of tumors (i.e., more than one tumor associated antigen) is the prevailing theory to explain the lack of clinical responses with ASI.

No tumor vaccine has been approved to date. There are ongoing multicenter phase III trials using ASI in treating malignant melanoma. It is unlikely, however, that a tumor vaccine will be approved within the next 5 years.

Throughout the discussion of these clinical trials, a description of side effects reported by the investigators was provided. To summarize, the variety in side effects appears to be determined by the adjuvant, which is either virus- or bacteria-based, depending on the study. Fatigue, nausea and vomiting (if a cytotoxic agent is added), very mild flu-like symptoms, and local reactions—such as pain, itching, granuloma, and ulceration—are common reactions.

Expansion of clinical trials to include hormone-dependent tumors has already begun. MacLean *et al.* (1993) recently published results on their experience with a synthetic epitope (sialyl-Tn) conjugated to a high molecular weight protein carrier (keyhole limpet hemocyanin). Sialyl-Tn (STn) is found on the majority of human carcinomas of diverse histologic types including breast, colon, lung, ovary, and pancreas. Early results evaluating administration of STn mixed with DETOX™ indicate that it is safe and well tolerated in ovarian and breast cancers. Early reports of a small cohort of patients indicate that this combination when given subcutaneously in divided doses may have efficacy in treatment of early metastatic breast cancer.

Mittelman *et al.* (1990) and Levy (Tao and Levy, 1993) each are conducting clinical investigations using anti-idiotype monoclonal antibodies in place of conventional ASI. The theory behind this approach is that anti-idiotypic monoclonal antibodies possess mirror images of tumor-associated antigens and may obtain or enhance anti-tumor-associated antigen immune responses. In an initial clinical trial, Mittelman *et al.* treated 15 patients with metastatic malignant melanoma, with three showing reductions in tumor size (Mittelman *et al.*, 1988).

Two other promising approaches are under investigation, one in the preclinical area and the other currently in clinical trials in India. The preclinical work of Kaufman *et al.* (1991) involves the development of a recombinant vaccinia virus expressing human carcinoembryonic antigen for the treatment of colon cancer. Work currently being done by Talwar *et al.* (1992) focuses on vaccines for controlling fertility and may have a crossover effect on lung cancer and other hormone-dependent cancers.

It should be emphasized that through clinical trials with ASI, much progress has been made in understanding tumor immunology. The eventual replacement of crude materials with well-defined antigens will enable investigators to achieve constant, reproducible results in large-scale trials (Mitchell, 1993).

References

Amery, W., and Bruynseels, J. 1992. Levamisole, the story and the lessons. *International Journal of Immunopharmacology* 143: 481–486.

Amery, W., Cosemans, J., Gooszen, H., *et al.* 1982. Four-year results from double-blind study of adjuvant levamisole treatment in resectable lung cancer. In Terry, W., and Rosenberg, S. (eds). *Immunotherapy of Human Cancer*. Amsterdam: Elsevier, pp. 123–133.

Askenase, P., Hayden, B., and Gershon, R. 1975. Augmentation of DTH by doses of cyclophosphamide which do not affect antibody response. *Journal of Experimental Medicine* 141: 697–702.

Berd, D., Maguire, H., McCue, P., *et al.* 1990. Treatment of metastatic melanoma with an autologous tumor-cell vaccine: Clinical and immunologic results in 64 patients. *Journal of Clinical Oncology* 8(11): 1858–1867.

Bier, J., Rapp, H., and Borsus, T. 1981. Randomized clinical study on intramural BCG-cell wall preparation (CWP) therapy in patients with squamous cell carcinoma in the head and neck region. *Cancer Immunological Immunotherapy* 12: 71–79.

Bonhomme, L., Fredj, G., and Averous, S. 1991. Topical treatment of epidermic Kaposi's Sarcoma with all-*trans*-retinoic acid. *Annals of Oncology* 2: 234–235.

Cassal, W., Murray, D., and Philips, H. 1983. A phase II study of the postsurgical management of stage II malignant melanoma with Newcastle disease virus oncolysate. *Cancer* 52: 856–860.

Chomienne, C., Balitrand, N., Cost, H., *et al.* 1986. Structure-activity relationships of aromatic retinoids on the differentiation of the human histiocytic lymphoma cell U–937. *Leukemia Research* 10: 1301–1305.

Currie, G. 1972. Eighty years of immunotherapy: A review of immunological methods used for the treatment of human cancer. *British Journal of Cancer* 26: 141–153.

DeBrabander, M., DeCree, J., Vandebroek, J., *et al.* 1992. Levamisole in the treatment of cancer: Anything new? (review). *Anticancer Research* 12: 177–188.

Dennert, G. 1985. Immunostimulation by retinoic acid. In Nugent, A., and Clark, S. (eds). *Retinoids, Differentiation and Disease*. London: Pitman, pp. 117–126.

Dennert, G., Crowley, C., Koula, J., *et al.* 1979. Retinoic acid stimulation of the induction of mouse killer T cells in allogeneic and syngeneic systems. *Journal of the National Cancer Institute* 62: 89–92.

DeVet, H. 1989. The puzzling role of vitamin A in cancer prevention (review). *Anticancer Research* 9: 145–152.

Epstein, J. 1986. All-*trans*-retinoid acid and cutaneous cancers. *Journal of the American Academy of Dermatology* 15: 772–778.

Foley, E. 1953. Antigenic properties of methylcholanthrene-induced tumors in mice of the same strain of origin. *Cancer Research* 13: 835–837.

Frankel, S., Eardley, A., and Lauwers, G. 1992. The "retinoic acid syndrome" in acute promyelocytic leukemia. *Annals of Internal Medicine* 1(117): 292–296.

Freeman, C., Harris, R., Geary, C., *et al.* 1973. Active immunotherapy used alone for maintenance of patients with acute myeloid leukemia. *British Medical Journal* 4: 571.

Freund, J. 1956. The mode of action of immunological adjuvants. *Advance Tubercle Research* 1: 130–148.

Greenspan, E. 1986. Is BCG an "orphan" drug suffering from chemotherapists' overkill? *Cancer Investigation* 4(1): 81–92.

Groenwald, S., Fisher, S., and McCalla, J. 1987. Biological response modifiers. In Groenwald, S. (ed). *Cancer Nursing: Principles and Practice.* Boston: Jones and Bartlett, pp. 385–404.

Gross, L. 1943. Intradermal immunization of C3H mice against a sarcoma that originated in an animal of the same line. *Cancer Research* 3: 326–333.

Hanna, Jr., M., DeJar, R., Giunan P., *et al.* 1992. Bacillus Calmette-Guérin (BCG) vaccine for tuberculosis: Antitumor effect in experimental animals and humans. *Vaccine Research* 1(2): 69–90.

Hanna, Jr., M., Snodgrass, M., Zbar, B., *et al.* 1972. Histopathology of tumor regression after intralesional injection of *Mycobacterium bovis.* IV. Development of immunity to tumor cells and to BCG. *Journal of the National Cancer Institute* 48: 245–257.

Hollinshead, A., Takita, H., Stewart, T., *et al.* 1988. Specific active lung cancer immunotherapy: Immune correlates of clinical responses and an update of immunotherapy trials evaluations. *Cancer* 62: 1662–1671.

Hong, W., Lippman, S., Itri, L., *et al.* 1990. Prevention of secondary primary tumor with isotretinion in squamous cell carcinoma of the head and neck. *New England Journal of Medicine* 323: 795–801.

Hoover, H., Surdyke, M., Dangel, R., *et al.* 1985. Prospectively randomized trial of adjuvant active-specific immunotherapy for human colorectal cancer. *Cancer* 55: 1236–1243.

Howard, J., Christie, G., and Scott, M. 1973. Biological effects of *corynebacterium parvum.* IV. Adjuvant and inhibitory activities on B lymphocytes. *Cellular Immunology.* 7: 290–301.

Jones, S., Grozen, P., Metz, E., *et al.* 1983. Improved complete remission rates and survival for patients with large cell lymphoma treated with chemoimmunotherapy: A Southwest Oncology Group Study. *Cancer* 51: 1083–1090.

Kaufman, H., Schlom, J., and Kantor, J. 1991. A recombinant vaccinia virus expressing human carcinoembryonic antigen (CEA). *International Journal of Cancer* 48: 900–907.

Klefstrom, P., Holsti, P., Grohn, P., *et al.* 1985. Levamisole in the treatment of stage II breast cancer. *Cancer* 55: 2753–2757.

Kessler, J., Jones, S., and Levine, N. 1987. Isotretinoin and cutaneous helper T-cell lymphoma (mycosis fungoides). *Archives of Dermatology* 123: 201–204.

Kuzel, T., Roenigk, H., and Rosen, S. 1991. Mycosis fungoides and the Sezary syndrome: A review of pathogenesis, diagnosis, and therapy. *Journal of Clinical Oncology* 9: 1298–1313.

Lamm, D., DeHaven, J., Shriver, J., *et al.* 1991. Prospective randomized comparison of intravesical and percutaneous bacillus Calmette-Guérin versus intravesical bacillus Calmette-Guérin in superficial bladder cancer. *Journal of Urology* 145: 738–740.

Lammer, E., Chen, D., and Hoar, R. 1985. Retinoic acid embryopathy. *New England Journal of Medicine* 313: 837–841.

Laurie, J., Moertel, C., Fleming, T., *et al.* 1989. Surgical adjuvant therapy of large bowel carcinoma: An evaluation of levamisole and the combination of levamisole and fluorouracil. *Journal of Clinical Oncology* 7: 1447–1456.

Levine, N., and Meyskens, F. 1980. Topical vitamin A acid therapy for cutaneous metastatic melanoma. *Lancet* 2: 224–226.

Lippman, S., Parkinson, D., Itri, L., *et al.* 1992a. 13-*cis*-retinoic acid and interferon alpha–2a: Effective combination therapy for advanced squamous cell carcinoma of the skin. *Journal of the National Cancer Institute* 84: 235–241.

Lippman, S., Kavanagh, J., Paredes-Espinoza, M., *et al.* 1992b. 13-*cis*-retinoic acid plus interferon-alpha–2a: Highly active systemic therapy for squamous cell carcinoma of the cervix. *Journal of the National Cancer Institute* 84: 241–245.

Lippman, S., Kessler, J., Al-Sarraf, M., *et al.* 1988. Treatment of advanced squamous cell carcinoma of the head and neck with isotretinion: A phase II randomized trial. *Investigational New Drugs* 6: 51–56.

Lippman, S., and Meyskens, F. 1987. Treatment of advanced squamous cell carcinoma of the skin with isotretinoin. *Annals of Internal Medicine* 107: 499–502.

Lippman, S., Kessler, J., Meyskens, J. 1987. Retinoids as preventive and therapeutic anticancer agents. *Cancer Treatment Reports.* 71: 391–405.

Lotan, R., and Dennert, G. 1979. Stimulatory effects of vitamin A analogs on induction of cell-mediated cytotoxicity in vivo. *Cancer Research* 39: 55–58.

MacLean, G., Reddish, M., Koganty, R., *et al.* 1993. Immunization of breast cancer patients using a synthetic sialyl-Tn glycoconjugate plus DETOX™ adjuvant. *Cancer Immunology Immunotherapy* 36: 215–222.

Mathé, G., Amiel, J., Schwarzenberg, L., *et al.* 1969. Active immunotherapy for acute lymphocytic leukemia. *Lancet* 1: 697.

McCulloch, P., Poon, M., Dent, P., *et al.* 1982. A randomized trial of 5-fluorouracil, doxorubicin (Adriamycin), and cyclophosphamide alone or with BCG in stage IV breast cancer. In Terry, W., and Rosenberg, S., (eds). *Immunotherapy of Human Cancer.* North Holland: Elsevier, pp. 183–186.

McCune, C., Schapira, D., and Henshaw, E. 1981. Specific immunotherapy of advanced renal carcinoma: Evidence for the polyclonality of metastases. *Cancer* 47: 1984–1987.

McKhann, C., Hendrickson, C., and Spitler, L. 1975. Immunotherapy of melanoma with BCG: Two fatalities following intralesional injection. *Cancer* 35: 514–520.

McKneally, M., Maver, C., and Kausal, H. 1977. Intrapleural BCG stimulation in lung cancer. *Lancet* 1: 593.

Miller, M. 1980. Use of levamisole in parasitic infections. *Drugs* 20: 122–130.

Mitchell, M. 1993. Active specific immunotherapy of cancer: Therapeutic vaccines ("theraccines") for the treatment of disseminated malignancies. In Mitchell, M., (ed). *Biological Approaches To Cancer Treatment: Biomodulation.* New York: McGraw-Hill, Inc., pp. 326–351.

Mitchell, M., Harel, W., Kempf, R., et al. 1990. Active-specific immunotherapy for melanoma. *Journal of Clinical Oncology* 8: 856–869.

Mitchell, M., and Murntz, R. 1979. Modulation of immunity by bacillus Calmette-Guérin (BCG). *Pharmacological Therapeutics* 4: 329.

Mittelman, A., Chen, Z., Kageshita, T., et al. 1990. Active specific immunotherapy in patients with melanoma: A clinical trial with mouse antiidiotypic monoclonal antibodies. *Journal of Clinical Investigations* 86: 2136–2144.

Mittelman, A., Kageshita, T., Kusama, K., et al. 1988. A clinical trial of murine antiidiotype monoclonal antibodies to high molecular weight melanoma associated antigens (HMW-MAA) in patients with malignant melanoma (meeting abstract). *Proceedings Annual Meeting American Society of Clinical Oncology* 7: A961.

Moertel, C., Fleming, T., MacDonald, J., et al. 1990. Levamisole and fluorouracil for adjuvant therapy of resected colon carcinoma. *New England Journal of Medicine* 322: 352–358.

Morales, A., Eidinger, D., and Bruce, A. 1976. Intracavity bacillus Calmette-Guérin in the treatment of bladder tumors. *Journal of Urology* 116: 180–183.

Morton, D., Eilber, F., Malmgren, R., et al. 1970. Immunological factors which influence response to immunotherapy in malignant melanoma. *Surgery* 68(1): 158–164.

Murahata, R., and Mitchell, M. 1976. Modulation of the immune response by BCG: A review. *The Yale Journal of Biology and Medicine* 49: 283–291.

Old, L., Clarke, D., and Benacerrat, B. 1959. Effect of bacillus Calmette-Guérin infection on transplanted tumors in the mouse. *Nature* 184: 231.

Parkinson, D., Smith, M., Cheson, B., et al. 1992. Trans-retinoic acid and related differentiation agents. *Seminars in Oncology* 19 (6): 734–741.

Prehn, R., and Main, J. 1957. Immunity to methylcholanthrene-induced sarcomas. *Journal of the National Cancer Institute* 18: 769–778.

Quirt, I., Shelley, W., Pater, J., et al. 1991. Improved survival in patients with poor-prognosis malignant melanoma treated with adjuvant levamisole: A phase III study by the National Cancer Institute of Canada Clinical Trials Group. *Journal of Clinical Oncology* 9: 729–735.

Renoux, G., and Renoux, M. 1971. *Effect immunostimulant d'un imidothiazole dans immunization des souris contre l'infection par Brucella abortus.* Academy of Science de Paris.

Ribi, E., Cantrell, J., Takayama, K., et al. 1984. Lipid A and immunotherapy. *Review of Infectious Diseases* 6: 567–572.

Sahasrabudhe, D., deKernion, J., Pontes, J., et al. 1986. Specific immunotherapy with suppressor function inhibition for metastatic renal cell carcinoma. *Journal of Biological Response Modifiers* 5: 581–594.

Sankowski, A., Janik, P., Jeziorska, M., et al. 1987. The results of topical applicaton of 13-*cis*-retinoic acid on basal cell carcinoma: A correlation of the clinical effect with histopathological examination and serum retinol level. *Neoplasma* 34: 485–489.

Scoggin, S., Sivanandham, M., Sperry, R., et al. 1992. Active specific adjuvant immunotherapy with vaccinia melanoma oncolysate. *Annals of Plastic Surgery* 28: 108–109.

Scott, M. 1975. Potentiation of tumor-specific immune response by *Cornebacterium parvum. Journal of the National Cancer Institute* 55: 65–72.

Smith, M., Parkinson, D., Cheson, B., et al. 1992. Retinoids in cancer therapy. *Journal of Clinical Oncology* 10(5): 839–864.

Snodgrass, M., and Hanna, Jr., M. 1973. Ultrastructural studies of histiocyte-tumor cell interactions during tumor regression after intralesional injection of *Mycobacterium bovis. Cancer Research* 33: 701–716.

Stone, R., and Mayer, R. 1990. The unique aspects of APL. *Journal of Clinical Oncology* 8: 1913–1921.

Symoens, J., DeCree, J., Van Bever, W., et al. 1979. Levamisole. In Goldberg, M. (ed). *Pharmacological and Biochemical Properties of Drug Substances,* Vol II. Washington, D.C.: American Pharmacology Association Academy of Pharmaceutical Sciences, pp. 407–463

Talwar, G., Singh, O., Pal, R., et al. 1992. Vaccines for control of fertility and hormone-dependent cancers. *International Journal of Immunopharmacology* 14(3): 511–514.

Tao, M., and Levy, R. 1993. Idiotype/granulocyte-macrophage colony-stimulating factor fusion protein as a vaccine for B-cell lymphoma. *Nature* 362: 755–758.

Van Wauwe, J., and Janssen, P. 1991. On the biochemical mode of action of levamisole: An update. *International Journal of Immunopharmacology* 13(1): 3–9.

Weill-Hallé, B. 1980. Routes and methods of administration: Oral vaccination. In Rosenberg, S.A., (ed). *BCG Vaccine: Tuberculosis-Cancer.* Littleton, MA: P.S.G. Publishing Co., pp. 165–170.

Windhorst, D., and Nigra T. 1982. General clinical toxicology of oral retinoids. *Journal of the American Academy of Dermatology* 6: 675–677.

Wood, W., Cosimi, A., Carey, R., *et al.*, 1982. Adjuvant chemoimmunotherapy in stage I and II melanoma, pp. 245–249, In Terry, W., and Rosenberg, S. (eds). *Immunotherapy of Human Cancer*. Amsterdam: Elsevier.

Zbar, B., Bernstein, I., Bartlett, G., *et al.* 1972. Immunotherapy of cancer: Regression of intradermal tumors and prevention of growth of lymph node metastases after intralesional injection of living *Mycobacterium bovis*. *Journal of the National Cancer Institute* 49: 119–130.

PART 3

Nursing Management and Future Perspectives

CHAPTER 10 | Patient Management

Paula Trahan Rieger, RN, MSN, OCN

The field of biotherapy has grown rapidly, because of the introduction of novel agents and therapies. For both the experienced and the novice oncology nurse, staying abreast of these changes represents a constant challenge. To maintain competency, nurses need an increased knowledge base regarding the biology of cancer and the immune system, an understanding of the mechanism of action for biological response modifiers (BRMs), and an awareness of diseases and conditions for which biological agents have received approval from the Food and Drug Administration (FDA). Managing toxic effects related to therapy, administering biological agents appropriately, teaching patients and families management of therapy in the home setting, and resolving reimbursement problems are necessary skills for achieving successful outcomes. Although the mode of action and patterns of toxicity for biotherapy differ from those for chemotherapy, oncology nurses can utilize their expertise in managing cancer patients to deal with side effects unique to biotherapy. At times the need to learn specifics regarding an entire new field of specialization may appear overwhelming, but it also represents a time of opportunity and growth. Nurses working in this area have the chance to be on the cutting edge in developing standards of care for patients receiving biotherapy.

This chapter covers management of patients receiving BRMs and includes (1) assessment and planning of therapy, (2) administration concerns, (3) handling issues, and (4) management of side effects. The flu-like syndrome, mental status changes, and the side effect of fatigue will be covered in detail in separate chapters. Additional chapters will focus on patient and family education and reimbursement issues. Where available, nursing research regarding care of patients receiving biotherapy will be highlighted.

THE NURSING PROCESS

The American Nurses' Association's *Standards of Clinical Nursing Practice* defines the scope of nursing practice and provides the minimum expectation of care to be received by clients. "Standards of care" describe a competent level of nursing care as exhibited by the nursing process: assessment, diagnosis, outcome identification, planning, implementation, and evaluation (ANA, 1991). *Standards of Oncology Nursing Practice* (Oncology Nursing Society and ANA, 1987) serves as a guide for implementing the generic standards described above and for caring for patients with cancer. Utilization of these two standards of nursing practice forms the cornerstone of managing patients who are receiving biotherapy.

ASSESSMENT

Nurses have a major responsibility in the multidisciplinary management of patients who are receiving biotherapy. Figure 10.1 provides a conceptual model for assessment of patient needs related to biotherapy (Tsevat and Lacasse, 1992). (For the purposes of this chapter, the word *patient* will be assumed to include the patient and family, where applicable). The process generally begins when the physician obtains a detailed history and conducts a physical examination before placing a patient on therapy. Explanation of the purpose of therapy and its appropriateness for the patient, the treatment schedule, associated side effects, and financial concerns should all occur at this point. At this time, the physician should also obtain informed consent for patients entering a clinical trial. It is important that nurses understand the ethical and legal foundations of informed consent, to help serve as both educator and advocate for the patient (Jassak and Ryan, 1989; Rieger and Weatherly, 1989; Varricchio and Jassak, 1989; Lynch, 1988). Within the scope of nursing practice, the nurse can do much to address patient concerns related to the clinical trial, reinforce information about biotherapy, and clarify misconceptions. Assessing whether pa-

tients understand the therapeutic plan and their responsibility to adhere to that plan is crucial. Any misconceptions should be relayed to other members of the health care team as appropriate, especially since the nurse is often in a position to answer many questions the patient is either too embarrassed or afraid to ask the physician.

Pretherapy Assessments

Prior to initiation of therapy, the nurse should use a body systems approach to perform a baseline assessment. This assessment should include a history of prior treatment; current symptoms related to the underlying disease process or prior treatment; history of chronic illnesses; functional status; psychosocial concerns; and hopes, fears, and expectations related to therapy (Brophy and Rieger, 1992). Examples of factors that place the patient at a higher risk for developing side effects associated with biotherapy include pre-existing cardiac problems, a history of psychiatric problems, poor functional status, poor nutritional status, or advanced age (Irwin, 1987). A medication and allergy profile should also be obtained. Medications such as aspirin, steroids, nonsteroidal anti-inflammatory drugs, or sedatives may be contraindicated with certain biological agents.

The needs of geriatric patients require special attention. Additional factors that may affect dosage and tolerance of biotherapy for these patients include alterations in hepatic and renal function; decreased cardiovascular function; alterations in neurosensory perceptual protective mechanisms (e.g., vision); and decreased integrity of tissue, skin, and mucous membranes (Rieger, 1994; Boyle *et al.*, 1992). Examination of the medication profile is of special importance in the elderly.

Recommended baseline physiological measurements include height, weight, temperature, pulse, blood pressure (including orthostatic measures for patients receiving agents known to cause hypotension), and respiratory rate. Results of baseline chest x-ray and electro-

Figure 10.1   Needs of Biotherapy Patients: A Conceptual Model.

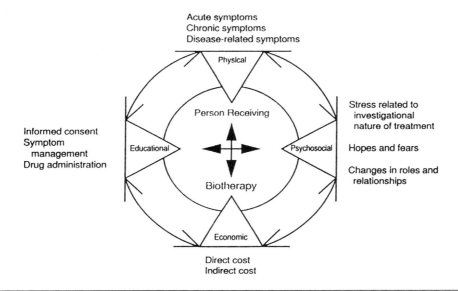

Source: Reprinted with permission from Tsevat, J., and Lacasse, C. 1992. Understanding the special needs of patients receiving biotherapy: A conceptual model. In Carroll-Johnson, R. (ed). *The Biotherapy of Cancer—V.* Pittsburgh: Oncology Nursing Press.

cardiogram should also be reviewed as should an initial laboratory profile to measure hematologic, renal, metabolic and hepatic functions. This profile may include

1. complete blood count, differential count, platelet and reticulocyte count, prothrombin time, and partial thromboplastin time;
2. blood urea nitrogen, creatinine, urinalysis;
3. electrolytes (sodium, potassium, chloride, carbon dioxide), calcium, magnesium, and phosphorus;
4. serum albumin, liver function tests (bilirubin, alkaline phosphatase, lactate dehydrogenase, serum aspartate aminotransferase, and serum alanine aminotransferase); and
5. TSH (thyroid-stimulating hormone), T3 (total serum triiodothyronine), T4 (total serum) (with interleukin–2 (IL–2) therapy) (Irwin, 1987; Lotze and Rosenberg, 1991).

Patients should be able to verbalize the rationale and nature of the therapy (e.g., commercial vs. investigational) they are to receive. The primary goal for chemotherapy is generally treatment of disease. However, due to the unique nature of biotherapy, several goals of treatment (investigational, therapeutic, diagnostic, or supportive) are possible. In most cases, biotherapy is used to treat disease and will be either conventional (FDA approved) or investigational. However, patients may also receive biotherapy for diagnostic purposes, as is the case with certain monoclonal antibodies (e.g., Onco-Scint®). Patients may receive biotherapy for supportive reasons as is evidenced by the post-chemotherapy use of hematopoietic growth factors to abrogate myelosuppression.

The therapeutic plan should also be assessed before treatment begins so that the oncology nurse can develop a care plan and intervene appropriately. Areas to consider include the following:

- Setting: Will therapy be given in the hospital, the ambulatory setting, or both? Determination of the patient's compliance with the treatment schedule is of prime importance in the ambulatory setting.
- Diagnostic tests: What types of laboratory tests (routine lab work, special lab work, or pharmacology studies) and diagnostic procedures are required?
- Toxicity: What agent(s) will the patient receive, and what are the associated side effects?
- Nature of therapy: Is the therapy approved by the FDA or investigational? If investigational, has consent been secured?
- Monitoring: Will special monitoring, such as orthostatic blood pressure, special vital signs, central venous pressure, or intake and output measurements, be required?

The initial assessment should also include evaluation of psychosocial concerns including the patient's usual coping patterns (Hogan, 1991; Madeya, 1990), support systems, financial status, and related concerns. Cultural factors such as race, religion, and belief system are also relevant and should be included in the initial assessment. Furthermore, the high percentage of biotherapy administered in the outpatient setting requires assessment of the home setting and the patient's ability to travel to and from the treatment center. Because many biotherapy trials are investigational, patients may receive therapy away from home and their usual support systems. Common concerns while patients are away receiving treatment include finances, appropriate housing, family, friends, and job. Patients may also feel lonely and fearful of the unknown outcome of their therapy. Allowing them to voice their concerns and assisting them with resolution of problems through appropriate referrals is an important

Table 10.1 Potential nursing diagnoses for patients receiving biotherapy

Prevention and Detection
  Health seeking behaviors
Information and Education
  Knowledge deficit
  Management of therapeutic regimen (individual), ineffective
Coping
  Anxiety
  Coping, ineffective individual
  Spiritual distress
  Body image disturbance
  Social interaction, impaired
  Role performance, altered
Discomfort
  Pain
Nutrition
  Nutrition, altered: less than body requirements
Protective Mechanisms
  Infection, high risk for
  Oral mucous membrane, altered
  Sensory/perceptual alterations
  Skin integrity, impaired
  Skin integrity, impaired, high risk for
  Body temperature, altered, high risk for
  Thought processes, altered
  Protection, altered
  Sleep pattern disturbance
Mobility and Activity
  Fatigue
  Activity intolerance
Elimination
  Diarrhea
  Urinary elimination, altered
Sexuality
  Sexuality patterns, altered
Ventilation
  Gas exchange, impaired
Circulation
  Fluid volume deficit, high risk for
  Tissue perfusion, altered (specify)

nursing intervention. Table 10.1 provides a list of potential nursing diagnoses for patients who are receiving biotherapy.

Assessment During Therapy

During therapy the nurse performs a significant role in assessment of the patient's adherence to the therapeutic plan and tolerance to therapy. Especially with BRMs that are investigational, information gained by the nurse can make a significant contribution to delineating side effects associated with an agent. A basic understanding of the mode of action and side effects (acute and chronic) associated with the agent(s) being administered forms the foundation for an ongoing assessment of biotherapy. This knowledge should be applied in a regular, systematic manner that includes monitoring of vital signs and review of body systems and pertinent laboratory values. Frequency should include every shift for hospitalized patients or every clinic visit for outpatients. This ongoing assessment assists in formulating and updating the patient's care plan.

Symptoms should be evaluated in the context of timing (onset, duration, and frequency), location, setting, quality, quantity, aggravating and alleviating factors, and associated symptoms. However, few scales exist that reliably quantify common symptoms associated with biotherapy (e.g., fatigue, anorexia, and mental status changes). Nevertheless, a symptom report form for self-reporting or a nursing care flow sheet can be designed to quantify and record the side effects experienced by patients. Quantification of severity of symptoms can range from as simple as noting numerical codes for mild, moderate, or severe, or can be more sophisticated as in the use of grading scales associated with clinical trials (White, 1992; Strauman *et al.*, 1988; Oken *et al.*, 1982; Miller *et al.*, 1981).

Post-Therapy Assessment

Once patients have completed or have been removed from therapy, routine follow-up examinations should continue. Toxic effects that were experienced during therapy should be reassessed for resolution. In addition, patients may continue to need assistance with managing symptoms associated with their disease.

Psychosocial Concerns

Psychosocial concerns are especially important at the time therapy is discontinued. A decision to stop therapy due to progression of disease often represents a time of crisis for patients. Previous responses to original diagnosis, prognosis, or possible failure of prior treatment may reoccur. Emotions may be intense, especially with the addition of disappointment and dashed hopes. It is critical that the patient not feel abandoned by the health care team. Often, the simplest measures such as touch and active listening can reassure patients that they will not be abandoned (Soeken and Carson, 1987). Even if cure is not possible, hope can be fostered that something, such as management of symptoms, can be done for the patient during the terminal phase of disease.

A study by Hunt Raleigh in 1992 identified and explored sources of hope in 90 patients with cancer or another chronic illness. In her study, no significant differences were found between patients with cancer and patients with other chronic illnesses. The most commonly reported sources for supporting hopefulness were family, friends, and religious beliefs. Patients were also able to describe specific cognitive or behavioral strategies used for maintaining hope. Strategies such as "getting busy," "talking to other people," the use of prayer or religious activities, and "thinking of other things" were employed to combat periods of lowered hope. Assessment of the need to refer the patient to the team psychologist, psychiatric clinical nurse specialist, clergy, or social workers should also be evaluated. The use of support groups, lay volunteers, or cancer survivors trained to provide support may also be helpful.

ADMINISTRATION OF BIOTHERAPY

Biotherapy may be administered by a variety of routes and schedules (see Chapters 4–9).

The most common routes are subcutaneous, intramuscular, or intravenous single bolus, and intermittent or continuous infusions. The nurse should be aware that patients receiving IL–2 are often at higher risk for catheter-related infections (Bock *et al.*, 1990). Potential reasons that this may occur include decreased neutrophil chemotaxis, transient impairment of T-cell immunity, and IL–2 skin toxicity. Strict aseptic technique should be used when caring for central catheters in patients receiving IL–2. In addition, many institutions use prophylactic antibiotics to prevent infection (Bock *et al.*, 1990; Snydman *et al.*, 1990). Other routes such as intraperitoneal (IP), intraarterial (IA), intrathecal (IT), intravesical, intralesional, or scarification may also be used. Dosage is usually calculated by body surface area (per m²), per kilogram (kg), or a predetermined standard dosage.

Several safety measures should be used when administering BRMS:

- Use proper aseptic technique during preparation and administration.
- Implement institutional procedures as appropriate for investigational agents.
- Identify the location of emergency equipment and supplies.
- Administer premedication (e.g., acetaminophen, meperidine) as ordered.
- Educate patients on expected side effects and on signs and symptoms that should be reported.
- Determine any special handling precautions or need for special equipment or supplies.
- Verify monitoring of special vital signs (e.g., every 15 minutes for 1 hour), orthostatic blood pressures, or assessment of injection sites.
- Use appropriate storage requirements. Many biological agents should be refrigerated—not frozen—at 36° to 46°F (2° to 8°C).

BRMs are manufactured by several companies; thus, characteristics of the particular drug to be used, such as available vial size, solubility, stability, compatibility, filterability, and storage requirements must be determined prior to administration. Any special considerations, such as mixing with albumin or the need for special pumps or tubing, must also be assessed. For example, with continuous infusions of IL–2, it is often difficult to simultaneously infuse vasopressor agents, concurrent fluids, and medications for control of symptoms; hence, a special intravenous tubing set-up may be required (Rieger, 1989). See Table 10.2 for a review of special considerations for commonly used BRMs. Pharmacy resource personnel and package inserts can also provide specific information on biological agents (Amgen, Inc., 1989; Chiron Therapeutics, 1994; Berlex, 1993; Knoll Pharmaceuticals, 1993; Ortho Biotech, 1993; Schering Corporation, 1992; Amgen, Inc., 1991; Genentech, 1991; Immunex Corporation, 1991; Janssen, 1990; Purdue Frederick, 1990; Roche Laboratories, 1990).

Handling and Disposal of Biological Agents

Policies and procedures governing safe handling of cytotoxic agents during preparation, administration, and disposal are well established nationwide (Dana and Anderson, 1990; Oncology Nursing Society, 1988). However, there has been no formal research to date regarding the safest way to handle biological agents. Although the majority of BRMs do not directly affect DNA and are therefore not considered genotoxic substances (Dana, 1988) and although no published recommendations exist, it is wise to avoid direct contact with skin and to avoid generating aerosols (Conrad and Horrell, in press). For simplicity, many institutions place BRMs in the category of cytotoxic products requiring special handling; nurses are advised to check institutional policy regarding handling of BRMs at their place of employment. The addition of chemotherapeutic agents or toxins to BRMs would necessitate special handling, and the addition of

Table 10.2 Characteristics of and dosage recommendations for commercially available BRMs

Agent	Vial sizes	Route	Dose	Characteristics and Stability	Distributor	Storage/ Special Guidelines
Intron®A (interferon alfa-2b recombinant)	3, 5, 10, 18, 25, and 50 MIU (powdered); Diluent included; 10 and 25 MIU (solution)	Intramuscular Subcutaneous Intralesional	Hairy Cell Leukemia 2 MIU/m²SC or IM 3x/week Kaposi's sarcoma 30 MIU/m²SC or IM 3x/week Hepatitis B 30–35 MIU/ week SC or IM QD or 10 MIU 3x/week for 16 weeks Hepatitis Non-A, Non-B/C 3 MIU SQ or IM 3x/week Condyloma acuminata 10 MIU/1.00 cc Inject 0.1 cc per lesion 3x/ week for 3 weeks	Multi-dose vial Reconstituted powder is stable 30 days when properly stored.	Schering Corporation (Kenilworth, NJ)	Refrigerate. Do not freeze or shake.
Roferon®-A (interferon alfa-2a recombinant)	3, 9, 18, 36 MIU liquid vials 18 MIU (powdered)	Intramuscular Subcutaneous	Hairy Cell Leukemia 3 MIU QD SC or IM x 16–24 weeks (induction) Kaposi's sarcoma 36 MIU QD SC or IM for 10–12 weeks (induction)	Multi-dose vial Reconstituted powder is stable 30 days when properly stored.	Roche Laboratories (Nutley, NJ)	Refrigerate. Do not freeze or shake.

Continued

Table 10.2 Continued

Agent	Vial sizes	Route	Dose	Characteristics and Stability	Distributor	Storage/ Special Guidelines
Alferon®N (interferon alfa-n3) Derived from human leukocytes	5 MIU (liquid)	Intralesional	Condyloma acuminata 250,000 IU/wart 2x/ week for up to 8 weeks	Multi-dose vial Stable 1 month after vial is punctured.	The Purdue Frederick Company (Norwalk, CT)	Refrigerate. Do not freeze or shake.
Actimmune® (interferon gamma 1b)	100-μg vials (liquid)	Subcutaneous	Chronic granulomatous disease (BSA > 0.5 m^2) 50 μg/m^2 SC 3x/week	Single-dose vial; discard unused portion. Stable for a maximum of 12 hours at room temperature.	Genentech, Inc. (San Francisco, CA)	Refrigerate. Do not freeze or shake.
Betaseron® (interferon beta 1B)	9.6 MIU powdered vial Diluent included	Subcutaneous	Multiple sclerosis 8 MIU SC every 48 hours	Single dose vial Discard unused portion Use within 3 hours of reconstitution	Berlex Laboratories (Richmond, CA)	Refrigerate. Do not freeze or shake.
Leukine® (sargramostim)	250 or 500 μg (powdered)	Intravenous infusion	Approved for the acceleration of myeloid recovery post autologous bone marrow transplant in patients with non-Hodgkin's lymphoma (NHL), acute lymphoblastic leukemia (ALL), and Hodgkin's disease. 250μg/m^2/day for 21 days as an intravenous infusion over 2 hours *Discontinue if ANC > 20,000/mm^3	Dilute in 0.9% sodium chloride solution for IV adminstration. Do not add other medications to infused solution. Preservative free, administer as soon as possible after reconstitution.	Immunex Corporation (Seattle, WA)	Refrigerate. Do not freeze or shake. If concentration is less than 10 mcg/ml, albumin should be added to saline.

Agent	Dosage Form	Route	Indication/Dosing	Preparation	Manufacturer	Storage
Neupogen® (filgrastim)	300 or 480 mcg (liquid)	Subcutaneous Intravenous	Approved to decrease incidence of infection in patients with non-myeloid malignancies receiving myelo-suppressive chemo-therapy and post bone marrow transplant in non-myeloid malignancies 5 μg/kg/day SC for 14 days or until ANC reaches 10,000 cells/mm³ Doses may be increased in increments of 5 μg/kg according to the duration and severity of neutropenia. Neupogen® should be administered no earlier than 24 hours after cytotoxic chemotherapy.	Dilute in dextrose 5% or 0.9% sodium chloride. Compatibility data not available. Single-dose vial; discard unused portions; Stable for a maximum of 6 hours at room temperature	Amgen Inc. (Thousand Oaks, CA)	Refrigerate. Do not freeze or shake.
Procrit® (epoetin alfa)	2000, 3000, 4000 or 10,000 units (liquid)	Intravenous Subcutaneous	Approved for the treatment of anemia in patients with chronic renal failure 50–100 U/kg 3x/week intravenous infusion until target hematocrit is reached May be given by subcutaneous route for non-dialysis patients Approved for the treatment of anemia in cancer patients on chemotherapy 150 U/kg 3x/week SC or by intravenous infusion until target hematocrit is reached	Do not administer in conjunction with other drugs. Single-dose vial; discard unused portions	Ortho-Biotech Ortho Pharma-ceutical Corporation (Raritan, NJ)	Refrigerate. Do not freeze or shake.

Continued

203

Table 10.2 *Continued*

Agent	Vial sizes	Route	Dose	Characteristics and Stability	Distributor	Storage/ Special Guidelines
			Approved for the treatment of anemia in AZT-treated HIV-infected patients (Epo level ≤ 500 mU/ml) 100 U/kg 3x/week SC or by intravenous infusion for 8 weeks			
Epogen® (epoetin alfa)	2000, 3000, 4000, or 10,000 units (liquid)	Intravenous Subcutaneous	Approved for the treatment of anemia in patients with chronic renal failure	Do not administer in conjunction with other drugs.	Amgen Inc. (Thousand Oaks, CA)	Refrigerate. Do not freeze or shake.
			50–100 U/kg 3x/week intravenous infusion until target hemotocrit is reached	Single-dose vial; discard unused portions		
			May be given by subcutaneous route for non-dialysis patients			
Proleukin® (aldesleukin)	22 million IU (powdered)	Intravenous bolus	Metastic renal cancer 600,000 IU/kg Q 8 hours by intravenous bolus x 14 doses	Do not mix with other drugs; do not use in-line filters.	Chiron Therapeutics (Emeryville, CA)	Refrigerate. Do not shake.
				Dilute with 5% dextrose; do not reconstitute with bacteriostatic agents.		
				Stable in solution 48 hours.		

| Ergamisol® (levamisole HCL) | 50 mg tablets | Oral | Adjuvant treatment of Duke's C colon cancer in combination with 5-fluorouracil (5-FU) post surgical resection 50 mg by mouth Q 8 hours for 3 days every two weeks for 1 year. | Stable at room temperature | Janssen Pharmaceutica (Piscataway, NJ) | Protect from moisture. |

MIU = million international units
IU = international units
U = units
SC = subcutaneous
IM = intramuscular
QD = every day
Q = every
BSA = body surface area
ANC = absolute neutrophil count

radioisotopes would further require the use of radiation safety precautions specific for the isotope in use. Appropriate precautions regarding blood and body fluids should also be adhered to per institutional policy, and patients should be taught these precautions.

Proper disposal of used vials and equipment used in biotherapy, especially in the home care setting, is a topic of increasing importance. Institutional and community policies regarding these concerns should be researched. The United States Environmental Protection Agency (1990) provides an educational card for disposal of equipment at home. In general, used vials, needles, and syringes should be disposed of in a sealed, puncture-resistant container. Patients should be taught not to recap needles. Occasionally, patients who are participating in a clinical trial may be required to return both empty and unused vials to the dispensing institution for accountability purposes (Hahn and Jassak, 1988).

MANAGEMENT OF SIDE EFFECTS

Managing side effects associated with biotherapy represents one of the primary challenges to the oncology nurse. Side effects unique to individual agents have been reviewed in Chapters 4–9. Side effects commonly associated with biotherapy include constitutional or flu-like symptoms, fatigue, anorexia, weight changes (increase or decrease), mental status changes, skin changes (erythema or rash), hypotension, and hematologic changes. This section will cover management strategies using a systems approach.

The pathophysiology underlying toxic effects associated with BRMs is now an active area of research and it is hoped, will guide future interventions (Sergi, 1991; Rieger, 1992). Though management of biotherapy-related side effects may require the acquisition of new knowledge and skills, utilization of existing expertise in the care of oncology patients forms a foundation on which to build. Nurses are in a pivotal position to advance the management of side effects by creatively manipulating the familiar to develop new solutions (Cunningham, 1989).

Characteristics of biotherapy-related side effects differ from those associated with chemotherapy. Most biotherapy toxicity is dose related, that is, with the intensity of effects increasing as the dose is elevated. Toxic effects are typically noncumulative in that there is not a ceiling dose beyond which a patient can receive no further therapy. Furthermore, most biotherapy-related side effects, myelosuppression included, are readily reversible upon cessation of therapy. Timing of side effects may also differ from that of chemotherapy. For example, certain side effects may occur early in therapy and are often termed acute. Others are manifested late in therapy and are classified as chronic. Although most side effects are not life-threatening, they often have tremendous impact upon the patient's quality of life. Physical side effects such as the flu-like syndrome (FLS), gastrointestinal effects, fatigue, and mental status changes may influence quality of life due to alteration of social, physiological, and psychological functions (Brophy and Sharp, 1991). Lastly, signs and symptoms deemed reportable by the health care team also differ for BRMs. See Table 10.3 for a list of critical indicators that should be reported.

Nursing interventions described in this section represent the author's experience as well as the expertise of nurses across the country who have worked with patients receiving biotherapy. The reader is referred to the following references for further information on care of the patient receiving biotherapy: Conrad and Horrell, in press; Rieger, 1994; Jassak, 1993; Brophy and Rieger, 1992; Rumsey and Rieger, 1992; White, 1992; Brophy and Sharp, 1991; Hood and Abernathy, 1991; Mayer, 1990; Dillman, 1989; Rieger and Weatherly, 1989; Collins and Thaney, 1988; Hahn and Jassak, 1988; Padavic-Shaller, 1988; Yarbro, 1993). In addition, many pharmaceutical companies provide educational resources for nurses to guide them in the care of patients who are receiving biotherapy. The local pharmaceutical sales representative for each company who

Table 10.3   Critical indicators in biotherapy

Excessive fatigue

Severe mental status changes
   Excessive somnolence
   Confusion
   Psychosis

Cardiac symptoms
   Chest pain
   Arrhythmias
   Symptomatic hypotension

Weight changes
   Losses greater than 10 lbs
   Gains greater than 10 lbs

Allergic reactions
   Anaphylaxis
   Hives and itching

Dyspnea

Oliguria

Severe local inflammatory reactions

Fever
   Uncontrolled with antipyretics
   Unrelated to normal patterns of response

markets oncology products is a valuable source of information on nursing support materials and patient support materials currently available from his or her company. See Table 10.4 for a list of some resources that are available. Guidelines from the Oncology Nursing Society are also available for specific nursing diagnoses to guide care of the oncology patient (McNally et al., 1991).

Gastrointestinal System

Maintenance of nutritional status during therapy is of prime importance because anorexia and associated weight loss are common side effects of many biological agents. Patients often complain of a decreased desire for food or lack of motivation to eat. Taste changes that negatively affect food intake are also commonly reported. Thus, baseline weight, nutritional status, and dietary intake should be assessed and documented. Measures used with other oncology patients—such as small, frequent meals and caloric supplements—are ap-

propriate with this patient population. Exploration of which foods remain appealing and emphasis on the foods the patient tolerates well rather than on foods the patient no longer finds appealing are often helpful. Educating the family to not expect the patient to eat three regular meals daily will assist in alleviating pressure on the patient to eat. Encouragement of socialization with meals may assist in increasing oral intake (Rust et al., 1990). A dietary consult should be utilized as needed, and if weight loss becomes significant (5% to 10% of body weight or greater) (Mayer et al., 1984), tube feedings or total parenteral nutrition may need to be considered.

Nausea and vomiting are uncommon with most biological agents, except for IL–2. With interferon therapy, nausea and vomiting usually occur in conjunction with FLS and are seen more consistently at higher doses (Quesada et al., 1986). The nausea and vomiting associated with IL–2 therapy more closely parallels that associated with chemotherapy. Patients tend to be sensitive to food odors and to be unable to eat due to nausea. Prophylactic, scheduled administration of antiemetics is often necessary to control this side effect. See Table 10.5 for a list of useful antiemetic medications. Nonpharmacological interventions might include relaxation therapy and guided imagery. Maintaining an odor-free environment and serving the patient cold foods are also practical measures.

Mucositis may also occur with biotherapy, most commonly with IL–2 therapy. Symptoms typically include a dry, inflamed oral mucosa without ulceration. The oral cavity should be assessed and its condition documented at regular intervals using a valid and reliable scale. A pretreatment oral assessment by the dental oncologist to identify and treat pre-existing oral disease may be recommended, especially when biotherapy will be given in conjunction with chemotherapy. Patients should have meticulous oral hygiene with saline and baking soda rinses and soft toothbrushes. Additional interventions include diet modification for comfort and avoidance of injury to the oral

Table 10.4   Available professional resources from pharmaceutical companies

Pharmaceutical Company	Resources
Amgen Inc. Thousand Oaks, CA	Professional Services Department 1–800–77–AMGEN • Filgrastim slide program • Hematopoiesis • Colony-stimulating factors • G-CSF • Neupogen®—Treatment and management of the neutropenic cancer patient • Management and education of the neutropenic cancer patient receiving Neupogen® therapy • Cancer, chemotherapy, and neutropenia • These programs are presented by the Amgen Clinical Support Specialist. Contact your Amgen Professional Sales Representative to schedule. Professional Speakers Bureau
Chiron Therapeutics Emeryville, CA	Professional Services Line (product and medical information) 1–800–244–7668 (1–800–CHIRON–8) Nurse Network 1–800–IL2NURSE Immuno-Primer Series (1987) R. B. Herberman series Editor Physician's and Nurse's Guidelines for Proleukin® (aldesleukin) Therapy (1993) Monograph Proleukin® (aldesleukin): Management of patients with metastic renal cell carcinoma (1993) Monograph Management guidelines for outpatient IL-2 therapy (available upon request) Professional Speakers Bureau
Immunex Corporation Seattle, WA	Professional Services Department 1–800–IMMUNEX Customer service 1–800–IMMUNEX • Leukine® slide curriculum • Hematopoiesis chart • The cells of the Hematopoietic Cascade—Video and monograph provides CE credit for nurses • Professional Speakers Program • Obtained via the local IMMUNEX oncology representative or via 1–800–IMMUNEX.
Ortho Biotech Ortho Pharmaceutical Corporation Raritan, NJ	Professional Speakers Bureau 1–800–2BIOTECH Therapy for anemia in cancer patients with nonmyeloid malignancies on chemotherapy: Procrit® (epoetin alfa)—Monograph 1993 Treatment of cancer-related anemias—Proceedings of an educational symposium held at ONS Congress, May 1992—monograph New therapies for the anemia of chemotherapy and hairy cell leukemia—based on a symposium held at the 18th annual ONS Congress, May 1993—monograph Peer-to-Peer Network 1–800–984–PEER (professional support for questions related to Procrit® administration) Dimensions of Caring 1–800–6ENABLE (professional support for questions related to fatigue and other related concerns)

Table 10.4 *Continued*

Pharmaceutical Company	*Resources*
Roche Laboratories Nutley, NJ	Professional Service Line 1–800–7ROFERON Professional Guidelines: Managing Roferon®-A therapy and self-administration instruction. The right combination—To increase survival and improve quality of life. Managing AIDS-Related Kaposi's Sarcoma Body Surface Area Calculator Managing Side Effects (videotape) Understanding the Immune System: A New Frontier in Medicine (videotape and workbook)
Schering Corporation Kenilworth, NJ	Drug Information Services (computerized data service) 1–800–526–4099 Intron®A: A practical guide for nurses. 3/94 The management of fatigue (slim Jim) Patient management techniques for interferon therapy (slim Jim) Chronic hepatitis B and Chronic hepatitis non-A, non-B/C: Two common forms one effective therapy. 6/92 Nursing Management of side effects of interferon-alpha—Videotape available in 1994

mucosa and avoidance of commercial mouthwash solutions that can exacerbate oral dryness. Artificial saliva and food with sauces may be helpful if oral dryness is extreme.

Diarrhea does not commonly occur with most biological agents, except for the severe diarrhea that occurs with IL–2 administration. Antidiarrheal medications will generally control this side effect. Careful assessment of hydration status and electrolyte balance of patients with diarrhea is an important nursing responsibility. Fluid replacement and dietary modifications, such as avoidance of foods high in roughage, are helpful suggestions for symptom management. It is also important that skin integrity in the perianal area be assessed in patients experiencing diarrhea. Hygienic measures and the use of prophylactic barrier creams to protect both damaged and intact skin are indicated.

Cardiovascular/Pulmonary Systems

A thorough assessment of cardiopulmonary parameters is important with administration of all BRMs, and is of extreme importance with IL–2 due to capillary leak syndrome (described in Chapter 5). Nursing measures critical for management of this syndrome include monitoring heart rate, blood pressure (including orthostatic checks), central venous pressure, and other cardiac indices. Accurate daily weights and strict fluid intake and output measures are of prime importance in evaluating fluid shifts (Lotze and Rosenberg, 1991; Sargent and Shelton, 1990; Padavic-Shaller, 1988; Simpson *et al.*, 1988) as is evaluation for edema and ascites. Daily measurement of abdominal girths may also be helpful in determining the quantity of fluid retention. Safety measures include teaching patients to rise slowly from a lying position to a sitting or standing position to avoid dizziness. Bed rest may be needed if systolic blood pressure consistently runs less than 80 mm Hg and the patient is symptomatic. Medical management includes the use of vasopressors to maintain blood pressure, judicious use of fluid boluses, and if cardiovascular parameters are unstable, transfer to the intensive care unit.

Table 10.5 Medications commonly used in the management of IL-2 toxicity

Antipyretic analgesic agents	*Antianxiety, antihallucinogen, and hypnotic agents*
acetaminophen	diphenhydramine
Antiinflammatory agents	diazepam
indomethacin	fentanyl
naproxen	flurazepam
sulindac	haloperidol
Histamine H₂ antagonist agents	*Diuretic agents*
cimetidine	furosemide
ranitidine	metolazone
Antiemetic agents	*Agents to control chills*
lorazepam	meperidine HCL
prochlorperazine maleate	indomethacin
promethazine HCL	dilaudid SL
droperidol	*Vasopressors and antiarrythmic agents*
ondansetron	dopamine HCL
ABH (lorazepam, diphenhydramine, haloperidol)	verapamil HCL
scopolamine patches	atropine SO₄
Antidiarrheal agents	*Antihypotensive measures*
codeine phosphate	0.9% sodium chloride boluses
kaolin and pectin	5% N serum albumin
opium tincture	
diphenoxylate HCL with atropine SO₄	*Antipruritic agents*
	hydroxyzine hydrochloride
	diphenhydramine
	colloidal oatmeal

Source: Revised and reprinted with permission from Padavic-Shaller, K. 1988. Nursing applications in a developing science. *Seminars in Oncology Nursing* 4(2): 142–151.

Pulmonary complications with biotherapy are most commonly associated with fluid shifts related to IL–2 therapy or allergic reactions to a monoclonal antibody. Assessment for such complications includes auscultation of breath sounds, monitoring oxygenation, and evaluating complaints of shortness of breath or altered breathing patterns (Farrell, 1992). Nursing measures include positioning patients for minimal respiratory effort, adjusting the patient's physical activities, and reporting significant changes to the physician. Medical management includes administration of oxygen or diuretics or interruption of therapy. In extreme cases, with patients on high-dose IL–2 therapy, intubation and mechanical ventilation may be required.

Renal System

Among the various biotherapies, renal toxicity is most frequently seen with IL–2 therapy, although renal changes may also be seen in patients receiving interferon therapy. Assessment for elevations in BUN, creatinine, decreased urine output, and significant weight gains should be made, and changes reported to the physician. With IL–2, fluid shifts will cause urine output to decrease over time. Intake and output will not balance; therefore, it is helpful if the physician defines a minimum fluid output (10–30 ml/hr, for example) (Hynes *et al.*, 1990) that can be used as a guideline for reporting changes. Medical management includes judicious administration of fluids, diuretics, and low doses of vasopressors to maintain blood flow to the kidneys.

Hematologic

Hematologic changes are not typically problematic in patients receiving biotherapy; however, white blood cell count (including differential and platelets), coagulation profile, and reticulocyte count should be monitored to detect significant lowering of counts. Should myelosuppression or thrombocytopenia develop, cessation of therapy will generally lead to rapid recovery of blood cell counts. The patient should be taught the signs and symptoms and appropriate precautions for thrombocytopenia, neutropenia, and anemia should they occur. Replacement therapy with blood and platelets should be administered as ordered (Rostad, 1991). There are no specific therapeutic interventions that are related to the rise in eosinophils that is seen with IL–2 administration.

Hepatic Function

Changes in measures of hepatic function are common in patients who receive biotherapy, although the precise pathophysiology is unknown. Nursing measures include assessing patients for changes in liver function tests, hyperbilirubinemia, jaundice or hepatomegaly, and reporting significant changes to the physician.

Metabolism

Metabolic changes such as hypothyroidism, hypomagnesemia, hypophosphatemia, and hypocalcemia may also be seen during treatment with BRMs, especially for patients receiving IL-2. Lab values should be monitored and significant changes reported to the physician. Medical interventions such as replacement therapy should be instituted as ordered.

Integument

Skin changes most frequently experienced are erythema, rashes, dryness with resultant desquamation and inflammatory reactions at injection sites. Rashes are commonly seen with IL-2 and may also occur with interferon and GM-CSF. The baseline assessment of skin condition should include evaluation for a history of underlying skin conditions such as psoriasis and any pre-existing rashes or lesions. Skin should be carefully inspected for signs of breakdown or infection. Therapeutic measures for dry, pruritic skin include application of water-based lotions or creams several times daily, especially after bathing. Bath oils and mild soaps should be used. Cleansing should be gentle (avoid scrubbing the skin), and bath water should be tepid rather than hot. Clothing should be of soft cotton. Perfumed lotions are to be avoided as they can further irritate already sensitive skin. Additional measures for treating pruritus include aggressive use of antipruritic medications such as diphenhydramine or hydroxyzine hydrochloride (often on a scheduled basis), and colloidal oatmeal baths (Dangel, 1986). For some patients room humidifiers help relieve pruritic skin conditions (Rieger and Weatherly, 1989). Patients who receive IL-2 should be cautioned against the use

of topical steroids, which are contraindicated in most cases due to interference with the biological effects of IL-2. Patients experiencing severe skin changes in addition to other related IL-2 side effects such as edema and weight gain often experience profound alterations in appearance. The resulting changes in body image can cause significant distress for patients. Nursing interventions include encouraging patients to express their feelings and providing reassurance that changes will resolve when therapy is completed (Becker and Koutlas, 1990).

Inflammation with resultant erythema and swelling may occur at subcutaneous injections sites. These reactions generally resolve within 24 to 48 hours, but may be upsetting to patients. Further injections at inflamed sites must be avoided until healing is complete. Treatment is usually not necessary, but if applications of cold or heat are considered, their use should be verified with the physician as they may alter medication absorption patterns. With subcutaneous injections of IL-2, knots may persist at the injection site for several months. If pruritus occurs at the injection site, premedication with diphenhydramine may be helpful. Occasionally patients complain of pain associated with subcutaneous injections. Topical applications of cream containing 50% lidocaine and 50% prilocaine (Emla® Astra Pharmaceutical Products, Inc., Westborough, MA) may be useful.

Although rare, alopecia may occasionally be experienced by patients who are receiving biotherapy. Patients will report a thinning of hair rather than actual hair loss. Use of wigs, scarves, and headwraps would be appropriate with this population should thinning cause noticeable changes. Patients may be reassured that hair will regrow when therapy is complete.

Allergic Reactions

Allergic reactions are most commonly associated with monoclonal antibody (MAB) infusions (Dillman, 1988). Symptoms may include fever, chills, hives, pruritus, shortness of breath, or hypotension. Patients should be monitored regularly for vital signs, often as frequently as every 15 minutes for the first hour, and observed closely when therapy is initiated. Emergency drugs such as epinephrine, hydrocortisone, and diphenhydramine should be kept at the bedside and a crash cart should be close at hand. Ideally, MAB should be administered via a side port so that if a severe allergic reaction occurs, the MAB infusion can be stopped and intravenous fluids initiated immediately. To avoid rapid bolus infusions, which tend to cause more side effects, an infusion pump should be used. An injection port should also be available on the intravenous tubing so that emergency drugs can be injected if an allergic reaction occurs. To prevent or alleviate chills, fever, or urticaria, medication (e.g., meperidine) may need to be administered before or during therapy. With certain MABs, especially those used in treating the hematologic malignancies, fever is common, and its relationship to the course of therapy (early versus late) should be evaluated (Dillman, 1988).

RADIATION PRECAUTIONS

With radiolabeled MABs, appropriate radiation safety precautions including the principles of time, distance, and shielding to minimize radiation exposure to the health care team (Hassey, 1987), should be observed. These will be determined by the isotope utilized and the dose the patient is to receive. Patients should be educated regarding the need for isolation with higher doses of radionuclides until radiation levels fall to state-regulated minimums. Any special precautions to be utilized while in isolation, such as using disposable food trays, flushing the toilet three times after voiding, sitting while urinating (men), and avoiding bathing for 24 hours after administration of the isotope, should all be reviewed. Patients are often fearful of radiotherapy and may voice reluctance to be near family members once they are discharged

from the hospital. To allay patient concerns, appropriate discharge precautions and issues related to sexuality should all be discussed prior to discharge.

SEXUALITY

Although nurses are often aware of the need to address sexual concerns, many are reluctant to do so because they or the patient feel uncomfortable discussing this issue. Patients who are receiving biotherapy may experience changes in sexuality due to factors such as fatigue, dryness of mucous membranes, FLS, and change in body image. The PLISSIT model is frequently used for sexuality counseling or nursing interventions. The success of each step of this counseling will depend on the nurse's knowledge and comfort level.

- P = *permission*. Discussion of patient concerns is promoted and the couple is encouraged to continue in their present pattern of sexual activity.
- LI = *limited information*. New information is included to address sexual concerns.
- SS = *specific suggestions*. New activities or techniques for the couple may be included.
- IT = *intensive therapy*. If necessary, the couple is referred to a therapist or counselor for more intensive treatment (Annon, 1976).

Examples of interventions include advising the use of the supine position or a side-lying position during intercourse when patients are experiencing fatigue or the use of other expressions of intimacy such as cuddling or caressing, the use of water-based lubricants for patients experiencing vaginal dryness, or strategies such as long periods of foreplay, showering or bathing together, or use of different rooms for lovemaking to help stimulate desire (Shell, 1994). The American Cancer Society books on sexuality for both men and women with cancer provide excellent resources (Schover, 1988a and 1988b).

SPECIAL ISSUES

Of special note are two issues relevant to nurses caring for patients who are receiving biotherapy: (1) the focus of the media on new or novel therapies, and (2) nurse stress related to care of patients who are receiving biotherapy, especially investigational biotherapy. Novel treatments or approaches are frequently heralded by the media before efficacy has been truly determined. Oncology nurses must be aware of information presented by the media so that they can serve as a resource for patient questions. Patients are often quite knowledgeable regarding ongoing clinical investigations across the country and frequently have questions about the efficacy of those therapies. For example, unconventional therapies that capitalize on the idea of manipulating the immune system may sometimes sound similar to certain types of biotherapy. By actively listening to patient concerns and consulting with other members of the multidisciplinary team, the nurse can help to clarify misconceptions (Fletcher, 1992).

McCaffrey (1992) reviewed the issue of nurse stress associated with care of patients receiving investigational biological agents. Patients who enter clinical trials are faced with a host of coping challenges: resolution about feelings of prior aggressive, unsuccessful therapies; reactions of hope and fear surrounding the proposed therapy; learning new information and self-care skills; experiencing often difficult side effects, and concern about financial issues. The nurse is responsible for administering the agents that cause distressing side effects that may greatly impact the patient's quality of life and may feel powerless to impact or lessen the severity of these side effects. Furthermore, personal values regarding decisions to continue with therapy may be in conflict with those of the patient. In addition, the nurse may experience feelings of failure when therapy is unsuccessful. These elements all create stress for the nurse. Strategies for managing stress include assessment and understanding of the problem (e.g., separating patient-related stress from nurse-related stress) and identifying measures to reduce both patient and personal stress. See Table 10.6.

AMBULATORY CARE

Current trends in health care have mandated changes in the way care has traditionally been provided. Issues shaping these changes are varied: shortened length of stay, a move towards more ambulatory care, and scrutiny by third-party payors of services provided all influence the manner in which care is provided. In addition, consumers are increasingly aware of costs and have a desire to control health care costs (Yasko, 1988). As a result of these trends, many biotherapies are administered in the outpatient setting, and work is in progress to revise current inpatient therapies so that they may be safely administered in the outpatient setting. All of these changes will continue to affect the role of the oncology nurse (Buchsel and Yarbro, 1993).

Considerations important to safe care of patients in the ambulatory setting also apply to preparing patients for discharge so that therapy may be continued in an outpatient setting. A primary goal for the patient with cancer is to develop or regain independence so that therapy may be successfully managed at home. Thus, discharge planning should begin on admission to the hospital so that adequate plans can be formulated for the patient to achieve self-sufficiency upon discharge. In the ambulatory setting, planning begins immediately following the decision to start therapy so that the goal of self-sufficiency may be achieved. Major areas that need to be addressed include monitoring the patient reaction to the initial administration of treatment, consistent assessment of tolerance to and compliance with therapy, patient education, use of support systems and referrals as appropriate, and financial concerns. Patient education and

Table 10.6   Reduction of nurse stress

Patient-Centered	Nurse-Centered
Set priorities with patients: • What bothers you the most right now? • What can I do to help you get through this difficult time?	Critically examine the personal issues you bring to work and their coexistence in the health care setting.
Use symptom distress scales to quantify the effect of nursing interventions.	Determine the extent of possible codependency: • Self-esteem derived heavily from patient interaction. • "Only I can do it well" phenomenon • Puts others' needs before own • Represses feelings, then acts passive/aggressively • Seldom asks for help
Implement a formal review process with peers of current caseload: • What went well? • What could we have done differently? • Extend mutual support and acknowledge the professional friend's contribution.	Delineate problems within the cancer care team and the patient and use strategy to resolve difficult relationships. Personally identify mechanisms to "recharge your batteries": • List 30 stress reducers • Use one daily. Reflect daily on successes in practice versus focusing on the "I should have."

Source: Reprinted with permission from McCaffrey, D. 1992. Cancer nurse stress: A paradigm with relevance to investigational biotherapy. In Carroll-Johnson, R. (ed.) *The Biotherapy of Cancer—V.* Pittsburgh: Oncology Nursing Press, pp. 22–27.

reimbursement issues will be covered in detail in Chapters 14 and 15, respectively.

When therapy is initiated in the outpatient or home setting, patients should be monitored for tolerance to the first dose. The agent(s) being administered and the dose used will determine the length of time patients need to be monitored and the frequency by which vital signs should be checked. It is helpful if medical orders specify any necessary premedications, any parameters that should be reported to the physician (e.g., blood pressure < 90 mm Hg), and discharge criteria.

Patients will generally require regular clinic follow-up visits or home nursing visits to assess tolerance to therapy. The use of symptom flow sheets, either as a self-reporting form or nursing documentation form, can facilitate assessment and management of outpatients (White, 1992). Patient diaries or logbooks of symptoms experienced can also be useful (Brophy and Sharp, 1991). In this manner, toxic effects can be reliably quantified and documented, and patient response to interventions can be assessed.

Scheduled follow-up visits allow for determining patient adherence to and compliance with the therapeutic regimen (e.g., the medication schedule and laboratory and diagnostic tests). Any misunderstandings or problems can then be addressed.

Evaluation of patient or caregiver support systems is of the utmost importance in planning outpatient therapy. Problems such as lack of financial resources or social support will need to be addressed by the multidisciplinary team to ensure successful implementation of therapy. Available resources such as home care, the local physician's office, support groups, community financial assistance programs, and community agencies such as the American Cancer Society or Meals on Wheels are just a few of the many resources that should be considered.

NURSING RESEARCH

Administration of biotherapy differs from that of chemotherapy: therapy may be given daily and often lasts for months to years. The associated toxic effects are complex, frequently chronic, tend to be subjective in nature, and often have a major effect on the patient's quality of life. These areas are of major importance in the field of biotherapy nursing, and quality of life and symptom management consistently have been ranked as high priority items in the Oncology Nursing Society research priorities survey (Mooney *et al.* 1991).

The field of biotherapy, including clinical biotherapy trials, is full of possibilities for nursing research. Symptom management is beginning to be researched, but further nursing research is needed on this subject. One of the major problems in doing so has been the difficulties in accurately measuring symptoms experienced by patients. Although observer-rated toxicity scales used in clinical trials have been adapted to accommodate symptoms associated with BRMs, they are often not sensitive enough for research purposes (Oken *et al.*, 1982; Strauman *et al.*, 1988). The subjective nature of most BRM-associated symptoms also makes their measurement a challenge. Two potential avenues exist: tools specific to biotherapy can be designed or existing tools can be adapted (Strauman, 1988). Although desirable, the formulation of tools specific to biotherapy requires a major investment of researcher time to validate scales. Numerous questionnaires and tools are already available to assess symptoms, quality of life (Till, 1992; Varricchio and Ferrans, 1990), functional status, fatigue, and depression in the general oncology population. It may be possible to adapt many of these instruments, such as the Symptom Distress Scale (McCorkle and Young, 1978), the Sickness Impact Profile (Bergner *et al.*, 1981) or the Functional Living Index Cancer (Schipper *et al.*, 1984) for use in patients who are receiving biotherapy. Nursing research efforts need means to quantify side effects before interventions to prevent and control them can be studied. *Instruments for Clinical Nursing Research* (Frank-Stromberg, 1992) is an excellent resource for those desiring more quantitative measures of symptoms. A clearer understanding of the

etiology of biotherapy-related side effects will also assist in the development of management strategies that can be tested.

Research studies related to biotherapy, especially quality of life issues, are beginning to appear in the literature. An exploratory, descriptive study of 30 patients by Longman *et al.* (1992) reported the care needs of home-based cancer patients receiving external-beam radiotherapy, biotherapy, or both, and the needs of their caregivers. For the purposes of the study, home-based care needs of ambulatory cancer patients were defined as the physical, psychological, and health service requirements necessary to maintain normal functioning at home. The caregivers' needs were reported in relation to the patients' situations. Data were presented for the group as a whole and were not separated according to individual therapeutic modalities. Scales were developed to assess patients' and caregivers' needs. All 30 patients reported needs in the areas of personal care, actual health care, activity management, and interpersonal interaction. Areas reported by patients as requiring nursing attention (rated very important (9 or 10 on a scale of 1 to 10 by > 50% of patients) included use of safe technique; competent and timely implementation of orders; being listened to by nurses; being kept informed about their condition, symptoms, and treatment in an understandable way; and being treated in a pleasant, cheerful, respectful manner. Caregivers valued help in getting physician orders, being assured the patient was comfortable, and being assured of the availability of emergency help and of the option for patient admission to the hospital. Although these results can not be generalized to the cancer population at large, they can provide direction and guidance for oncology nurses whose patients are receiving biotherapy. It would be interesting to repeat the study with a larger population of patients who were receiving only biotherapy. Laizner *et al.* (1993) provide a review of research efforts regarding the needs of family caregivers of persons with cancer.

The long-term biological, psychological, and social effects of IL–2 therapy were reported by Jackson *et al.* (1991). Data were collected at baseline, during the treatment period; and at 1, 6, and 12 months after the completion of therapy. Measures for the various aspects of quality of life were the Sickness Impact Profile (SIP), the Inventory of Current Concerns (ICC), the Symptom Distress Scale (SDS), the Acute Physiology and Chronic Health Evaluation Scale (APACHE), and the Therapeutic Intervention Scoring System (TISS). Severity of illness, as measured by APACHE and TISS scores, showed a considerable increase during therapy, with a decline in severity beginning upon cessation of therapy. This pattern reflected an increased need for nursing care during therapy. Emotional concerns, as measured by the ICC, and symptom distress also increased significantly during therapy but returned to baseline by the one month after the completion of therapy. Because of poor survival rates, analysis of quality of life, as measured by the SIP, was only possible at one month after completion of therapy. Mean SIP scores at the one-month time point did not differ significantly from pretherapy scores. This study presents important data regarding the biological, psychological, and social effects of IL–2 therapy. Increasingly, questions about the economic cost, changes in quality of life, and discomfort related to therapy are being viewed as equally as important as the effects of therapy on the tumor.

A retrospective, descriptive study by Rieker *et al.* (1992) reported perceptions of quality of life and quality of care for patients with cancer who were receiving biological therapy. The sample was drawn from patients with advanced cancer who had completed biological therapy from January 1986 through June 1988 at two biotherapy treatment centers in the southern United States or from significant relatives of patients who had died. For the purposes of the study, quality of care and

quality of life were evaluated subjectively and were considered to be multidimensional constructs. Quality of life was evaluated only for the patients alive at the end of data collection and was measured by the Profile of Mood States (POMS) and the Linear Analogue Self-Assessment. Quality of care was measured by a self-report questionnaire previously used in studies of survivors of cancer and was tailored to each of the sample subsets. The final sample consisted of 33 patients (response rate, 60%) and 71 relatives (response rate, 70%). Despite the uncertainty concerning treatment outcomes, patients who had received biological therapy reported a relatively good quality of life. Available data indicated that the psychological status of the patient sample, as measured by the POMS, was similar to that of other groups of patients with advanced cancer and was within the range reported for healthy (e.g., noncancer) samples. The majority of patients and relatives gave positive reports about the quality of care that they had received; relatives of the deceased patients gave less positive reports about quality of care than did surviving patients and their relatives. The findings indicated that four components—symptom control, availability of support services, communication with the medical team, and adequate information about how medical care was proceeding—were significant in both patients' and family members' assessment of quality of care. These concerns should help provide direction for future research areas to help target interventions by the health care team. Findings from the study are limited due to recall bias and a small, single-setting sample. However, the need to initiate prospective studies on quality of life and quality of care with patients receiving biotherapy should be an area of focus.

Fazio and Glaspy (1991) assessed quality of life in ten patients with chronic neutropenia who were receiving therapy with recombinant granulocyte colony-stimulating factor (rG-CSF). The Ferrans & Powers Quality of Life Index was used to assess quality of life. Measurements were taken at three time points:

pretherapy, after 4 months of therapy, and after 10 months of therapy. The mean overall quality of life had improved significantly by the second time point and was maintained through the third time point. Subjects reported feeling "more healthy" after treatment with rG-CSF. The major limitations of this study were the small sample size, the lack of a control group, and the use of the quality of life index in the pediatric population. However, the study illustrates the importance of measuring both the efficacy and the impact on quality of life of a particular therapy.

There are many patient management issues to be addressed through nursing research of biotherapy. Efforts should focus on the development of tools to measure side effects and symptom distress, determination of the most effective time of drug administration to alleviate side effects, development of interventions to control or prevent toxicity, and evaluation of patient education methods. Studies measuring quality of life have gained increasing importance in the field of oncology and should be incorporated into biotherapy research and clinical trials. It is exciting that nursing research is also beginning to explore issues of concern to those caring for patients who are receiving biotherapy. However, a great deal of work remains to be completed.

SUMMARY

Biotherapy nursing represents an expanding area of specialization within the field of oncology nursing. Due to the rapid introduction of novel agents, approaches, and combination therapies, nurses are needed who have a desire to learn about new therapeutic modalities and the creativity to develop new standards of care for patients who are receiving these therapies. By building on prior oncology experience, integrating new knowledge specific to biotherapy, and conducting research to generate innovative approaches for new problems, nurses who care for cancer patients who are receiving this exciting new treatment modality will be able to meet the challenge.

References

American Nurses Association. 1991. *Standards of Clinical Nursing Practice.* Washington, D.C.: American Nurses Publishing.

Amgen, Inc. 1991. Neupogen® (filgrastim) Package insert. Thousand Oaks, CA: Amgen, Inc.

Amgen, Inc. 1989. Epogen® (epoetin alfa) Package insert. Thousand Oaks, CA: Amgen, Inc.

Annon, J. 1976. *Behavioral treatment of sexual problems: Brief therapy.* Hagerstown, PA: Harper & Row.

Astra Pharmaceutical Products, Inc. 1993. Emla® Cream (lidocaine 2.5% and prilocaine 2.5%). Package insert. Westborough, MA: Astra Pharmaceutical Products, Inc.

Becker, K., and Koutlas, J. 1990. Alteration in body image for the patient undergoing RIL–2/LAK cell therapy. *Oncology Nursing Forum* 17(6): 965.

Bergner, M., Bobbitt, R., Carter, W., *et al.* 1981. The sickness impact profile: Development and final revision of a health status measure. *Medical Care* 19(8): 787–805.

Berlex Laboratories. 1993. Betaseron® (interferon beta 1B) package insert. Richmond, CA: Berlex Laboratories.

Bock, S., Lee, R., Fisher, B., *et al.* 1990. A prospective randomized trial evaluating prophylactic antibiotics to prevent triple-lumen catheter-related sepsis in patients treated with immunotherapy. *Journal of Clinical Oncology* 8(1): 161–169.

Boyle, D., Engelking, C., Blesch, K., *et al.* 1992. ONS position paper on cancer and aging. *Oncology Nursing Forum* 19(6): 913–933.

Brophy, L., and Rieger, P. 1992. Biotherapy. In Clark, J. and McGee, R. (eds). *Core Curriculum for Oncology Nursing.* 2nd ed. Philadelphia: W.B. Saunders, pp. 346–358.

Brophy, L., and Sharp, E. 1991. Physical symptoms of combination biotherapy: A quality-of-life issue. *Oncology Nursing Forum* 18(1) (Suppl): 25–30.

Buchsel, P., and Yarbro, C. (eds). 1993. *Oncology Nursing in the Ambulatory Setting.* Boston: Jones and Bartlett.

Chiron Therapeutics. 1994. Proleukin® (aldesleukin) package insert. Emeryville, CA: Chiron Corporation.

Collins, J., and Thaney, K. (eds). 1988. Biotherapy: A nursing challenge. *Seminars in Oncology Nursing* 4(2): 83–150.

Conrad, K., and Horrell, C. (eds.). (in press). *Recommendations for Nursing Practice Related to Biotherapy* 2nd ed. Pittsburgh, PA: The Oncology Nursing Press.

Cunningham, M. 1989. Putting creativity into practice. *Oncology Nursing Forum* 16(4): 499–505.

Dana, W., and Anderson, R. 1990. Handling of cytotoxic agents. *Cancer Bulletin* 42(6): 399–404.

Dana, W. 1988. Procedure for handling biological response modifiers. *Pharmacy Bulletin* 6: 2. Houston, TX: The University of Texas M. D. Anderson Cancer Center.

Dangel, R. 1986. Pruritus and cancer. *Oncology Nursing Forum* 13(1): 17–21.

Dillman, J. 1989. New antineoplastic therapies and inherent risks: Monoclonal antibodies, biologic response modifiers, and interleukin–2. *Journal of Intravenous Nursing* 12(2): 103–113.

Dillman, J. 1988. Toxicity of monoclonal antibodies in the treatment of cancer. *Seminars in Oncology Nursing* 4(2): 107–111.

Farrell, M. 1992. The challenge of adult respiratory distress syndrome during interleukin–2 therapy. *Oncology Nursing Forum* 19(3): 475–480.

Fazio, M., and Glaspy, J. 1991. The impact of granulocyte colony-stimulating factor on quality of life in patients with severe chronic neutropenia. *Oncology Nursing Forum* 18(8): 1411–1414.

Fletcher, D. 1992. Unconventional cancer treatments: Professional, legal, and ethical issues. *Oncology Nursing Forum* 19(9): 1351–1354.

Frank-Stromberg, M. (ed) 1992. *Instruments for Clinical Nursing Research*. Boston: Jones and Bartlett.

Genentech. 1991. Actimmune® (interferon gamma 1B) package insert. San Francisco, CA: Genentech, Inc.

Hahn, M., and Jassak, P. 1988. Nursing management of patients receiving interferon. *Seminars in Oncology Nursing* 4(2): 95–101.

Hassey, K. 1987. Principles of radiation safety and protection. *Seminars in Oncology Nursing* 3(1): 23–29.

Hogan, C. 1991. Coping with biotherapy: Physiological and psychosocial concerns. *Oncology Nursing Forum* 18(1) (Suppl): 19–23.

Hood, L., and Abernathy, E. 1991. Biological response modifiers. In Baird, S., McCorkle, R. and Grant, M. (eds). *Cancer Nursing: Comprehensive Textbook*. Philadelphia: W.B. Saunders, pp. 321–343.

Hunt Raleigh, E. 1992. Sources of hope in chronic illness. *Oncology Nursing Forum* 19(3): 443–448.

Hynes, M., Bournes, L., Brich, A., et al. 1990. Managing side effects associated with IL–2 therapy. *Oncology Nursing Forum* 17(6): 963.

Immunex Corporation. 1991. Leukine® (sargramostim) package insert. Seattle, WA: Immunex Corporation.

Irwin, M. 1987. Patients receiving biological response modifiers: Overview of Nursing Care. *Oncology Nursing Forum* 14(6) (Suppl): 32–37.

Jackson, B., Strauman, J., Frederickson, K., et al., 1991. Long-term biopsychosocial effects of interleukin–2 therapy. *Oncology Nursing Forum* 18(4): 683–690.

Janssen Pharmaceutica, Inc. 1990. Ergamisol® (levamisole hydrochloride) Package insert. Piscataway, NJ: Janssen Pharmaceutica, Inc.

Jassak, P. 1993. Biotherapy. In Groenwald, S., Hansen Frogge, M., Goodman, M., and Yarbro, C. (eds). *Cancer Nursing: Principles and Practice*. 3rd ed. Boston: Jones and Bartlett, pp. 366–392.

Jassak, P., and Ryan, M. 1989. Ethical issues in clinical research. *Seminars in Oncology Nursing* 5(2): 102–108.

Knoll Pharmaceutical. 1993. Onco Scint® CR/OV (satumomab pendetide), Package insert. Whippany, NJ: Knoll Pharmaceutical.

Laizner, A., Shegda Yost, L., Barg, F., et al. 1993. Needs of family caregivers of persons with cancer: A review. *Seminars in Oncology Nursing* 9(2): 114–120.

Longman, A., Atwood, J., Sherman, J., et al. 1992. Care needs of home-based cancer patients and their caregivers. *Cancer Nursing* 15(3): 182–190.

Lotze, M., and Rosenberg, S. 1991. Interleukin–2: Clinical applications. In DeVita, V., Hellman, S., Rosenberg, S. (eds). *Biologic Therapy of Cancer*. Philadelphia: J.B. Lippincott, pp. 159–177.

Lynch, M. 1988. The nurse's role in the biotherapy of cancer: Clinical trials and informed consent. *Oncology Nursing Forum* 15(6) (Suppl): 23–27.

Madeya, M. 1990. Coping with investigational therapy. *Oncology Nursing Forum* 17(6): 965.

Mayer, D. 1990. Biotherapy: Recent advances and nursing implications. *Nursing Clinics of North America* 25(2): 291–308.

Mayer, D., Hetrick, K., Riggs, C. et al. 1984. Weight loss in patients receiving recombinant leukocyte-A interferon (IFNrA): A brief report. *Cancer Nursing* 7(1): 53–56.

McCaffrey, D. 1992. Cancer nurse stress: A paradigm with relevance to investigational biotherapy. In Carroll-Johnson, R. (ed). *The Biotherapy of Cancer—V*. Pittsburgh: Oncology Nursing Press, pp. 22–27.

McCorkle, R., and Young, K. 1978. Development of a symptom distress scale. *Cancer Nursing* 1(3): 373–378.

McNally, J., Somerville, E., Miaskowski, C., et al. 1991. *Guidelines for Cancer Nursing Practice*. Philadelphia: W.B. Saunders.

Miller, A., Hoogstraten, B., Staquet, M., et al. 1981. Reporting results of cancer treatment. *Cancer* 47: 207–214.

Mooney, K., Ferrell, B., Nail, L., et al., 1991. 1991 Oncology Nursing Society research priorities survey. *Oncology Nursing Forum* 18(8): 1381–1388.

Oken, M., Creech, R., Tormey, D., et al., 1982. Toxicity and response criteria of the Eastern Cooperative Oncology Group. *American Journal of Clinical Oncology* 5(6): 649–655.

Oncology Nursing Society. 1988. Cancer Chemotherapy Guidelines. Pittsburgh: Oncology Nurse Press.

Oncology Nursing Society and American Nurses' Association. 1987. *Standards of Oncology Nursing Practice*. Pittsburgh: Oncology Nursing Press.

Ortho Biotech. 1993. Procrit® (epoetin alfa) Package insert. Raritan, NJ: Ortho Pharmaceutical Corporation.

Padavic-Shaller, K. 1988. Nursing applications in a developing science. *Seminars in Oncology Nursing* 4(2): 142–151.

Purdue Frederick. 1990. Alferon® N (interferon-alfa N–3) Package insert. Norwalk, CN: Purdue Frederick.

Quesada, J., Talpaz, M., Rios, A., *et al.* 1986. Clinical toxicity of interferons in cancer patients: A review. *Journal of Clinical Oncology* 4(2): 234–243.

Rieger, P. 1994. Biotherapy. In Otto, S. (ed). *Oncology Nursing.* 2nd ed. St. Louis: Mosby Year Book, pp. 526–560.

Rieger, P. 1992. The pathophysiology of selected symptoms associated with BRM therapy, monograph. Emeryville, CA: Cetus Corporation.

Rieger, P. 1989. Infusing interleukin–2 and dopamine. *Oncology Nursing Forum* 16(2): 276.

Rieger, P., and Weatherly, B. 1989. Can your nursing skills meet the challenge of a patient receiving IL–2? *Dimensions in Oncology Nursing* 3(3): 9–19.

Rieker, P., Clark, E., and Fogelberg, P. 1992. Perceptions of quality of life and quality of care for patients with cancer receiving biological therapy. *Oncology Nursing Forum* 19(3): 433–440.

Roche Laboratories. 1990. Roferon®-A (interferon-alfa 2A) Package insert. Nutley, NJ: Hoffmann-LaRoche, Inc.

Rostad, M. 1991. Current strategies for managing myelosuppression in patients with cancer. *Oncology Nursing Forum* 18(2) (Suppl): 7–15.

Rumsey, K., and Rieger, P. 1992. *Biological Response Modifiers: A self-instructional module for health care professionals.* Chicago: Precept Press.

Rust, D., Bell, D., Colao, D., *et al.* 1990. Symptom management for patients receiving biotherapy. *Oncology Nursing Forum* 17(6): 964.

Sargent, C., and Shelton, B. 1990. Cardiotoxicities of interleukin–2 (IL–2): The nursing challenge. *Oncology Nursing Forum* 17(6): 964.

Schering Corporation. 1992. Intron®-A (interferon-alfa 2b) package insert. Kenilworth, NJ: Schering Corporation.

Schipper, H., Clinch, C., McMurray, A., *et al.* 1984. Measuring the quality of life of cancer patients—FLIC: Development and validation. *Journal of Clinical Oncology* 2(5): 472–483.

Schover, L. 1988a. *Sexuality and cancer: For the man who has cancer, and his partner.* New York: American Cancer Society.

Schover, L. 1988b. *Sexuality and cancer: For the woman who has cancer, and her partner.* New York: American Cancer Society.

Sergi, J. 1991. The physiology of the flu-like syndrome and the cardiopulmonary and renal symptoms associated with BRM therapy, monograph. Emeryville, CA: Cetus Corporation.

Shell, J. 1994. Impact of cancer on sexuality. In Otto, S. (ed). *Oncology Nursing,* 2nd ed. St. Louis: Mosby Year Book, pp. 737–760.

Simpson, C., Seipp, C., and Rosenberg, S. 1988. The current status and future applications of interleukin–2 and adoptive immunotherapy in cancer treatment. *Seminars in Oncology Nursing* 4(2): 132–141.

Snydman, D., Sullivan, B., Gill, M., *et al.,* 1990. Nosocomial sepsis associated with IL–2. *Annals of Internal Medicine* 112(2): 102–107.

Soeken, K., and Carson, V. 1987. Responding to the spiritual needs of the chronically ill. *Nursing Clinics of North America* 22(3): 603–611.

Strauman, J. 1988. The nurse's role in the biotherapy of cancer: Nursing research of side effects. *Oncology Nursing Forum* 15(6) (Suppl): 35–39.

Strauman, J., Brady, P., and Harwood, K. 1988. Development of a self-report side effect scale for assessing symptoms associated with biologic response modifiers. Pilot study. Eastern Cooperative Oncology Group.

Till, J. 1992. Quality of life measurements in cancer treatment. In DeVita, V., Hellman, S., and Rosenberg, S. (eds). *Important Advances in Oncology.* Philadelphia: J.B. Lippincott, pp. 189–204.

Tsevat, J., and Lacasse, C. 1992. Understanding the special needs of patients receiving biotherapy: A conceptual model. In Carroll-Johnson, R. (ed). *The Biotherapy of Cancer—V.* Pittsburgh: Oncology Nursing Press, pp. 5–9.

United States Environmental Protection Agency. 1990. *Disposal Tips for Home Health Care.* Washington, D.C.: Office of Solid Waste, United States Environmental Protection Agency.

Varricchio, C., and Ferrans, C. (eds). 1990. Quality of life assessment in clinical practice. *Seminars in Oncology Nursing* 6(4): 247–308.

Varricchio, C., and Jassak, P. 1988. Informed consent: An overview. *Seminars in Oncology Nursing* 5(2): 95–98.

White, C. 1992. Symptom assessment and management of outpatients receiving biotherapy: The application of a symptom report form. *Seminars in Oncology Nursing* 8(4) (Suppl 1): 23–28.

Yarbro, C. (ed) 1993. Management of patients receiving interleukin–2 therapy. *Seminars in Oncology Nursing* 9(3) (Suppl 1): 1–35.

Yasko, J. 1988. Biological response modifier treatment reimbursement: Present status and future strategies. *Oncology Nursing Forum* 15(6) (Suppl): 28–34.

CHAPTER 11 | Fatigue

Karen A. Skalla, RN, MSN

Paula Trahan Rieger, RN, MSN, OCN

Fatigue represents a unique nursing challenge in management of the patient with cancer. Many times, nurses are the only patient care providers to give serious consideration to the symptom of fatigue because so little is known about its etiology and treatment (Potempa, 1989). Fatigue, as a subjective experience, may not be clearly evident when assessing the oncology patient. However, many studies report fatigue as the most commonly cited symptom in patients with cancer and indicate that some level of fatigue exists in nearly all patients, especially those actively undergoing treatment with biological response modifiers (Winningham *et al.*, 1994). Fatigue has been documented in the literature with all modes of cancer treatment: chemotherapy, radiation therapy, surgery, and biotherapy.

For many patients, fatigue may become a critically important issue. It potentially influences sense of well being, daily performance, activities of daily living, relationships with family and friends, and compliance with treatment (Pickard-Holley, 1991). The impact of this symptom becomes apparent when one considers that it can be a dose-limiting toxicity of biological therapy (Quesada *et al.*, 1986) Quesada *et al.* found fatigue, in patients receiving interferon, to frequently result in job absenteeism, social withdrawal, a rise in the total hours of sleep per day, and in extreme cases caused impairment of all physical activities. The social implications of fatigue, therefore, may be profound. Financial resources may become limited as patients are forced into disability programs, or worse, out of a job. Patient outcomes may then become compromised due to difficulties in maintaining health insurance, problems in gaining access to care, or the erection of financial barriers toward pursuing aggressive treatment. A thorough understanding of fatigue, consequently, may lead to initiation of effective interventions that ultimately improve patient outcomes.

Fatigue may have particular significance to some patients. In today's society, it has become increasingly necessary for all eligible family members to be employed. The experience of fatigue may be especially difficult for those who place a special significance on their role as primary breadwinner or caregiver (Davis, 1984). The deterioration in level of functioning may be mildly bothersome to some, while intolerable to others, especially for those formerly independent individuals who must now surrender to the "sick role" (Davis, 1984).

The essence of the nursing role is to facilitate self-care in the patient. Nail *et al.* (1991) documented fatigue as the most commonly reported symptom (81%) in a sample of outpatient chemotherapy patients. They suggest that the current trend in oncology for chemotherapy to be delivered on an outpatient basis necessitates a shift in responsibility for control of side effects from nurse to patient. It is imperative that we empower patients to develop the self-care abilities necessary to cope with fatigue. This proves a challenge as fatigue has been shown to interfere with self-care activities (Davis, 1984; Rhodes *et al.*, 1988).

Despite the serious consequences of this symptom, little is known about the patterns or mechanisms of fatigue in patients treated with chemotherapy, and especially in those treated with biological response modifiers (BRMs). Several problems become evident when examining research related to fatigue. The examination of fatigue in a variety of clinical situations by several disciplines other than nursing has hindered efforts in establishing both a universal definition and theory of fatigue. Furthermore, ambiguous literature and a lack of specific tools to measure fatigue have created difficulties in establishing assessment and management guidelines.

This chapter will address the current level of understanding about the clinical nature of fatigue. Definitions of fatigue, its pathophysiology, and clinical presentation in treatment with BRMs will be discussed. Research which has guided development of nursing assessment and intervention techniques will be presented. A broad understanding of fatigue as a biotherapy-related problem will facilitate development of effective nursing interventions, thereby enabling patients to develop self-care abilities and improve the outcomes of their cancer treatment.

DEFINITION OF FATIGUE

A standard definition of fatigue remains elusive. Many similar definitions exist but they differ depending on perspective or discipline. Fatigue may be characterized by a condition of physical, psychological, or spiritual well-being, disrupted by tiredness or weakness which prevents an individual from functioning at expected potential. Fatigue has been described using such terms as tiredness, exhaustion, weakness, lack of energy, lack of purpose, sleepiness, and changes in ability to concentrate. Many different factors appear to influence fatigue in cancer patients. Table 11.1 provides a compilation of early work that delineated factors contributing to fatigue. Several definitions are presented here which represent different philosophical viewpoints.

Piper *et al.* (1987) proposed a definition for fatigue from which a conceptual model, similar to the existing pain model, was developed. From a nursing perspective, fatigue is defined as a subjective feeling of tiredness that is influenced by circadian rhythm. Piper divides fatigue into two categories: acute and chronic. Acute fatigue is perceived as normal or expected tiredness characterized by localized intermittent symptoms, rapid onset, and short duration. Acute fatigue serves a protective function. Chronic fatigue, in contrast, is perceived as abnormal or excessive generalized tiredness. It is constant or recurrent, for least a month, with an insidious onset and cumulative effect. The function of chronic fatigue is unknown. Additional research is needed to further support Piper's definition and model.

Pickard-Holley (1991) defines fatigue as a condition characterized by the subjective feeling of increased discomfort and decreased

Table 11.1   Factors contributing to fatigue in cancer patients

Physiological	Psychological	Situational
Accumulation of toxic waste products secondary to radiation, chemotherapy, or the tumor (Britton, 1983; Haylock and Hart, 1979)	Anxiety (Kellum, 1985; Britton, 1983; Minden and Reich, 1983)	Sensory deprivation due to disturbance of sleep pattern (Britton, 1983)
Hypermetabolic state associated with active tumor growth, infection, fever, or surgery (Britton, 1983)	Depression (Kellum, 1985; Britton, 1983; Minden and Reich, 1983)	Immobility (Britton, 1983)
	Anticipatory nausea and vomiting	Crisis (Kellum, 1985; Britton, 1983)
Competition of the tumor with the body for nutrients (Britton, 1983; Cushman, 1986; Gold, 1974; Theologides, 1972)	Grief (Minden and Reich, 1983)	Problems with relationships (Britton, 1983)
Inadequate intake of nutrients secondary to anorexia, nausea, vomiting, gastric obstruction (Britton, 1983; Cushman, 1986; Gold, 1974; Theologides, 1972)		Drugs—antibiotics, antidepressants, alcohol, nicotine, antianxiety agents, long-acting sleeping agents, analgesics, medications, caffeine (Kellum, 1985; Minden and Reich, 1983)
Chronic pain (Britton, 1983)		Sleep deprivation (Britton, 1983; Minden and Reich, 1983)
Impairment of aerobic energy metabolism secondary to dyspnea and anemia due to various causes (Haylock and Hart, 1979; Maxwell, 1984)		Diagnostic tests (Donovan and Giston, 1984)
		Loss

Source: Reprinted with permission Aistars, J. 1987. Fatigue in the cancer patient: A conceptual approach to a clinical problem. *Oncology Nursing Forum* 14(6): 25–30.

functional status related to a decrease in energy. Factors involved may be physical, mental, emotional, environmental, physiological, and pathological, with a voluntary component. Fatigue is characterized as a state of increased discomfort and decreased efficiency which may be experienced as tiredness or weakness usually resolved by rest or sleep.

Aistars (1987) defines fatigue as subjective feelings of generalized weariness, weakness, exhaustion, and lack of energy resulting from prolonged stress that is directly or indirectly attributable to the disease process. Fatigue results from exertion or stress and leads to increased discomfort and decreased efficiency. It causes deterioration of both mental and physical activities. These commonalities are also expressed by Rhoten (1982). Rhoten's model combines attitude, speech patterns, general appearance, subjective description, concentration, and activity level to reflect the many different aspects encompassed by the word *fatigue*.

Many factors may contribute to both the mechanism and manifestation of fatigue, which hinders attempts at a universal definition. This is particularly true for biotherapy-related fatigue. It is often easier, therefore, to understand fatigue as a concept rather than a definition.

THEORETICAL FOUNDATIONS

Fatigue theory is diverse in both focus and philosophy. Historically, goals in theory development have been to establish theory in healthy populations and then progress towards ill populations. Early studies examining fatigue were performed in order to investigate optimal worker productivity (Yoshitake, 1971; Grandjean, 1968) and these have laid the foundation for the current investigation of fatigue in oncology populations.

Grandjean (1968) was one of the pioneers in development of fatigue theory on the physiological level. In studying fatigue in industrial workers, he developed a theory to explain the fatigue produced by "monotonous surroundings." He believed that the activation and inhibition systems of the brain were on opposite ends of a continuum. The reticular activating system (RAS) is responsible for activation of the organism into an alert state using sensory afferent stimulation. Pathways exist from the RAS to the cortex to provide a feedback mechanism. Inhibition from the cortex takes two forms: active or passive. Active inhibition results from increased inhibitory impulses from the brainstem whereas passive inhibition is achieved from decreased sensory input or decreased cortical feedback. Depending on which system input predominates, the organism feels either aroused or fatigued. Grandjean proposed that in monotonous surroundings there was a decrease in both afferent sensory impulses and feedback from the cortex resulting in fatigue.

In keeping with the philosophy of the profession, nursing, has focused on development of a holistic theory for fatigue. Although additional research is needed to support these models, they are important to review for their historical significance. Piper et al. (1987) proposed a "fatigue framework" (see Figure 11.1). Biological and behavioral factors are modified by the perception of fatigue. Thirteen patterns are thought to influence fatigue: accumulation of metabolites, changes in energy and energy substrate patterns, activity/rest patterns, sleep/wake patterns, disease patterns, treatment patterns, symptom patterns, psychological patterns, oxygenation patterns, changes in regulation/transmission patterns, and other related patterns (e.g., environment, life events, unique circadian rhythms).

Aistars (1987) utilizes the "stress response" as a model for fatigue. The basis for her hypothesis is that prolonged stress causes fatigue. People with cancer frequently suffer from extreme stress over a long period of time. Activation of both the RAS system and sympathetic nervous system as a result of stress results in the release of stress hormones, which ultimately leads to depletion of energy stores. Consequently, these people experience a high level of fatigue.

Energy and the relationship to fatigue has been explored by several authors (Koeller, 1989; Mayer et al., 1986) interested in cancer cachexia. Patients receiving interferon often experience significant weight loss and fatigue. This concept must be compared to findings in another study (Kaempfer and Lindsey, 1986) which demonstrated that cancer patients vary in their energy requirements. Something other than energy requirements alone must be functioning to produce fatigue. Winningham et al. (1994) describe the Winningham Psychobiological-Entropy Model (PEH) for fatigue. This model expands on the concept of energy requirements and the possible relationship in producing fatigue. In this model, fatigue is defined as an energy deficit and relational associations between fatigue and disease, treatment, activity, rest, symptom perception, and functional status are proposed (see Figure 11.2). The PEH uses the energetic approach to determine the optimal balance between restorative rest and restorative activity or exercise. Because the PEH is directive in terms of conceptual relationships, it provides suggestions for the development of nursing interventions to manage fatigue.

Few nursing models exist which describe fatigue in physiological detail. One model has been proposed which is based on neurophysiological principles and evaluates the interaction of both central and peripheral components. This model incorporates the peripheral system (muscles and nerves) and central component (psyche/brain and spinal cord) that

Figure 11.1   Piper Integrated Fatigue Model

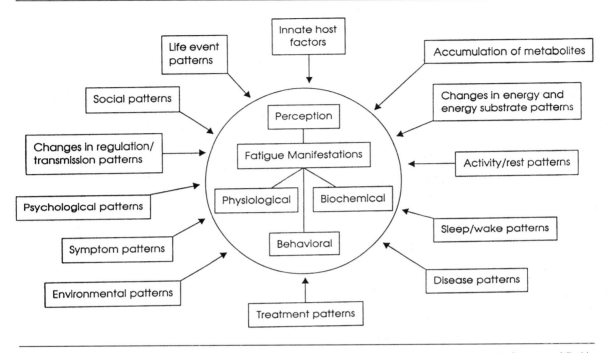

Source: Reprinted from the *Oncology Nursing Forum* with permission from the Oncology Nursing Press, Inc. Piper, B., Lindsey, A., and Dodd, M. 1987. Fatigue mechanisms in cancer patients: Developing nursing theory. *Oncology Nursing Forum* 14(6): 17–23.

may influence perception of fatigue. Impairment of central components causes lack of motivation, impaired spinal cord transmission, and exhaustion or malfunction of brain cells in the hypothalamic region. Damage to the peripheral component can cause impaired peripheral nerve function in transmission at the neuromuscular junction, thereby affecting muscle fiber activation. Both are hypothesized to play a role in chronic fatigue. The central mechanism may be the key to explaining the extreme fatigue of biotherapy-treated patients (Piper *et al.*, 1989a).

The development of clinically-based models to examine fatigue and design interventions to manage fatigue offers exciting prospects. Nursing theory is only beginning to identify proposed models for fatigue. To date, these models are concerned with fatigue as a general concept, and are not specific for bio-

therapy-related fatigue. Several researchers studying biological therapy have proposed mechanisms for biotherapy-related fatigue which will be reviewed in the following section.

PRESENTATION AND PATHOPHYSIOLOGY OF FATIGUE

Interferon

The two most difficult effects of interferon to manage are fatigue and alterations in the central nervous system (Quesada *et al.*, 1986). Fatigue is profound at doses equal to or greater than 20 MIU daily. This potentially therapeutic drug was reduced or discontinued in 50–100% of patients within 2 to 4 weeks when given in high doses. In addition, older patients

Figure 11.2   The psychobiological-entropy model

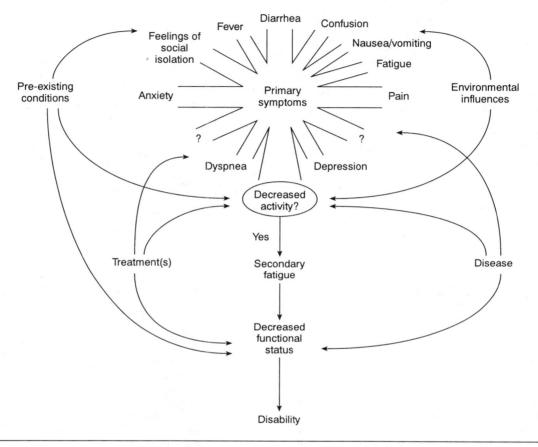

or those with poor performance status are often more severely affected. Mayer *et al.* (1984) examined interferon-induced weight loss in a phase I clinical trial. The prevalence of fatigue among patients studied was 70%, making it the most commonly reported side effect of therapy. Another study (Wadler *et al.*, 1989) documented fatigue at interferon doses of 6–18 MIU per day as being dose dependent (the higher the dose, the higher the level of fatigue). Fatigue has been reported at doses of interferon-alpha as low as 2 MIU daily (Gastl *et al.*, 1989). In the same study, fatigue was not reported when interferon was administered at doses of .2 to .6 MIU daily. A dose-dependent relationship does not become evident until approximately 2–3 MIU daily are administered.

Exacerbation of fatigue becomes apparent (Piper *et al.*, 1989b) when interferon is used in combination with other modalities. A study by Wadler *et al.* (1989) demonstrated that with administration of 5-fluorouracil and interferon-alpha patients developed fatigue or malaise during the second week of therapy. Daily administration of interferon-alpha produced more fatigue than intermittent administration.

The level of fatigue varied from none to extreme (requiring dose reduction) in the patients participating in the study. Interleukin–2 (IL–2) combined with interferon-alpha was shown (Lee *et al.*, 1989) to produce two dose-limiting toxicities: hypotension and chronic fatigue (associated with a decrease in performance status). Although fatigue improved between cycles, a decrease of up to 30 points in the Karnofsky Performance Status was seen in patients receiving high doses of IL–2 and interferon.

Quesada *et al.* (1986) and Adams *et al.* (1984) have suggested that interferon-induced fatigue, decreases in appetite, and cognitive-emotional disorders may be caused by central nervous system or frontal lobe neurotoxicity. Postulated causes of this toxic encephalopathy are direct effects of interferon on the frontal lobe or on deeper brain structures. Interferon may impede neurotransmitters, cause an alteration of cholinergic balance, or cause the release of other substances that affect frontal lobe functions. Other BRMs cause similar symptoms therefore enabling this theory to be applied to other biological treatments. The central or peripheral release of substances such as cytokines (e.g., tumor necrosis factor) affects sensations of appetite and fatigue. This humoral effect is supported by a study described by Grandjean (1968) where the cerebral spinal fluid of sleep-deprived animals, when injected into other animals, produced fatigue. Repeated administration of BRMs may cause fatigue to become a chronic toxicity along with weight loss, anorexia, and malaise (Koeller, 1989). Patients diagnosed with Chronic Fatigue Syndrome are also thought to be influenced by a central mechanism triggered by peripheral stimulation (Potempa *et al.*, 1986).

Davis (1984) was one of the first nurses to conduct research on interferon-induced fatigue. She designed a correlational study to identify the impact of fatigue on the functional status of 16 melanoma patients who received a cumulative dose of interferon-alpha ranging from 100 MIU to 2000 MIU. Fatigue was mea-sured by the Pearson-Byars Scale (Pearson and Byars, 1956) and the Fatigue Symptom Checklist (Yoshitake, 1969). The impact of fatigue on physical performance status was measured with an adapted Sickness Impact Profile (Gilson *et al.*, 1975). Results from this study suggested a relationship between interferon therapy and fatigue. Specific symptoms related to fatigue reported were walking slower (70%); sleeping more or sitting during most of the day (50%); decreased sexual activity (50%); eating less (43%); and engaging in fewer social activities (43%). Positive correlations between fatigue measures and reported symptoms suggested a statistically significant relationship ($p \leq 0.001$). Statistical significance was also found between fatigue scores and cumulative dose of interferon ($r = .537$; $p = 0.001$). There was no relationship between length of therapy and amount of fatigue. Mean dysfunctional scores correlated positively with cumulative interferon dose ($p \leq 0.005$), especially in sleep and socialization activities. The most common symptoms reported were leg weakness, a need to lie down, difficulty thinking, and impatience with others.

A study by Rieger (1987) described changes in fatigue level, functional status, and muscular strength as experienced by patients with cancer who received treatment with interferon-alpha and interferon-gamma, alone, together, or in combination with ampligen (an interferon inducer). Fatigue was measured pre, at 1 week, and at 1 month of therapy using the Pearson-Byars Scale and the Jamar handheld dynamometer, which assessed muscle strength. Functional quality of life was measured by the Functional-Living Index for Cancer (FLIC) (Schipper *et al.*, 1984). Over time, there was no significant difference demonstrated for fatigue, functional quality of life, or muscle strength. Grip strength did decrease significantly only in the group receiving interferon-alpha alone. Significant negative correlation was found between fatigue scores and quality of life. Complaints of fatigue, as documented in the medical record, increased from approximately 47% baseline to 74% at the 1-month time point. This suggests that fatigue measures used were not sufficiently sensitive to adequately measure fatigue experienced. Limitations of this study include a small sample size and comparison of groups receiving different types of therapy.

Skalla (1992) examined correlates of fatigue in patients treated with interferon. The purpose of this descriptive study was to investigate the behavioral, physiological, and biochemical factors that might affect subjective ratings of fatigue and simultaneously to question how fatigue may be different in patients with cancer versus healthy populations. This was a pilot study that addressed the feasibility of extending the research to a larger population. The convenience sample consisted of three groups: five medical oncology patients receiving treatment with interferon (group 1), five oncology patients matched to the first group for primary malignancy and stage of disease (group 2), and five health subjects matched for age and sex to the first group (group 3). The use of normal controls is unique in the fatigue literature.

The level of fatigue was expected to be highest in the interferon group and negligible in the health control group. Correlates of fatigue were classified and examined according to the framework developed by Piper *et al.* (1987) and included physiological variables, biochemical factors, and behavioral factors. Physiological variables included disease status, stage of disease, duration of illness, and performance status. Behavioral variables as measured by the Profile of Mood States (POMS) included mood, social support, marital status, and sleep changes. Many biochemical factors could be measured as potential correlates to fatigue such as medications, liver function tests, and chemistries; however, this study was limited in examining only a complete blood count.

The researcher briefly interviewed patients and completed a chart review for pertinent information including: performance status, employment, marital status, sex, race, presence of pain, sleep patterns, date of diagnosis, perceived social support, disruption of social activities, current hematological laboratory values, and current cancer therapy. The tool chosen to measure fatigue was a ten centimeter visual analogue scale (VAS). Patients were asked to measure both the amount of fatigue they were experiencing today and their usual amount of fatigue. Measures for other variables included the short form of the POMS and a brief questionnaire.

The interferon group scored highest in the categories of fatigue level, pain ratings, duration of illness, and hours of sleep per night. Group 1 had the highest mean score for fatigue (x = 43.80 mm, sd = 27.76). The score for Group 2 was slightly lower (x = 40.20 mm, sd = 25.85), with Group 3 experiencing the least amount of fatigue (x = 20.40 mm, sd = 23.13). These differences were not statistically significant, and may have been limited by the small sample size. It is important to note that in this study some level of fatigue was reported in all groups.

Biochemical variables, as measured by the complete blood count, were all lower in the interferon group than in the disease control group. This may have affected the fatigue rating. The effect of interferon altering hematological values is well documented (Radin *et al.*, 1989; Silver *et al.*, 1985) and was consistent with the findings of this study.

The physiological variables of disease status, duration of illness, performance status, and pain may be difficult to evaluate as separate entities. Most of the cancer patients studied (80%) had metastic disease. The highest mean for duration of illness was found in the interferon group and may support Aistars' (1987) theory that prolonged stress causes fatigue. Performance status, as measured by the Karnofsky scale, was rated at 90 for all of the patients with cancer. These results differ from those of Davis, 1984 who found significant differences in performance status among patients receiving interferon. This study also did not find that interferon dose correlated with the level of fatigue as was found in Davis's study at cumulative doses greater than 100 MIU.

The primary limitation of this study was the small sample size. Data collection of fatigue correlates was limited by the documentation of laboratory values in the chart and the sensitivity of the tool used to measure performance status.

Interleukin–2

Fatigue is a prevalent side effect in patients receiving interleukin–2 (IL–2) therapy and is dose and schedule dependent. In general, higher doses and more prolonged therapy will intensify the level of fatigue (Piper et al., 1989b). Other side effects experienced by the patient receiving therapy with IL–2, such as nausea and vomiting, anemia, diarrhea, mental status changes, hypotension, and fever, will increase perceived levels of fatigue. Numerous medications (e.g., antinausea and antipruritic medications) used to control IL–2-related side effects may also contribute to the intensity of fatigue experienced by the patient. Therapy combining IL–2 with other agents known to cause fatigue such as interferon and chemotherapy can also result in increased levels of fatigue (Viele and Moran, 1993; Siegel and Puri, 1991; Farrell et al., 1990; Janisch, 1990).

Limited information exists about patterns of fatigue in patients receiving therapy with IL–2. In reports from clinical trials evaluating the efficacy of IL–2, fatigue is frequently described in association with the flu-like symptoms. When described, it is characterized solely as present in a given percentage of patients. When fatigue is frequent and severe (e.g., with interferon and IL–2-related fatigue) it is often characterized as a dose-limiting toxic effect. In clinical trials, fatigue is generally measured on grading scales of 1 to 4, which identify the degree of fatigue as none, mild, moderate, or severe. Measures of performance status may also be used to characterize

fatigue. Data presented from a phase II clinical trial conducted by the National Biotherapy Study Group (NBSG) that evaluated continuous infusion IL–2 in patients with advanced malignancies reported fatigue as a predominant side effect. Over 90% of patients spent greater than 12 hours per day in bed (Sharp, 1993). Fatigue is a common occurrence in patients receiving outpatient administration of IL–2, whether IL–2 is administered by the subcutaneous route, or as a bolus or continuous intravenous infusion. The degree of fatigue is dose- and schedule-dependent (Viele and Moran, 1993). Fatigue is often more severe in patients receiving IL–2 therapy than in those receiving interferon. Patients frequently spend the majority of the day in bed and are unable to perform self-care activities. It may take up to 6–8 weeks for fatigue to resolve post completion of therapy (Piper et al., 1989).

Hodges (1992) investigated the pattern of fatigue, as measured by the Zubrod Scale, in patients with metastatic malignant melanoma during their first course of treatment with IL–2 alone or IL–2 in combination with interferon-alpha. Therapy consisted of a 4-day continuous infusion of IL–2 which started on day 1. In the group receiving interferon (group 2) injections were given days 1 through 4. All patients were given a break from therapy on days 6 and 7. During the study, this cycle was repeated for 4 weeks for the IL–2 group (group 1) and for 3 weeks for group 2. Each 3- or 4-week cycle constituted a course of therapy. This study used a retrospective record review to yield data which was grouped by biotherapy treatment. Limitations were secondary analysis of existing data, the use of the Zubrod Scale as a measure of fatigue, and a lack of data on analysis of fatigue status between courses of IL–2.

In both groups, the percentage of fatigue increased during treatment with the highest levels of fatigue occurring on the last full day of treatment. Although slight recovery did occur during the break period each week, Zubrod scores never returned to pretreatment levels. During treatment, approximately 25%

of patients in group 1 experienced fatigue severe enough to require assistance with activities of daily living. Patients in group 2 experienced a greater degree of fatigue than those in group 1. No significant relationship between fatigue and the selected toxicity criteria was found for both groups during all weeks of treatment, however, anorexia did correlate significantly with the level of fatigue in patients in group 2. Although this study cannot be generalized to all populations, it does provide information on the patterns and level of fatigue experienced by patients receiving therapy with IL–2 and IL–2/interferon-alpha.

The mechanisms which cause IL–2-related fatigue remain unknown. Both central and peripheral mechanisms may be involved in biotherapy-related fatigue states. It has been hypothesized that the release of cytokines such as tumor necrosis factor (TNF) may affect the sensations of fatigue and appetite. In patients receiving IL–2 therapy, the release of cytokines such as interferon-gamma and TNF, combined with the capillary leak syndrome may cause alterations in neuroendocrine secretion, brain electrical activity, and blood-brain barrier permeability (Piper et al., 1989b). It is likely that the significant number of systemic side effects experienced with IL–2 both impact and have a causal relationship in the development of IL–2-related fatigue.

Tumor Necrosis Factor

Fatigue is also common in patients receiving therapy with TNF, although patterns are not as well documented. In the majority of phase I trials evaluating TNF, hypotension is reported as the dose-limiting side effect, although fatigue is occasionally mentioned in this context. Reports of fatigue in patients receiving TNF range from approximately 50% to 92% (Alexander and Rosenberg, 1991; Moldawer and Figlin, 1988). The route of administration does not appear to affect the level of fatigue. When TNF is given in combination with other biological agents known to cause fatigue, its severity generally increases (Martin, 1991).

The precise mechanism responsible for TNF-related fatigue remains unknown. It is possible that TNF-related fatigue may result from biochemical and morphologic changes in skeletal muscle (St. Pierre et al., 1992). These pathologic changes in muscle would require a patient to exert an additional amount of effort to perform physical activity and maintain body posture, hence resulting in fatigue. It has been hypothesized that the muscle wasting associated with cachexia is mediated by TNF. Although there are experiments linking TNF and skeletal muscle wasting, the precise mechanisms remain unclear. Tumor necrosis factor may affect both the synthesis and degradation rate of protein stores in muscle. The ultimate effect probably depends on other variables including tumor type, tumor status, and general condition of the patient. Nevertheless, the involvement of muscle in the occurrence of TNF-related fatigue will play a role in determining the level of patient's self-care abilities or the ability to participate in an exercise program.

Hematopoietic Growth Factors

Fatigue is more consistently reported as a side effect of granulocyte-macrophage colony-stimulating factor (GM-CSF) than with other hematopoietic growth factors. In general GM-CSF-associated fatigue is mild in nature and resolves readily upon cessation of therapy. The ability of GM-CSF to activate monocytes, which in turn leads to the expression of TNF and interleukin–1 may be the mechanism behind this fatigue. Fatigue was the most commonly reported side effect in patients with acquired immune deficiency syndrome receiving GM-CSF, although it is difficult to separate the effects of therapy from the underlying effects of the disease (Lynch et al., 1988).

Interleukin–3 (IL–3) is generally well tolerated, but there have been reports of debilitating fatigue following its administration. Reilly and McKeever (1993) reported significant levels of fatigue in patients with aplastic anemia or myelodysplastic syndrome receiving therapy with IL–3 in a phase I/II clinical trial. Patients reported a decreased ability to perform daily activities, decreased job performance, and time lost from work as a result of fatigue. The onset of fatigue occurred 3 hours after receiving IL–3 with a duration up to 8 hours. Owing to this pattern of fatigue, it was recommended that patients receive IL–3 in the evening so that they might sleep through the fatigue episode. The authors report diminished levels of fatigue with this intervention. This abstract does not discuss the tools used to measure fatigue. In addition, symptoms associated with the conditions of aplastic anemia and myelodysplastic syndrome and that may cause fatigue, such as anemia, are not reviewed.

The occurrence of fatigue is uncommon with administration of granulocyte colony-stimulating factor or erythropoietin. Because anemia is known to cause both fatigue and impact the level of fatigue, the administration of erythropoietin to treat anemia may actually decrease fatigue in some patients.

Monoclonal Antibodies

Fatigue is not a side effect commonly associated with the administration of monoclonal antibodies. Malaise is more common and occurs in association with fever, chills, and diaphoresis. This constellation of symptoms occurs most frequently in patients with hematologic malignancies during the removal of circulating target cells, and resolves quickly upon the cessation of therapy (Dillman, 1988).

MEASUREMENT OF FATIGUE

A variety of tools, reflective of the diversity of definitions for fatigue, exist to measure the phenomenon of fatigue in patients receiving biotherapy. It is measured, with few exceptions, using a modified tool for other aspects of fatigue such as psychological or physical symptom distress, rather than as a tool specific for fatigue. Measurements exist which describe either subjective or objective parameters of fatigue, some measures have been used in a temporal fashion, while others capture fatigue at a certain moment in time. Reliability and validity data are beginning to accrue regarding the use of these tools to measure fatigue in cancer populations.

Tools which measure subjective fatigue are visual analogue scales, the Pearson-Byars Fatigue Feeling Tone Checklist (Pearson and Byars, 1956), The Fatigue Symptom Checklist (Yoshitake, 1969), various symptom distress scales (original and adapted) (McCorkle and Young, 1978), and the Profile of Mood States (short and long forms) (Shacham, 1983; McNair et al, 1971). Objective parameters have been measured by behavioral indicators such as alterations in general appearance, level of activity, communication patterns, attitudes, and functional performance status.

Physiological indicators to measure fatigue may include changes in levels of neurotransmitters, electromyograms, heart rate, oxygen consumption rate, degree of anemia, temperature, blood glucose, thyroid function, electrolyte levels, and indirect calorimetry. Biochemical indicators used in measuring fatigue are changes in Ph, lactate and pyruvate measurements, the proportion of fast twitch to slow twitch fibers (determined by muscle biopsy), and levels of metabolic end products (determined by magnetic resonance spectroscopy).

Two specific measures of fatigue have been developed: the Rhoten Fatigue Scale (Rhoten, 1982) and the Piper Fatigue Scale (Piper et al., 1989a). The Rhoten Fatigue Scale was designed to assess post-surgical fatigue and has not been proven reliable and valid for use in cancer populations. The Piper Fatigue Scale remains in developmental stages (Winningham et al., 1994).

The two most frequently used tools for measuring fatigue are a visual analogue scale (VAS) and the Profile of Mood States (POMS). The VAS is simple and lends itself easily to clinical practice with endpoints expressing the two ends of the fatigue continuum. The POMS is the most reliable and valid tool to date. The original POMS measures various aspects of mood in a 64-item questionnaire. Descriptive adjectives are rated on a zero (not at all) to four (extremely) scale. Adjectives are grouped into six subscales to give subscale scores. These emotional dimensions are tension-anxiety, depression-dejection, anger-hostility, vigor-activity, fatigue-inertia, and confusion-bewilderment. The shortened version of the POMS has been used by Jamar (1989), Oberst et al. (1991), and Blesch et al. (1991) to study fatigue in patients with cancer. The shortened POMS was developed by Shacham (1983) with a sample of oncology patients and was designed specifically for use on ill populations. The short version has been reduced to 37 items, but retains high correlation scores for mean subscale scores. The POMS (both short and long forms) is available through Educational and Industrial Testing Service, San Diego, California.

Tools such as those presented here may be used in conjunction with measurements of physiological parameters to identify patients who may be at risk for or are experiencing significant fatigue while being treated with biological response modifiers. Some tools may be more useful and realistic for the clinical setting, while others may be more appropriate for research purposes.

MANAGEMENT OF BIOTHERAPY-RELATED FATIGUE

Fatigue represents one of the most commonly occurring side effects in patients receiving biotherapy. Therapy with agents such as interferon or interleukin–2 that are known to cause debilitating levels of fatigue often affects quality of life. As with many quality of life issues, the management of fatigue is frequently relegated to nursing. Nursing research is only beginning to formulate theory that explains the nature of fatigue and develop tools that adequately measure fatigue. Over the past ten years, studies have begun to emerge that describe patterns and intensity of biotherapy-related fatigue. To date, few commonly recommended interventions suggested for management of fatigue have been evaluated by research to confirm efficacy or risk (Winningham et al., 1994). As the state of the knowledge regarding fatigue continues to progress, empirically based interventions should begin to emerge.

Assessment

A thorough assessment of fatigue that obtains both subjective and objective data provides the foundation for managing the symptom of fatigue. Fatigue should be assessed pretherapy to provide baseline information, during therapy to evaluate severity and determine effectiveness of interventions, and post therapy to determine when fatigue is resolved. Both the analysis of a symptom criterion described in Chapter 10 and theoretical models of fatigue described earlier in this chapter will provide a framework from which to assess fatigue.

Before therapy, determination of the patient's risk for development of fatigue should occur. Knowledge of biological agents known to cause the highest levels of fatigue will result in preplanning of strategies to combat fatigue. Cofactors which either predispose the patient to fatigue, or influence the level of fatigue experienced, are important to assess (see Figures 11.1 and 11.2). Examples include disease patterns, activity and rest patterns, energy patterns (nutritional intake), sleep and rest patterns, treatment patterns, symptoms patterns such as anemia, nausea, and pain, and oxygenation patterns (Nail and Winningham, 1993; Piper et al., 1987). An inventory of the patient's medications may also detect substances that contribute to or influence fatigue levels (e.g., alcohol, caffeine, narcotics, sedatives, hypnotics, or antihypertensives) (Piper, 1991a).

The patient's perception of fatigue provides subjective data. Important areas to assess include usual patterns of functioning and any changes that have resulted due to treatment, the meaning of fatigue, how distressing the symptom of fatigue is (Rhodes and Watson, 1987), and the physical, emotional, and psychological symptoms experienced (Piper *et al.*, 1989a). Physical symptoms may include expressions about whole body tiredness, feeling "drained," "weary," "listless," "pooped," or feeling tired in the eyes, arms or legs. Emotionally, fatigue may be described as unpleasant or as a lack of motivation. Behaviorally, patients or family members may notice that it takes longer to perform physical activities or that more effort is required. Some activities may no longer be attempted as they are viewed as requiring "too much energy." Mental or cognitive symptoms may include difficulty concentrating or reading, or in the ability to think clearly (Piper, 1993).

In clinical practice, one of the simplest ways to assess fatigue is to have the patient rate the level of fatigue on a scale of 1 to 10, with 1 being "no fatigue" and 10 being "the most possible fatigue" (Winningham *et al.*, 1994). Having the patient maintain a fatigue diary or journal can yield a significant amount of information on fatigue patterns. Determination of temporal levels of fatigue (e.g., when fatigue levels are highest) and which types of factors aggravate and alleviate fatigue will guide interventions.

Objective indicators of fatigue include physiological, biochemical, and behavioral factors. In the clinical setting, behavioral factors are the most easily assessed. Examples include performance status (Karnofsky and Zubrod are the most frequently used), physical appearance, and affect (Piper, 1991b).

It is also important to assess social support systems. Patients often need assistance from family or friends during periods of acute or chronic fatigue. The patient with limited support systems may need referrals initiated to provide other options for assistance. Evaluation of support from the patient's place of employment should also occur, as work schedules may need to be altered during periods of significant levels of fatigue. Support systems should be reassessed regularly during therapy, as increased role demands can lead to fatigue and strain of caregivers (Jensen and Givens, 1991) and social isolation for the patient and family.

Management Strategies

Medications
There are few published reports addressing the use of medications to decrease fatigue in patients receiving biotherapy. Piper (1993) summarizes the few studies that have tested the effects of medications on subjective fatigue, however, none were conducted in patients with cancer. A summary on fatigue in cancer patients by Bruera and MacDonald (1988) reviews the use of methylprednisolone and various amphetamines and their derivatives (e.g., methylphenidate) on patients with cancer and reports varying responses. There have been anecdotal reports (Quesada *et al.*, 1986) on the use of methylphenidate in patients receiving therapy with interferon-alpha with varying success rates. The use of medications to alleviate biotherapy-related fatigue remains an area that requires further investigation. When possible, medications that may cause decreased energy and tiredness (e.g., hypnotics, antihistamines) should be eliminated.

Manipulation of Treatment
The alteration of dose and schedule of biological agents may provide a means to diminish fatigue. Few published reports exist, but additional research may begin to delineate patterns of fatigue associated with different doses of biological agents (e.g., high doses versus low doses), different routes of administration (e.g., subcutaneous versus intravenous bolus versus intravenous continuous infusion), and combinations of biological agents. The information may provide a basis for modifying dosing schedules such that equal clinical outcomes are achieved using regimens that cause lower levels of fatigue and less toxic effects. Nurses, because of their role in ongoing assessment of tolerance of therapy, should work

collaboratively with physicians in designing dosing schedules that are best tolerated by the patient.

Most biological agents at lower doses, tend to cause less fatigue than at higher doses, although this will vary depending on the patient's clinical status. It has been reported that intermittent scheduling (two to three times per week) of interferon is better tolerated, with less fatigue (Quesada *et al.*, 1986). Others have reported that evening administration of interferon is better tolerated, with less fatigue and side effects (Abrams *et al.*, 1985). A recent pilot study by Dean *et al.* (1993) evaluated this question. Patients with metastatic melanoma were randomized to receive either morning (8 AM) or evening (5 PM) administration of interferon-alpha. Symptom distress was measured by the Symptom Distress Scale (McCorckle and Young, 1978) and the Piper Fatigue Scale (Piper *et al.*, 1989) before treatment began and every 2 weeks for 2 months. Early results demonstrated less symptom distress with evening administration than with morning administration at the 4-week time point. Although there was no statistical difference in fatigue ratings between the two groups, a plot of mean scores for the morning group showed a trend for the scores to increase over time, while the evening group seemed to plateau at 4 weeks.

To achieve higher doses, stepwise escalation of the dose over time has been reported to assist in reaching higher doses with better tolerance (Talpaz, personal communication). Patients treated with interferon and interleukin–2 will respond to brief rest periods with resolution of fatigue prior to the next cycle or course of therapy. The optimal best dose, route, and schedule is yet to be determined for most biological agents, therefore, future research efforts should focus on regimens that are tolerated with less fatigue and symptom distress while maintaining clinical efficacy.

Nursing Measures
Several publications have reviewed clinical interventions for cancer-related fatigue (Nail and Winningham, 1993; Piper, 1993, 1991a, 1991b; Clark *et al.*, 1992; Skalla and Lacasse, 1992a; 1992b; Brophy and Sharp, 1991; Rieger, 1988; Aistars, 1987). To date, the majority of clinical interventions used for fatigue in patients with cancer, and specifically for biotherapy-related fatigue, do not have an empirical foundation (Winningham *et al.*, 1994). However, the prevalence of this side effect and its impact on patient's quality of life provide a unique opportunity for nurses to initiate clinical research in this arena. See Table 11.2 for an overview of recommendations for clinical practice regarding cancer-related fatigue.

A useful analogy for assisting patients to cope with fatigue is to have them think about personal energy stores as a bank (Skalla and Lacasse, 1992a; Piper, 1991a). "Deposits" and "withdrawals" are made over time to achieve a balance between activities that are energy-restoring and those that are energy-depleting. Several studies have reported useful activities for managing fatigue (Robinson and Posner, 1992; Piper and Dodd, 1991; Rhodes *et al.*, 1988). In patients receiving therapy with either interleukin–2 or interferon-alpha (Robinson and Posner, 1992), self-care interventions identified by patients as helpful included rest or sleep, maintaining their usual routine, or exercising lightly. Patients reported that interventions which assisted them in reducing fatigue were "helping me with household chores" or "driving me to work." A surprising finding of the study was that only 31% of family member's recommendations for alleviating fatigue corresponded with those of the patients, and only 46% of nurses's suggestions corresponded with those of the patient. Although the sample size was limited, the results of this study suggest that nurses need to be more attuned to assessing fatigue, and both nurses and family members should verify the effectiveness of suggested interventions with the patient.

Energy Restoration   Numerous interventions have been suggested in the literature to assist

Table 11.2   Recommendations for clinical practice regarding cancer-related fatigue

Assessment	Education	Interventions
• Differentiate fatigue from depression. • Evaluate patterns of activity and rest during the day and over time. • Assess for the presence of correctable correlates or contributors to fatigue (e.g., dehydration, anemia, electrolyte imbalance). • Determine the patient's attentional ability. • Monitor the effects of fatigue on perception of quality of life. • Evaluate the efficacy of self-care fatigue interventions on a regular and systematic basis.	• Provide anticipatory guidance regarding the likelihood of experiencing fatigue and of the fatigue patterns associated with particular treatments. • Educate patients and families regarding deleterious effects of prolonged bedrest and too much inactivity. • Educate patients and families about expectancies of fatigue related to disease and treatment.	• Help patients and families identify what fatigue-promoting activities they can modify and how to modify them. • Encourage patients to maintain a journal to identify fatigue patterns. • Establish priorities for safe activities based on usual social role and cultural values. • Encourage activity within individual limitations; make goals realistic by keeping in mind state of disease and treatment regimens. • Suggest individualized environmental or activity changes that may offset fatigue. • Maintain adequate hydration and nutrition. • Promote an adequate balance between activity and rest. • Recommend physical therapy referral for patients with specific neuromusculoskeletal deficits. • Schedule important daily activities during time of least fatigue and eliminate nonessential, unsatisfying activities. • Address the negative impact of psychological and social stressors and how to modify or avoid them.

Source: Adapted with permission from Winningham, M., Nail, L., Barton Burke, M., et al., 1994. Fatigue and the cancer experience: The state of the knowledge. *Oncology Nursing Forum,* 21(1): 23–36.

patients in replenishing energy stores. Napping and resting are the most frequently used and frequently suggested interventions. Patients may need to take short naps during the day following periods of activity, or take a nap prior to a period of planned activity in order to ensure adequate energy levels. However, the majority of patients experiencing biotherapy-related fatigue experience chronic fatigue and should be cautioned to avoid too much rest, as this can negatively impact fatigue levels. Maintenance of normal sleep patterns at night is encouraged.

Despite anorexia being a common problem in patients receiving biotherapy, adequate hydration and nutrition are important in maintaining or restoring energy levels. Fluids are hypothesized to assist with excretion of cell destruction end-products that may be associated with fatigue. Adequate energy stores are necessary for optimal muscle functioning. See Chapter 10 for suggestions for enhancing nutritional intake.

Relaxation or diversional activities such as visiting friends, reading, listening to music, watching a movie, or involvement in a hobby may also be energy-enhancing. Cimprich (1992) tested an intervention aimed at increasing subjects' participation in activities thought to maintain or restore directed attention. Post-surgical patients were randomly assigned to set aside a minimum of 30 minutes, 3 times a week for restorative activities. Compared to a control group, the experimental group showed higher rates of returning to work and of engaging in newly initiated, purposeful activities. Although not a proven intervention for patients receiving biotherapy, this study provides a basis for future research and intervention efforts that could certainly prove useful.

Management of correlates of fatigue such as anemia, nausea and vomiting, and pain can also enhance energy stores. In theoretical models described earlier in this chapter, these factors are proposed to influence or cause fatigue. Successful interventions for management of these factors are available, therefore, they should be assessed and treated when present.

Although limited, a research base does exist for using exercise as an intervention to combat fatigue. Winningham proposes the idea of a fatigue-inertia spiral (Winningham, 1992). Symptoms, such as fatigue, can lead to an actual or perceived need for bed rest and limited activity (hypodynamia). This results in physiologic changes, which in turn lead to lower energetic capacity and heightened feelings of fatigue. The more fatigued a patient feels, the more he or she tends to rest, which leads to more physiologic changes. Over time, this spiral can result in profound decreases in functional status (see Figure 11.3). An individualized endurance exercise training program might serve as the foundation of an effective energy restoring regimen.

Winningham (1983) reported results from a rehabilitation project involving patients with breast cancer who were receiving chemotherapy. Patients placed on the Winningham Aerobic Interval Training (WAIT) protocol for 10 weeks exhibited increases in objective measures of functional capacity, and reported increased feelings of internal control as com-

Figure 11.3   The fatigue/inertia spiral

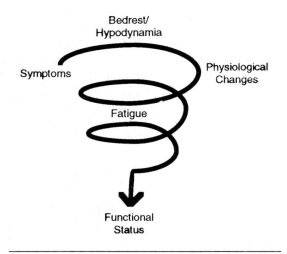

Source: © 1991, 1994 Maryl L. Winningham, RN, PhD, FACSM. Used with express written consent of the author. Graphics by Linda Bishop.

pared to a control group that did not exercise. Subsequent work using the same exercise program documented a decreased perception of fatigue as measured by the Profile of Mood States (POMS) fatigue subscale (MacVicar and Winningham, 1986). Mock *et al.* (1994) evaluated a modified version of the rhythmic walking program in patients with breast cancer. This exercise protocol, described in the booklet *Rhythmic Walking: Exercise for People Living with Cancer* (Winningham *et al.*, 1990) is a low-intensity, self-care walking program that is lower risk and lower cost than the WAIT protocol. In this study, the non-exercise group reported twice the fatigue of the exercise group. Although these studies are not generalizable to biotherapy-related fatigue, they do provide a sound rationale for the use of exercise to diminish sensations of fatigue. Serendipitously, many patients who exercise regularly and are receiving biological agents such as interferon, report less problems with fatigue.

Any exercise program should be individualized to the patient's clinical status. Risk factors such as lytic bone lesions, thrombocytopenia, fever, or neutropenia may be contraindicated (Piper, 1991a). Guidelines and precautions for the use of exercise as an intervention have been reported (Winningham, 1991). In addition, St. Pierre (1992) cautions that in patients who are cachectic or receiving tumor necrosis factor as therapy, nurses should be concerned that the development of fatigue may involve changes in skeletal muscle protein stores. The involvement of muscle in the occurrence of fatigue may be a factor in determining if the patients can successfully participate in an exercise program. Physiologic factors may exist that predispose patients with cancer to develop fatigue or to experience an adverse response to exercise.

Energy Conservation/Utilization   Other interventions designed to limit or relieve fatigue center on effective utilization of existing energy stores. Measures such as modification of the environment, scheduling activities for times when energy levels are at their peak, pacing activities, eliminating nonessential activities, requesting assistance from family members or friends, and the use of energy saving equipment to do household chores can be helpful. The nurse can assist patients to cope with fatigue by jointly reviewing a normal day's activities and obligations and making adjustments to fit current energy levels. Frequent follow-up assessments will assist in verifying the effectiveness of these changes. Nurses should also assist with scheduling laboratory tests and diagnostic studies so that patient energy stores are not depleted by repeated trips to the hospital or clinic setting.

Stress Reduction   The Aistars Organizing Framework (1987), based on energy and stress theory, implicates physiologic, psychological, and situational stressors as contributing to fatigue. By educating patients on effective coping strategies and facilitating their use of existing coping strategies, nurses can help patients to decrease experienced stressors. Although not well researched, this may be useful in decreasing fatigue levels. Participation in support groups may also help patients to decrease

fatigue levels through reduction of stress. Depression and anxiety also influence fatigue, therefore, these symptoms should be recognized and treated when present. Several studies have demonstrated that patients' perceived ability to manage symptoms correlates with fatigue distress (Jones, 1993; Pickard-Holley, 1991). Patient education on fatigue-management strategies can empower the patient to more effectively cope with therapy (Skalla and LaCasse, 1992b).

Patient Education   Johnson *et al.* (1988) reported that perception of fatigue may be reduced by providing the patient with information that prepares them to view fatigue as an expected part of treatment rather than a sign of disease progression. Other researchers investigating fatigue have also noted the importance of anticipatory guidance and counseling for symptom management (Yeager *et al.*, 1993; Holland, 1991). Teaching should include a definition of what fatigue is, the types of symptoms that may be experienced with biotherapy agents the patient is to receive, and when symptoms are expected to occur. Patients should also be aware of the expected duration of fatigue (e.g., acute or chronic), and should be assured that chronic fatigue does not necessarily signal a recurrence of disease, progression of disease, or a lack of response to therapy. Discussing what other individuals have found useful in preventing and eliminating fatigue is helpful. Patients should be instructed to report early signs and symptoms of fatigue so that interventions can be instituted immediately in an attempt to prevent fatigue from worsening (Skalla and Lacasse, 1992a; Piper, 1991a). Reportable signs and symptoms of severe chronic fatigue include spending all day in bed or on a couch, being able to perform only minimal activities of daily living, and decreased ability to concentrate.

RESEARCH ON FATIGUE

Winningham *et al.* (1994) summarize future directions for research regarding cancer-related fatigue. Important areas include developing a research-based definition of fatigue, clarification of concepts related to fatigue (e.g., weakness or tiredness), differentiating acute versus chronic fatigue, determination of the mechanisms of fatigue, delineation of predictors of fatigue and patterns of fatigue associated with different types of therapy, and the testing of interventions to alleviate fatigue. These issues are all relevant for research on biotherapy-related fatigue.

Critical review of fatigue literature is problematic. The lack of consistent research tools and theory have created a body of literature that must be carefully reviewed for bias before drawing conclusions. As an early pioneer of fatigue, Grandjean (1968) initially makes an important point that must be considered when studying fatigue in patients treated with BRMs. During the assessment of fatigue, the testing process itself is a stress that alerts the organism which may mask a previous state of fatigue. As a result of this response, tests that measure fatigue may provide results which report lower fatigue levels than were actually experienced. Current investigations (Cimprich, 1992) address "attentional fatigue" as a concept applied to cancer patients. This type of fatigue is another theoretical bias that could be introduced into a study which administers lengthy tools to measure fatigue. Thought must be given to these factors when revieweing the results of any study that investigates fatigue.

One of the earliest nursing fatigue studies was initiated by Freel and Hart (1977) and examined fatigue in patients with multiple sclerosis. In 1979, Hart and Haylock completed a study of fatigue in oncology patients who were receiving radiation therapy. Since then, nursing has documented fatigue in cancer patients receiving biotherapy (Hodges, 1992; Skalla, 1992; Rieger, 1987; Davis, 1984; Mayer et al., 1984) as well as chemotherapy (Blesch et al., 1991; Nail et al., 1991; Pickard-Holley, 1991; Jamar, 1989), radiation therapy (Oberst et al., 1991), and surgery (Rhoten,

1982). A review by Irvin et al. (1991) provides a concise overview of the research literature investigating fatigue in patients with cancer. Current research efforts are focused on attempts to characterize the clinical nature of fatigue in patients with cancer.

The study of biotherapy-related fatigue remains at an early stage. Few studies have been published that document patterns of fatigue associated with BRMs. Precise mechanisms for fatigue experienced with biological agents have yet to be determined.

St. Pierre et al. (1992) looked at the relationship between fatigue, cachexia, and tumor necrosis factor. Cachexia was found in earlier research (Mayer et al., 1984), to be associated with interferon administration and may play a role in fatigue associated with muscle wasting. St. Pierre has expanded this concept to create a cause-effect relationship by proposing a biochemical mechanism that causes changes in skeletal muscle physiology which may affect fatigue. The research by St. Pierre provides critical groundwork in nursing research from a physiological perspective. It would be useful and relatively easy to include measurements such as albumin and blood pH, in an expanded form of this study, to provide data that may support this type of theory. The data provided by this type of research may also provide physiological data to support the Piper et al. (1987) theoretical model for fatigue. Questions which address the physiological relationship between fatigue and other symptoms which contribute to fatigue must be explored.

Investigation of the relationship between fatigue and BRMs could be enhanced in many ways. Due to the subjective nature of fatigue, qualitative research should be combined with quantitative research to steer further research efforts in appropriate directions. Biological response modifiers seem to have a particular dose-relationship with fatigue; studies which examine the physiological relationship of this phenomenon may yield specific information about the clinical nature of fatigue which could then guide efforts to focus on other treatment modalities. Healthy control populations are important to include in these studies to differentiate effects of disease and treatment on fatigue. Additional questions may be answered by comparing two patient populations; for example, one receiving interferon for treatment of a malignancy and one receiving interferon treatment for a non-malignant disease such as hepatitis. Finally, a critical need for research efforts is to concentrate on the development of tools that adequately measure fatigue. Measures specific for fatigue must be developed which are reliable, valid, and easily applied in the clinical setting.

SUMMARY

Fatigue is recognized as a significant symptom in patients receiving biotherapy. At times, fatigue may be so severe that it becomes the dose-limiting side effect. Patients may request to stop effective therapy due to the negative impact of fatigue on quality of life. Nurses are responsible for management of this challenging side effect, and they are in the position of being able to advance the science of fatigue research.

The study of fatigue has progressed over the past decade, but there are many questions that remain unanswered. Research examining functional aspects of fatigue is important. This information could potentially strengthen justification for research funding. Specific details on functional impact would lay the foundation for studies testing interventions to alleviate fatigue. This information could be used in cancer rehabilitation to improve the quality of life of the cancer patient. A substantial impact on the outcomes of patients with fatigue may result, particularly on those patients receiving interferon and other biological response modifiers. Nurses caring for patients receiving biotherapy have a unique opportunity to conduct research that adds to existing the body of knowledge.

References

Abrams, P., McClamrock, E., and Foon, K. 1985. Evening administration of alpha interferon. *New England Journal of Medicine* 312: 443–444.

Adams, F., Quesdad, J., and Gutterman, J. 1984. Neuropsychiatric manifestations of human leukocyte interferon therapy in patients with cancer. *Journal of the American Medical Association* 151: 938–941.

Aistars, J. 1987. Fatigue in the cancer patient: A conceptual approach to a clinical problem. *Oncology Nursing Forum* 14(6): 25–30.

Alexander, R., and Rosenberg, S. 1991. Tumor necrosis factor: Clinical applications. In DeVita, V., Hellman, S., Rosenberg, S. (eds). *Biologic Therapy of Cancer*. Philadelphia: J.B. Lippincott, pp. 378–392.

Blesch, K., Paice, J., Wickham, R., *et al.* 1991. Correlates of fatigue in people with breast or lung cancer. *Oncology Nursing Forum* 18(1): 81–87.

Britton, D. 1983. Fatigue. In Yasko, J. (ed.). *Guidelines for Cancer Care: Symptom Management*. Reston, VA: Reston Publishing Company, Inc., pp. 33–37.

Brophy, L., and Sharp, E. 1991. Physical symptoms of combination biotherapy: A quality-of-life issue. *Oncology Nursing Forum* 18(1 Suppl): 25–30.

Bruera, E., and MacDonald, R. (1988). Overwhelming fatigue in advanced cancer. *American Journal of Nursing* 88: 99–100.

Cimprich, B. 1992. Attentional fatigue following breast cancer surgery. *Research in Nursing and Health* 15: 199–207.

Clark, J., McGee, R., and Preston, R. 1992. Nursing management of responses to the cancer experience. In Clark, J., and McGee, R. (eds). *Oncology Nursing Society Core Curriculum for Oncology Nursing*, 2nd ed. Philadelphia: W.B. Saunders, pp. 67–155.

Cushman, K. 1986. Symptom management: A comprehensive approach to increasing nutritional status in the cancer patient. *Seminars in Oncology Nursing* 2(1): 30–35.

Davis, C. 1984. *Interferon Induced Fatigue*. Unpublished masters thesis. Yale University, New Haven, CT.

Dean, G., Spears, L., Quan, W., *et al.*, 1993. Evening administration of interferon-alpha significantly reduces symptom distress in patients with metastatic melanoma. *Society for Biological Therapy 8th Annual Meeting Programs and Abstracts:* 82(abstract).

Dillman, J. 1988. Toxicity of monoclonal antibodies in the treatment of cancer. *Seminars in Oncology Nursing* 4(2): 107–111.

Donovan, M., and Girton, S. 1984. *Cancer Care Nursing*. 2nd ed. Norwalk, CT: Appleton-Century-Crofts.

Farrell, M., Gray, P., and Creekmore, S. 1990. Long-term biological therapy using interleukin-2 plus cyclophosphamide as a treatment for patients with melanoma: Nursing responsibilities. *Oncology Nursing Forum* 17(2 Suppl): 239 (abstract).

Freel, M., and Hart, L. 1977. Fatigue phenomena of multiple sclerosis patients. Grant No. 5R02–NM–00524–02. Washington, DC: United States Department of Health, Education and Welfare (USDHEW) Division of Nursing, pp. 118.

Gastl, G., Werter, M., De Pauw, B., *et al.* 1989. Comparison of clinical efficacy and toxicity of conventional and optimum biological response modifying doses of interferon alpha–2C in the treatment of hairy cell leukemia: A retrospective analysis of 39 patients. *Leukemia* 3(6): 453–460.

Gilson, B., Gilson, J., Bergner, M., *et al.*, 1975. The sickness impact profile: development of an outcome measure of health care. *American Journal of Health Care* 65(12): 1304–1310.

Gold, J. 1974. Cancer cachexia and gluconeogenesis. *Annals of the New York Academy of Sciences* 230: 103–110.

Grandjean, E. 1968. Fatigue. *American Industrial Hygiene Association Journal* 31: 401–411.

Haylock, P., and Hart, L. 1979. Fatigue in patients receiving localized radiation therapy. *Cancer Nursing* 2(6): 461–469.

Hodges, C. 1992. *A preliminary study of fatigue in patients receiving IL–2 biotherapy.* Unpublished master's thesis, University of Texas Health Science Center School of Nursing, Houston, Texas.

Holland, J. 1991. Fatigue in the patient with cancer during the week following a chemotherapy treatment. *Oncology Nursing Forum* 18(2): 54 (abstract).

Irvine, D., Vincent, L., Bubela, N., *et al.* 1991. A critical appraisal of the research literature investigating fatigue in the individual with cancer. *Cancer Nursing* 14(4): 188–199.

Jamar, S. 1989. Fatigue in women receiving chemotherapy for ovarian cancer. In Funk, S., Tornquist, E., Champagne, M., Copp, L., and Weise, R. (eds). *Key Aspects of Comfort.* New York: Spring Hill Publishing, pp. 224–233.

Janisch, L. 1990. Nursing management of side effects of interleukin–2 and interferon alfa–2a administered as subcutaneous injections. *Oncology Nursing Forum* 17(2 Suppl): 102 (abstract).

Jensen, S., and Given, B. 1991. Fatigue affecting family caregivers of cancer patients. *Cancer Nursing* 14(4): 181–187.

Johnson, J., Nail, L., Lauver, D., *et al.*, 1988. Reducing the negative impact of radiation therapy on functional status. *Cancer* 61: 46–51.

Johnson, D., Hande, K., Hainsworth, J., *et al.* 1983. Neurotoxicity of interferon. *Cancer Treatment Reports* 67: 958–961.

Jones, L. 1993. *Correlates of fatigue and related outcomes in individuals with cancer undergoing treatment with chemotherapy.* Unpublished doctoral dissertation. Buffalo: State University of New York, Buffalo, New York.

Kaempfer, S., and Lindsey, A. 1986. Energy expenditure in cancer. *Cancer Nursing* 9(4): 194–199.

Kellum, M. 1985. Fatigue. In Jacobs, M., Feels, W. (eds.). *Signs and Symptoms in Nursing: Interpretation and Management.* Philadelphia: JB Lippincott Company, pp. 103–118.

Koeller, J. 1989. Biologic response modifiers: The interferon alpha experience. *American Journal of Hospital Pharmacy* 46(2) Suppl: S11–15.

Lee, K., Talpaz, M., Rothberg, J., *et al.*, 1989. Concomitant administration of recombinant human interleukin–2 and recombinant interferon alpha–2a in cancer patients: A phase I study. *Journal of Clinical Oncology* 7(11): 1726–1732.

Lynch, M., Yanes, L., and Todd, K. 1988. Nursing care of AIDS patients participating in a phase I/II trial of recombinant human granulocyte-macrophage colony-stimulating factor. *Oncology Nursing Forum* 15: 463–469.

Lever, A., Lewis, D., Bannister, B., *et al.* 1988. Interferon production in postviral fatigue syndrome. *Lancet* 7: 101.

MacVicar, M., and Winningham, M. 1986. Promoting the functional capacity of cancer patients. *Cancer Bulletin* 38: 235–239.

Martin, G. 1991. TNF and IL–2. *Oncology Nursing Forum* 18(2): 307 (abstract).

Maxwell, M. 1984. When the cancer patient becomes anemic. *Cancer Nursing* 7(4): 321–326.

Mayer, D., Hetrick, K., Riggs, C., *et al.* 1984. Weight loss in patients receiving recombinant leukocyte A interferon (IFLrA) A brief report. *Cancer Nursing* 7(1): 53–56.

McCorkle, R., and Young, K. 1978. Development of a symptom distress scale. *Cancer Nursing* 1: 373–378.

McNair, D., Lorr, M., and Doppelman, F. (eds.). 1971. Manual for the Profile of Mood States. San Diego, CA: Educational and Industrial Testing Service, pp. 3–29.

Minden, S., and Reich, P. 1983. Nervousness and fatigue. In Blacklow, R. (ed.). *MacBryde's Signs and Symptoms.* Philadelphia: J.B. Lippincott Co., pp. 591–621.

Mock, V., Burke, M., Sheehan, P., *et al.*, (in press). A nursing rehabilitation program for women with breast cancer receiving adjuvant chemotherapy. *Oncology Nursing Forum* 21(5): 899–907.

Moldawer, N., and Figlin, R. 1988. Tumor necrosis factor: Current clinical status and implications for nursing management. *Seminars in Oncology Nursing* 4(2): 120–125.

Nail, L., and Winningham, M. 1993. Fatigue. In Groenwald, S., Frogge, M., Goodman, M., *et al.* (eds). *Cancer nursing: principles and practice,* 3rd ed. Boston: Jones and Bartlett, pp. 608–619.

Nail, L., Jones, L., Greene, D., *et al.* 1991. Use and perceived efficacy of self-care activities in patients receiving chemotherapy. *Oncology Nursing Forum* 18(5): 883–887.

Oberst, M., Chang, A., and McCubbin, M. 1991. Self-care burden, stress appraisal, and mood among persons receiving radiotherapy. *Cancer Nursing* 14(2): 71–78.

Pearson, R., and Byars, G. 1956. *The development and validation of a checklist for measuring subjective fatigue.* Randolph AFB, Texas School of Aviation Medicine: United States Air Force,(Report # 56–115).

Pickard-Holley, S. 1991. Fatigue in cancer patients: A descriptive study. *Cancer Nursing* 14: 13–19.

Piper, B. 1993. Fatigue. In Carrieri-Kohlman, V., Lindsey, A., and West, C. (eds). *Pathophysiological Phenomena in Nursing: Human Responses to Illness* (2nd ed). Philadelphia: W.B. Saunders, pp. 279–302.

Piper, B. 1991a. Alteration in comfort: Fatigue. In McNally, J., Somerville, E., Miaskowski, C., *et al.* (eds). *Guidelines for oncology nursing practice* (2nd ed). Philadelphia: W.B. Saunders, pp. 155–162.

Piper, B. 1991b. Alterations in energy: The sensation of fatigue. In Baird, S., McCorckle, R., and Grant, M. (eds). *Cancer Nursing: A Comprehensive Textbook.* Philadelphia: W.B. Saunders, pp. 894–908.

Piper, B., and Dodd, M. 1991. Self initiated fatigue interventions and their perceived effect. *Oncology Nursing Forum* 18(2): 391 (abstract).

Piper, B., Lindsey, A., Dodd, M., *et al.*, 1989a. Development of an instrument to measure the subjective dimension of fatigue. In Funk, S., Tornquist, E., Champagne, M., *et al.*, (eds). *Key Aspects of Comfort: Management of Pain, Fatigue and Nausea.* New York: Springer Publishing Co., pp. 199–208.

Piper, B., Rieger, P., Brophy, L., *et al.* 1989b. Recent advances in the management of biotherapy side effects: Fatigue. *Oncology Nursing Forum* 16(6) Suppl: 27–34.

Piper, B., Lindsey, A., and Dodd, M. 1987. Fatigue mechanisms in cancer patients: Developing nursing theory. *Oncology Nursing Forum* 14(6): 17–23.

Potempa, K. 1989. Chronic fatigue: Directions for research and practice. In Funk, S., Tornquist, E., Champagne, M., Copp, L., and Weise, R. (eds). *Key Aspects of Comfort.* New York: Spring Hill Publishing, pp. 229–231.

Potempa, K., Lopez, M., Reid, C., *et al.* 1986. Chronic fatigue. *Image* 18(4): 165–169.

Quesada, J., Talpaz, M., Rios, A., *et al.*, 1986. Clinical toxicity of interferons in cancer patients: A review. *Journal of Clinical Oncology* 4(2): 234–243.

Radin, A., Grant, B. Anderson, J. *et al.* 1989. Toxicity of interferon-alpha in the chronic myeloproliferative disorders: preliminary results of a collaborative phase II trial. *Blood* 74(7 Suppl 1): 236a.

Reilly, L., and McKeever, S. 1993. Fatigue management in the patient treated with the biological response modifier interleukin–3. *Oncology Nursing Forum* 20(2): 218 (abstract).

Rhodes, V., Watson, P., and Hanson, B. 1988. Patients' descriptions of the influence of tiredness and weakness on self-care abilities. *Cancer Nursing* 11: 186–194.

Rhodes, V., and Watson, P. 1987. Symptom distress—the concept: past and present. *Seminars in Oncology Nursing* 3: 242–247.

Rhoten, D. 1982. Fatigue in the postsurgical patient. In Norris C. (ed). *Concept Clarification in Nursing* Rockville: Aspen Systems Corporation, pp. 277–295.

Rieger, P. 1988. Management of cancer-related fatigue. *Dimensions in Oncology Nursing* II(3): 5–8.

Rieger, P. 1987. Interferon-induced fatigue: A study of fatigue measurement. *Sigma Theta Tau International 29th Biennial Convention Book of Proceedings*: A163.

Robinson, K., and Posner, J. 1992. Patterns of self-care needs and interventions related to biologic response modifier therapy: Fatigue as a model. *Seminars in Oncology Nursing* 8(4 Suppl 1): 17–22.

Schipper, H., Clinch, C., McMurray, A., *et al.*, 1984. Measuring the quality of life of cancer patients: the functional living index-cancer: development and validation. *Journal of Clinical Oncology* 2(5): 472–483.

Shacham, S. 1983. A shortened version of the profile of mood states. *Journal of Personal Assessment* 47(3): 305–306.

Sharp, E. 1993. Case management of the hospitalized patient receiving interleukin–2. *Seminars in Oncology Nursing* 9(3 Suppl 1): 14–19.

Siegel, J., and Puri, R. 1991. Interleukin–2 toxicity. *Journal of Clinical Oncology* 9: 694–704.

Silver, H., Connors, J., and Salinas, F. 1985. Prospectively randomized toxicity study of high-dose versus low-dose treatment strategies for lymphoblastoid interferon. *Cancer Treatment Reports* 69(7–8): 743–750.

Skalla, K. 1992. Correlates of fatigue in patients treated with interferon: A pilot study. Unpublished master's thesis, MGH Institute of Health Professions. Boston, MA.

Skalla, K., and Lacasse, C. 1992a. Fatigue and the patient with cancer: What is it and what can I do about it? *Oncology Nursing Forum* 19: 1540–1541.

Skalla, K., and Lacasse, C. 1992b. Patient education for fatigue. *Oncology Nursing Forum* 19: 1537–1539.

St. Pierre, B., Kasper, C., and Lindsey, A. 1992. Fatigue mechanisms in patients with cancer: Effects of tumor necrosis factor and exercise on skeletal muscle. *Oncology Nursing Forum* 19(3): 419–425.

Theologides, A. 1972. Pathogenesis of cachexia in cancer: A review and a hypothesis. *Cancer* 29(2): 484–488.

Viele, C., and Moran, T. 1993. Nursing management of the nonhospitalized patient receiving recombinant interleukin–2. *Seminars in Oncology Nursing* 9(3 Suppl 1): 20–24.

Wadler, S., Lyver, A., and Wiernik, P. 1989. Clinical toxicities of the combination of 5-fluorouracil and recombinant interferon alpha–2a: An unusual toxicity profile. *Oncology Nursing Forum* 16(6) Suppl: 12–15.

Winningham, M., Nail, L., Barton Burke, M., *et al.* 1994. Fatigue and the cancer experience: The state of the knowledge. *Oncology Nursing Forum* 21(1): 23–36.

Winningham, M. 1992. How exercise mitigates fatigue: Implications for people receiving cancer therapy. In Carroll-Johnson, R. (ed) *The Biotherapy of Cancer-V* (monograph). Pittsburgh: Oncology Nursing Press, pp. 16–21.

Winningham, M. 1991. Walking program for people with cancer: Getting started. *Cancer Nursing* 14: 270–276.

Winningham, M., Glass, E., and MacVicar, M. 1990. *Rhythmic Walking: Exercise for People Living with Cancer.* Columbus: Ohio State University, Arthur G. James Cancer Hospital and Research Institute.

Winningham, M. 1983. Effects of a bicycle ergometry program on functional capacity and feelings of control in women with breast cancer. Columbus: Ohio State University, Doctoral dissertation.

Yeager, K., Dibble, S., and Dodd, M. 1993. The experience of fatigue among patients receiving chemotherapy. *Oncology Nursing Forum* 20(2): 297 (abstract).

Yoshitake, H. 1971. Relations between the symptoms and feelings of fatigue. *Ergonomics* 14: 175–196.

Yoshitake, H. 1969. Rating the feelings of fatigue. *Journal of Science and Labour* 45(7): 422–432.

CHAPTER 12 | The Flu-Like Syndrome

Douglas Haeuber, RN, MSN, MA, OCN

The use of biotherapy in the treatment of cancer, both alone and as a supportive adjunct to other modalities has become increasingly widespread. Still, the identification of side effects associated with various biological response modifiers (BRMs) in clinical trials has kept pace with this increase in their utilization. Whereas the side effects of each agent vary, the so-called "flu-like syndrome" (FLS), to a greater or lesser degree has appeared consistently.

Flu-like syndrome may be defined as a cluster of constitutional signs and symptoms that may include fever, **chills**, **rigors**, **myalgias**, headache, **malaise**, upper respiratory symptoms (e.g., cough and nasal congestion) and gastrointestinal symptoms (e.g., anorexia, nausea, vomiting, and diarrhea). Within this broad array of potential effects, those that have become most closely associated with FLS are the first five.

This syndrome is often characterized as a mild, yet troublesome, toxic effect. Although not itself life-threatening, FLS is nonetheless significant for several reasons. First, it can contribute substantially to the debilitation of a population of patients who may already be physically compromised. The side effects mentioned above are not without physiologic sequelae; expert clinicians know that fever, rigors, or both can sap a patient's precious strength. Second, an episode of influenza is a miserable experience for anyone; once a winter is more than enough. Anticipation of a flu-like episode, following every treatment with certain BRMs, may exact from the patient a high emotional and psychological price in his or her efforts to continue therapy.

Flu-like syndrome has the potential to significantly affect quality of life. Among health care providers, nurses are perhaps the most conscious of and committed to quality-of-life

Table 12.1   The interferons

Symptom/ Side Effect	Interferon-alpha	Interferon-beta	Interferon-gamma
Fever	• T_{max} approx. 6 hours • Duration 4 to 8 hours • Dose dependent • Tolerance develops with daily doses	• Fever pattern similar to that for IFN-α • Frequently higher than 39.4°C	• T_{max} in 10 to 12 hours • Longer duration, up to 18 hours • Dose-dependent • No tolerance develops with daily doses
Chills/Rigors	• Precede fevers	• Precede fevers • Dose dependent	• Within first hour • Duration related to T_{max}
Myalgias	• Occur with fevers	• Common • Mild to moderate in severity	• Common • Experienced by 30–80% of all patients
Headache	• Occur with fevers	• Common • Generally mild to moderate	• Common • May be severe

T_{max} = Peak temperature.

issues for the persons for whom they care. Addressing and managing the side effects of cancer therapies and therefore enhancing the physical and psychological well-being (i.e., the quality of life) of patients represents the heart of oncology nursing. Therefore, acquiring a thorough understanding of FLS and developing strategies to help patients cope with it is an important role of the nurse who administers biotherapy.

In this chapter, patterns of FLS in biotherapy will be discussed in relation to pathophysiologic mechanisms. These mechanisms are closely tied to the processes of fever causation, an area that has seen intense research activity in recent years as the study of cytokines has progressed. Finally, nursing management of FLS and applicable areas of nursing research will be addressed.

PRESENTATION OF THE FLU-LIKE SYNDROME

Because the pattern and severity of FLS will vary with most agents, recognizing these patterns is important for nurses administering BRMs. This recognition will allow nurses to better distinguish between FLS as a side effect of biotherapy and an infection for which the

patient may need treatment and to prepare the patient and family for their experience with a particular biotherapy regimen.

Interferons

Interferons (IFNs) tend to cause flu-like symptoms that are dose-dependent in occurrence and severity, particularly for the elderly, the very young, or those with concomitant illnesses. Within this particular category of BRMs, variations in side effects seen with specific types of IFN are probably due to the differing effects of each agent on components of the immune system (See Table 12.1).

Interferon-alpha (IFN-α) and interferon-beta (IFN-β) produce fevers of rapid onset (2 to 4 hours), typically lasting 4 to 8 hours. These fevers may be preceded by mild chills and accompanied by headache and myalgias. In contrast, interferon-gamma (IFN-γ) causes fevers that tend to peak at 6 to 12 hours and last substantially longer. With each IFN, the symptom profile may also vary, depending on the route and schedule of drug administration. Another interesting difference is that patients who receive IFN-α or IFN-β tend to develop tolerance to FLS with continued administration over time, whereas those who

Table 12.2 The hematopoietic growth factors

Symptom/ Side Effect	EPO	G-CSF	GM-CSF	IL-3
Fever	• None	• None or low grade	• Generally low grade but may rise to 40°C	• Nearly 100% of all patients have low-grade fever (≤40°C)
Chills/Rigors	• None	• Uncommon	• Absent or mild	• Very common with fevers
Myalgias	• None	• Uncommon	• Common • General muscle aches, esp. in the thighs • May be severe enough to require analgesia	• Not reported
Headache	• None	• Uncommon	• Experienced by 50% of all patients • Transient and mild	• Common, esp. at higher doses • Usually mild, but may require analgesia • May be accompanied by neck stiffness

receive IFN-γ do not. This development of tolerance to certain toxic effects is known as **tachyphylaxis**.

Hematopoietic Growth Factors

Hematopoietic growth factors (HGFs), which make up another category of BRMs, have seen increasing use in the past five years. Although they generally have a benign symptom profile, FLS is associated with some of these agents (e.g., granulocyte-macrophage colony-stimulating factor (GM-CSF) and interleukin–3 (IL–3)) when administered in high doses (See Table 12.2). The difference in occurrence of symptoms within this category is most likely accounted for by the point in the sequence of hematopoietic events at which a given HGF has impact and by the cytokines produced and released in response to these actions.

Single Lineage Hematopoietic Growth Factors

Erythropoietin and granulocyte colony-stimulating factor (G-CSF) are primarily single-lineage HGFs that affect more mature precursor cells in the erythrocyte lineage and the granulocyte lineage, respectively. Cells stimulated by these HGFs tend not to produce cytokines involved in the production of FLS. (See the section on Pathophysiology of the Flu-Like Syndrome). Therefore, it is not surprising that these HGFs are associated only rarely with FLS. Erythropoietin has been associated with FLS in a small number of patients when given by intravenous bolus (Tabbara, 1993). Because G-CSF does have some impact on early, multilineage progenitor cells, it may occasionally cause a low-grade fever.

Multi-Lineage Hematopoietic Growth Factors

Granulocyte-macrophage colony-stimulating factor affects both the granulocyte and macrophage/monocyte lineages at higher levels in the hematopoietic sequence of events. Cells in the macrophage/monocyte line are well established as the source of many cytokines involved in fever causation and thus in the symptom pattern of FLS. Granulocyte-macrophage colony-stimulating factor is generally associated with low-grade fevers (≤ 38°C), although it may cause fevers to rise to 40°C. Patients who receive GM-CSF may also experience mild chills, transient headache, and on occasion, severe myalgias. These side effects may be more pronounced and more common with intravenous administration of the agent, although they can also appear with subcutaneous administration.

Interleukin–3, sometimes known as multi-CSF, is a multi-lineage HGF that promotes the

Table 12.3   Interleukin-2

Symptom/ Side Effect	Interleukin 2

Fever	• Experienced by 80–100% of all patients
	• Dose-dependent T_{max}
	• Delayed onset:
	  (a) Bolus infusion: T_{max} in 6 hours with slow decline
	  (b) Continuous intravenous infusion Elevated throughout, resolved 2 to 3 days after end of infusion

Chills/Rigors	• Common, precede fever • May be more frequent and more severe when IL-2 is given with LAK and TIL cells
Myalgias	• May accompany fever
Headache	• May accompany fever

Table 12.4   Monoclonal antibodies

Symptom/ Side Effect	Monoclonal Antibodies

Fever	• Common (Experienced by 20–100% of all patients
	• Two patterns:
	  (a) During first hour of infusion
	  (b) 1 to 2 hours after infusion

Chills/Rigors	• Occur with fever
Myalgias	• Arthralgias are reported rather than myalgias
Headache	• Not reported

proliferation and differentiation of early multipotential progenitor cells. Although fewer clinical trials have been conducted with IL–3 than GM-CSF, side effects caused by IL–3 are well characterized and appear to be caused in much the same manner as with GM-CSF. Nearly all patients who receive IL–3 experience low-grade fevers accompanied by chills and, at higher dose levels, these side effects have been accompanied by mild headaches (Kurzrock *et al.*, 1991).

Interleukin–2

Interleukin–2 (IL–2) stimulates the proliferation, differentiation, and activation of T and B lymphocytes, natural killer cells, and thymocytes. It has been administered in clinical trials alone and in combination with other BRMs (e.g., IFNs), lymphokine-activated killer cells (LAK cells) and tumor-infiltrating lymphocytes (TIL). Whether IL–2 is administered alone or in combination with other agents, FLS is a common side effect. Fever, chills, and rigors, sometimes accompanied by myalgias and headache, are nearly universal and appear within 2 to 4 hours after initiation of IL–2 therapy. (See Table 12.3.) With the addition of LAK cells or TIL to IL–2 therapy, mild to severe chills and rigors tend to occur within 30 minutes to 4 hours after the first infusion. Although it is difficult to separate the side effects of this treatment from those of the treatment with IL–2 alone, there appears to be an additive effect. Symptoms of FLS are similar for these two forms of treatment (Margolin *et al.*, 1989; Kintzel and Calis, 1991). When IL–2 is administered by continuous infusion for several days, FLS symptoms become more intense (Thompson *et al.*, 1988). Furthermore, tolerance to symptoms does not appear to develop over successive courses of IL–2 therapy (Kintzel and Calis, 1991). Thus, the effects of dosage, dosage interval, rate of infusion, and duration of IL–2 therapy and of IL–2 containing regimens on FLS are even more pronounced than is the case with other BRMs.

Monoclonal Antibodies

Monoclonal antibodies (MABs) have been studied both as a diagnostic tool and as a therapeutic modality. Their use is associated with the development of FLS and the symptom profile includes chills and rigors, fever, diaphoresis and **arthralgias** rather than myalgias. (See Table 12.4.) With intravenous infusion, two distinct side-effect patterns emerge: those appearing within the first hour of infusion and those appearing within a couple of hours of its completion.

Mechanisms causing these two patterns of MAB-associated FLS are distinct not only from each other but also differ from mechanisms causing other BRM-related FLS. These mechanisms will be discussed in the section on Pathophysiology.

Tumor Necrosis Factor

Tumor necrosis factor (TNF), a secretory cytokine of activated monocytes/macrophages and lymphocytes, has a significant role in modulation of both the immune response and the inflammatory response. This agent's early promise as an antitumor therapy has yet to be realized, however, in part because of its severe and wide-ranging side effects. In fact TNF may be a prime cause of the development of FLS which results from treatment with other BRMs.

In clinical trials, TNF has been associated with moderately severe FLS (Table 12.5). When TNF is administered intravenously, rigors occur within 10 to 15 minutes. Fever generally occurs within an hour or two after initiation of therapy, with a maximum temperature of 39°C to 40°C. When TNF is administered subcutaneously or intramuscularly, side effects are somewhat milder and delayed in appearance, with temperatures peaking between 2 and 10 hours after injection and remaining elevated up to 20 hours. With both routes of administration, headaches and myalgias frequently accompany the development of fevers (Gamm *et al.*, 1991; Aulitzky *et al.*, 1991).

PATHOPHYSIOLOGY OF THE FLU-LIKE SYNDROME

The pathophysiology of FLS as manifested during therapy with BRMs shares many of the same mechanisms as fever caused by illness. In the past several years, advances in understanding the physiology of fever have paralleled research in BRMs and cytokines. Biological agents are key components in the causa-

Table 12.5 Tumor necrosis factor

Symptom/ Side Effect	Tumor Necrosis Factor
Fever	• Common (Experienced by 40–80% of all patients) • Dose-dependent severity • Continuous intravenous infusion: Temperature elevated for 24 hours then returns to baseline • 30-minute intravenous infusion: Fever peaks at 1 hour, returns to baseline after 4 to 6 hours • Subcutaneous/intramuscular injection: Temperature peaks at 2 to 10 hours, remains elevated for up to 20 hours
Chills/Rigors	• Common • Appears within 15 minutes of start of intravenous infusion • Follows fever pattern
Myalgias	• Common
Headache	• Common

Source: Tables 12.1 through 12.5 are adapted with permission from Haeuber, D. 1989. Side effects of Biotherapy: Flu-like syndrome. *Oncology Nursing Forum* 16(6 Suppl): 35–41.

tion of fever and its accompanying signs and symptoms. While there remain numerous gaps in the scientific understanding of fever, many aspects of the febrile condition and its associated symptoms are now clear.

Fever can be defined as a condition in which the thermoregulatory "set point" governing the temperature of the body is raised above the normal level. Core body temperature may or may not be raised to this same level, although the thermoregulatory ability remains intact. This condition should be distinguished from hyperthermia, in which core temperature is increased above the set point and which can be caused by the inability to dissipate heat efficiently or rapidly enough (Kluger, 1991; Holtzclaw, 1992).

Thermoregulatory Set Point

The thermoregulatory set point is a narrow range of temperatures around 37°C, the optimal temperature for cellular metabolism and body function. When body temperature rises above or falls below the set point, compensatory cooling or warming mechanisms are initiated to return body temperature to set point range. The site of temperature control is an area of the brain called the preoptic anterior hypothalamus (PO/AH). It is here that incoming thermal information is processed and compared to the set point range. Signals are then sent to initiate appropriate compensatory temperature-regulating mechanisms.

Pyrogens

The thermoregulatory set point rises in response to contact with substances called **pyrogens**, of which there are two basic types. **Exogenous** pyrogens are those produced outside the body, and they include bacterial endotoxins, fungi, viruses, neoplastic cells, and antigenic substances such as certain drugs. Although some exogenous pyrogens may directly influence the thermoregulatory set point in the PO/AH, their effects are typically mediated via **endogenous** pyrogens (EPs) (Dascombe, 1986; Bligh, 1982).

As implied, EPs are synthesized and released by host cells. Interleukin–1 (IL–1) has long been considered a prime example of an EP, with a tremendous amount of scientific research having been directed toward elucidating its nature. Interleukin–1 is produced primarily by phagocytic cells such as monocytes and tissue macrophages and is secreted in response to contact with bacterial endotoxins or other antigenic substances. Once released into the circulation, it initiates a multitude of effects including (1) increased numbers and immaturity of circulating neutrophils; (2) increased muscle proteolysis, causing greater availability of amino acids for synthesis of new proteins (e.g., immunoglobulins); (3) B-cell proliferation and enhanced antibody production; (4) T-cell activation with concomitant lymphokine production; (5) clonal expansion of various T-cell and natural killer cell subsets; and (6) fever (Dinarello *et al.*, 1986).

Kluger (1991; 1992b) has persuasively argued that although IL–1 may be an EP, it is not the only one. In a review of the subject (1991), he suggests that other cytokines, such as TNF, the IFNs, and interleukin–6 (IL–6), are also involved in the inflammatory response and may therefore meet one or more of the criteria that define an EP. Kluger (1992b) suggests that varying cytokine combinations may be responsible for altering the thermoregulatory set point and so may account for varying fever patterns.

Production of Fever

Figure 12.1 depicts an overview of the process by which EPs produce fever. These inflammatory cytokines can stimulate numerous cell types (e.g., fibroblasts and monocytes) to release prostaglandins, particularly prostaglandin E_2 (PGE$_2$), which may mediate many effects of EPs. Once secreted, EPs travel via the circulatory system to the organosum vasculosum lamina terminalis, an area in the hypothalamic endothelium where the production of PGE$_2$ is stimulated. Subsequently, PGE$_2$ upregulates the temperature set point in the PO/AH (Coceani *et al.*, 1986; Dinarello *et al.*,1988). The question of whether EPs such as IL–1 also have a <u>direct</u> effect on the thermoregulatory set point remains to be answered (Hashimoto *et al.*, 1991). Once the thermoregulatory set point is reset, efferent signals are transmitted to activate both autonomic and behavioral compensatory mechanisms, causing increased body temperature. The first phase of fever, known as the chill or cold stage, represents the body's effort to bring core temperatures up to the new, higher set point. Chills are described as shivering accompanied by the sensation of cold, and are the forerunner of fever. The muscular contractions that result in shivering serve to generate heat. Simultaneously, vasoconstriction conserves heat through decreased skin perfusion. Further-

Figure 12.1   The etiologies, characteristics, and consequences of fever.

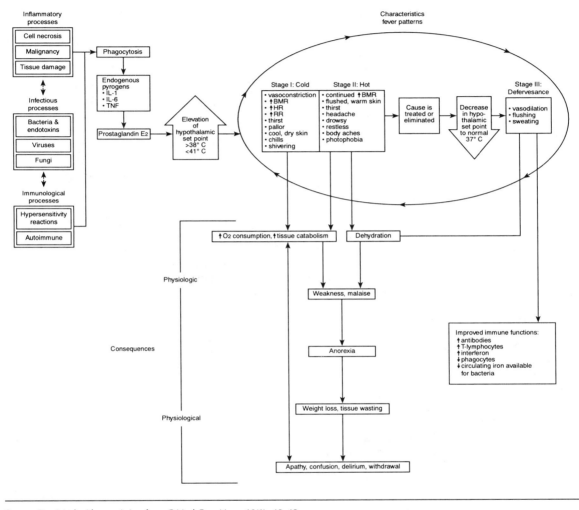

Source: Reprinted with permission from *Critical Care Nurse* 12(1): 40–49.

more, in response to the subjective sensation of cold, patients will dress warmly or huddle under the covers in bed in an attempt to conserve heat.

The second phase of a fever, the hot or plateau stage, occurs when the core temperature reaches or overshoots the new set point. The patient's skin will be warm and flushed, the basal metabolic rate will be elevated, and the patient will experience tachycardia and tachypnea. Headaches, myalgias, and thirst are also common sensations during this phase.

Once the underlying cause of the fever has been treated or antipyretic medications have been administered, the patient enters the defervescence stage. This stage is characterized by diaphoresis, vasodilation, and behavioral measures such as removal of clothes and covers (Bruce and Grove, 1992; Holtz-claw, 1992; Kluger, 1991).

As noted above, EPs may also cause increased muscle proteolysis. As with fever causation, this process is also mediated by the release of PGE_2 into muscle tissues. Because PGE_2 is known to stimulate pain receptors, one side effect of this process may therefore be the myalgias commonly associated with FLS (Baracos et al., 1983). Muscular activity involved in shivering during the cold phase of fever is also likely to exacerbate myalgias.

Fever Related to BRM Administration

What are the connections between the physiologic processes of fever causation and FLS associated with BRM administration? Some connections are obvious, others less obvious, and a few merely speculative. As is apparent from the above discussion, the pathophysiology of fever and its associated symptoms is still under investigation. It is clear that the varying patterns of FLS seen with BRM administration are most certainly related to their role as EPs themselves or to subsequent induction of purported EPs such as IL–1 and IL–6 (Hirano, 1992). Some BRMs, such as the IFNs and TNF, are probably themselves EPs and therefore initiate symptom patterns similar to those associated with IL–1 (Cerami, 1992; Dinarello et al., 1988; Dinarello et al., 1984; Kluger, 1991; Kluger, 1992b). If the IFNs and TNF are in fact EPs, this would explain the rapid onset of fever when these agents are administered, because as EPs they may directly stimulate PGE_2 synthesis (Bernheim, 1986). Interferons may also induce host cells to release IL–1 and TNF, causing a secondary initiation of FLS. Tumor necrosis factor is thought to be an EP by most researchers, who believe that it can, therefore, cause fever and other symptoms separately from its interactions with other EPs. Dinarello et al. (1988) observed in animal studies that a biphasic fever curve occurs with TNF administration. The initial rise in temperature is probably due to a direct effect of TNF on the hypothalamus,

as mediated by PGE_2, whereas the second temperature spike is related to a subsequent increase in circulation of other EPs such as IL–1. In a study of patients experiencing the paroxysms of chills and fevers due to malaria, Karunaweera et al. (1992) found that serum TNF levels closely paralleled the occurence of chills and the rise and fall in temperatures, preceding these events by 30 to 60 minutes. This parallel supports the hypothesis that TNF is an EP.

As indicated in Table 12.3, the onset of FLS after the administration of IL–2 is delayed, in contrast to the more immediate effects of IFN and TNF. Both in vitro and in vivo studies suggest that IL–2 itself is not pyrogenic but rather induces cells such as T lymphocytes and macrophages to release IFN-γ and TNF (Michie et al., 1988; Kintzel and Calis, 1991). Thus, FLS is caused either directly by these substances or by pathways mediated by other EPs.

Whether HGFs cause FLS depends on the point in the hematopoietic sequence of events at which they have their effect and on which types of cells they stimulate. It appears that they are not innately pyrogenic but rather cause FLS through indirect pathways. Granulocyte-macrophage colony-stimulating factor and IL–3, for example, are associated with chills, fevers, and in some cases, headaches and myalgias. It is now well established that GM-CSF can stimulate cells in the macrophage/monocyte lineage to release TNF, IL–1, and IL–6, all purported to be EPs (Kanz et al., 1991; Grant and Heel, 1992). Interleukin–3 has demonstrated enhancement of the release of TNF, which may account for its ability to cause FLS (Kanz et al., 1991; Kurzrock et al., 1991). Additionally, Gietema et al. (1992) found a dose-dependent increase in serum IL–6 after administration of IL–3, and they suggested that IL–6 may be responsible for the elevated temperatures associated with IL–3 therapy.

Finally, MABs most likely have an entirely different mechanism for inducing fever, thus accounting for the differences in symptoms observed during MAB therapy and therapy with other BRMs. Dillman *et al.* (1986) have suggested that FLS that appears with administration of MABs is probably related to the elimination of circulating target (tumor) cells during the infusion, and have compared this effect with the leukocyte agglutination induced fevers sometimes seen during blood transfusions. This interaction between MABs and circulating tumor cells may account for symptoms occasionally observed early in the infusion. In mice, delayed symptoms seem to be caused by the development of antibodies to MABs, indicating the possible importance of a hypersensitivity component in MAB therapy (Meeker *et al.*, 1985).

MANAGEMENT OF BRM-RELATED FLU-LIKE SYNDROME

Assessment

Assessment begins with a thorough analysis of FLS as experienced by the patient. This analysis should include determination of the timing (onset, duration, and frequency), setting, location, quality and quantity of the symptoms, associated symptoms, as well as factors that alleviate or aggravate symptoms. In addition, factors that may exacerbate the severity of FLS (e.g., co-existing illnesses, age, performance states, and nutritional status) should also be evaluated. This information will provide baseline data to be used later in judging the effectiveness of interventions and documenting patterns of symptoms.

Determination of the patient's understanding of the cause of the fever is important. Atkins (1984) outlined the longstanding association between fever and illness in many cultures. In a study of knowledge and attitudes toward fever in Norway, Eskerud *et al.* (1991) found misunderstandings regarding regulation of body temperature to be quite common. For example, many subjects thought that even moderate fevers in both adults and children were life threatening. Thus, it is important to assess the knowledge of the patient and fam-

ily members regarding the symptoms associated with FLS and provide information as needed.

It is not unlikely that some individuals receiving biotherapy may associate FLS with a worsening of their illness and suffer from anxiety as a consequence. Fletcher and Creten (1986) found that patients and family members were "overly" concerned about the bodily damage that could be caused by fever. They suggested that treatment of low-grade fevers may be initiated in order to allay the anxiety of patients, family members, and health care professionals. Reassurance that FLS is an expected side effect and not due to progression of disease can also serve to allay fears.

Assessment of the distress associated with FLS will assist with management of the symptoms and with explanation of the meaning of these symptoms to the patient. Physical comfort is subjective and will be perceived differently by patients. For example, a temperature of 38°C may be rated as extremely distressful by one patient and not distressing at all by another.

A final area that should be assessed in the patient who receives biotherapy is the risk of infection. Although BRMs cause fever and other flu-like symptoms, it should not automatically be assumed that all fevers in a particular patient are related to therapy. This issue has caused some controversy in the medical literature, especially with respect to HGFs. Vreugdenhil *et al.* (1992) offer a list of criteria for restricting the administration of antibiotics in neutropenic patients receiving GM-CSF, given the known propensity of that agent to cause fever and associated symptoms. On the other hand, Khwaja *et al.* (1992) argue that it would be "injudicious" to withhold antibiotic coverage from neutropenic patients receiving GM-CSF. For the nurse caring for patients who receive BRMs, it is important to realize that many of these patients are susceptible to infections from a variety of causes. Therefore, when symptoms appear, it is critical to study their pattern for conformity with

Table 12.6 Assessment related to FLS in the patient receiving BRMs

Age

Co-existing Illnesses
  Cardiac disease
  Pulmonary disease
  Diabetes mellitus
  Anemia

Performance Status

Nutritional State

Risk of Infection

Signs and Symptoms of Infection

Knowledge of FLS and its Relationship to BRM
  therapy

Anxiety Regarding Fever and its Relationship to
  Illness

Physical Comfort during FLS

patterns expected from the BRM administered. The nurse should at all times maintain a high index of suspicion that a fever may be of infectious etiology.

Assessment should be ongoing throughout the course of therapy to determine the patient's tolerance of the treatment, the success of interventions to lessen side effects, and to detect untoward events. Table 12.6 summarizes the most important elements involved in the assessment of the patient experiencing biotherapy-induced FLS.

Management

The first issue to consider with respect to the management of FLS associated with BRM therapy is whether to "manage" the symptoms at all, and if so, under which circumstances. Thereafter, potential strategies to address symptoms may be considered.

There has been a longstanding controversy regarding the potential therapeutic bene fits of fever. Once again, it is important to distinguish whether fevers result from conditions such as hyperthermia or heat stroke, in which case it is unquestionably essential to control temperature. In the case of infectious

or BRM-related fevers, the correct course of action is less clear. Blatteis (1986) and Banet (1986) question the assertion that fever itself has therapeutic value, arguing that insufficient evidence exists to draw conclusions regarding beneficial effects of fever in enhancing the natural and immune defenses of the infected host. Kluger (1992a; 1992b; 1986) has strongly argued that fever has an ancient, phylogenetic history suggestive of an important adaptive response that allows the infected host's immune defenses to respond more effectively to pathogens. In a review of the literature regarding the effects of fever on immunologic defenses, Roberts (1991) concludes that elevated temperatures appear to improve T-lymphocyte responses and increase the sensitization and activation of mononuclear leukocytes.

However, even if fever is an adaptive response to infection, it does not follow that it enhances the antineoplastic or immunomodulatory aspects of biotherapy (Dinarello, Conti, and Mier, 1986). Nevertheless, Kluger (1992a) questions the practice of identifying fever as a side effect of BRMs and automatically treating it. He wrote, "Since many tumours seem more sensitive to increases in temperature than normal cells are, I suggest that before fever in patients on treatment with biological response modifiers is 'treated,' careful consideration be given to the possibility that the fever may be helping the patient to rid himself or herself of the tumour." Gietema *et al.* (1992) suggest that fever associated with administration of IL–3 may be "interpreted as a sign of increase in host defenses rather than merely as an adverse effect." Those considerations argue for a measured response to FLS in biotherapy. Holtzclaw (1992), after studying fever in critically ill patients, advocates a "clarification of the therapeutic goal" before implementing a nursing response to fever. Certainly this is also sound advice for the nurse administering biotherapy. Styrt and Sugarman (1990) offer several indications for the suppression of fever. These include the risk of damage to the central nervous system, the potential for tissue hypoxia and cardiovascular compromise, and, finally, comfort of the patient. The first is of particular importance for the patient with neurological problems and in the case of a pediatric patient who is at known risk for febrile seizures.

The second indication for the therapeutic suppression of fever is especially relevant to cancer patients, many of whom are elderly and may have co-existent cardiovascular or pulmonary conditions. Aggravation of these conditions by the increased basal metabolic rate, tachycardia, and oxygen demand associated with fevers and chills caused by BRM administration is a potential problem. For every increase in temperature of one degree centigrade, it has been estimated that the metabolic rate increases by 10% with a proportionate increase in tissue oxygen requirements (Rosenthal and Silverstein, 1988). In a study of fever among Gambian children, Stettler et al. (1992) calculated that the caloric cost of fever is 11.7% for each one-degree (centigrade) rise in temperature. Strenuous shivering accompanying fever is a costly way to produce heat, subjecting patients to cardiovascular and musculoskeletal demands equivalent to riding a bicycle. In a study of shivering caused by administration of amphotericin B, Holtzclaw (1990) found that in patients monitored by pulse oximetry during the infusion, severe shivering caused a fall in oxygen saturation from approximately 98% to less than 80%. Dyspnea and labored breathing were seen among shivering patients.

An added consideration in the cancer patient population is the fact that fever appears to stimulate muscle protein degradation and causes a negative nitrogen balance (Baracos et al., 1983). This may be important when a person is in a debilitated or malnourished state and receives a BRM associated with a substantial incidence of FLS.

Comfort, the final consideration mentioned by Styrt and Sugarman (1990), is of prime importance in nursing. There are both psychological and physical components to comfort; however, neither the physical nor psychological aspects of comfort in relation to FLS and associated symptoms have been well-studied. Styrt and Sugarman (1990) point out the ambiguity of using antipyretics for the "symptomatic treatment" of fever, since exactly which symptoms are being treated is often unclear. Certainly, some elements of FLS, including myalgias and headaches, may cause patients discomfort. Whether fever, aside from the chills preceding it, is uncomfortable has not been examined. It is possible that the use of antipyretics may cause a cycle of chilling and diaphoresis that is ultimately more uncomfortable for the patient than experiencing a moderate fever. Until such issues receive scrutiny, assessment of physical comfort and associated distress as related to FLS remains a priority in determining if symptomatic relief of fever is warranted.

Approaches to Management of BRM-Related FLS

There are several complementary approaches to the management of FLS in persons receiving BRMs. (See Table 12.7.)

Manipulation of the Treatment. The first approach lies within the purview of the physicians involved in the specific treatment program, although nursing input can have a significant impact on deciding how to most effectively implement therapy. At times, however, alterations in treatments may be limited by the research protocol. Several examples will suffice to indicate the importance of treatment manipulation as an approach to managing FLS. Thompson et al. (1988) examined the toxicity of IL–2 given at different dose levels by either 24-hour continuous intravenous infusions or 2-hour intravenous bolus infusions. They found that independent of dose, side effects were substantially more severe with continuous infusions. Daily administration of either IFN-α or IFN-β is associated with decreasing incidence and severity of symptoms after 7 to 10 days. With intermittent (1 or 2 times/week) or cyclic (3 or 4 times/week) administration, however, tachyphylaxis may not

Table 12.7 Approaches to the management of BRM-related FLS

Treatment Manipulation
  Dose
  Schedule
  Route
  Rate of administration
Medications
  Prophylactic
  For Fever/Myalgias—prostaglandin inhibitors
    nonsteroidal anti-inflammatory drugs (ibuprofen,
    indomethacin)
    acetaminophen
    aspirin
  For Chills/Rigors, centrally acting agents
    meperidine
    other narcotics
  For Headache
    antihistamines
    prostaglandin inhibitors
Nursing Measures
  Extremity wraps
  "Bundling"
  Increase ambient temperature
  Hydration
  Relaxation and guided imagery techniques
  Patient/family education, reassurance

occur (Quesada *et al.*, 1986). Dillman *et al.* (1986) have noted that decreasing the rate of intravenous administration of MABs will also diminish side effects.

Nurses involved in the treatment of patients receiving BRMs should be cognizant of the potential for alleviating FLS through manipulation of the above-mentioned factors. They should closely observe patients for potential benefits from changes in administration route and schedule. Within the latitude allowed by the treatment protocol, nurses can then make appropriate and informed recommendations.

Medications. The administration of medications provides another approach to controlling BRM-related side effects, although this too may be limited by the treatment protocol. Certain categories of drugs, such as pros-

taglandin inhibitors and antihistamines, may be effective in the control of FLS (Milton, 1982). Antipyretics such as acetaminophen, aspirin (Kim *et al.*, 1982) and the nonsteroidal anti-inflammatory drugs such as indomethacin and ibuprofen may also be effective. These agents block the synthesis of prostaglandins both at the hypothalamus and in the muscle tissue. Through this mechanism, they may be effective in controlling the fever and associated symptoms of FLS.

To prevent side effects, many clinicians routinely prescribe premedications before BRMs are administered. Other clinicians use medications as "infrequently as possible" (Sriskandan *et al.*, 1986), either to allow for determination of toxic effects or to avoid a possible adverse effect on the desired biological activity of the BRM. In addition, there is evidence, as previously discussed, that the elevated temperatures that frequently occur with biotherapy may be intrinsically involved in the biological effect of the agent or may be important in activation of the agent (Dinarello *et al.*, 1986). Therefore, symptom management may be therapeutically counterproductive. Furthermore, even such seemingly innocuous medications as ibuprofen and acetaminophen may have adverse effects on the kidneys and liver (Murphy, 1992). Isaacs *et al.*, (1990) examined the general use of antipyretics in a university-based tertiary care center. They found that orders for the administration of antipyretics were often written imprecisely and without clear consideration of a therapeutic goal. This led to sporadic and inconsistent patterns of administration. Certainly, in caring for patients who receive biotherapy, nurses should approach the use of these medications in a clear, goal-directed manner.

Chills related to BRM administration can be quite uncomfortable. Meperidine is often effective in controlling this particular side effect (Thompson *et al.*, 1988). Drawing on the experience of using meperidine to control rigors associated with the administration of amphotericin B (Rutledge and Holtzclaw,

1988), it may also be possible to give meperidine either orally, as part of a prophylactic medication regimen, or intravenously, to quickly relieve chilling when it occurs. As with antipyretics, the decision to use meperidine should be based on the type of BRM administered, on its association with chills, and on a thorough assessment of the individual patient's experience with that BRM. On occasion, morphine sulfate may be used to control chills, and some institutions are experimenting with the use of sublingual hydromorphone for the same purpose (Jassak, personal communication, 1993).

Nursing Measures. Nursing care of the individual who is experiencing FLS as a result of biotherapy should be directed toward determination of effective nonpharmacologic means of symptom management. It may be possible, for example, to forestall the development of such untoward side effects as chills by applying warmed blankets, encouraging the patient to wear warmer clothes, or increasing the ambient air temperature during and after BRM administration. These measures may reduce the sensed temperature gradient between the core temperature and the hypothalamic set point, thereby preventing the shivering response.

Abbey *et al.* (1973) and Rutledge and Holtzclaw (1988) have evaluated wrapping the extremities with several layers of terrycloth towels to diminish the shivering response in different populations in which shivering would be expected to occur. The proposed effectiveness of this intervention is based on the abundance in the hands and feet of thermosensory nerve endings that are involved in the initiation of shivering (Holtzclaw, 1992). Although bundling the patient who is febrile may appear counterintuitive, it is important to remember that the fever caused by BRMs is self-limiting, that shivering usually increases temperatures, that truly dangerous fevers are extremely rare (Styrt and Sugarman, 1990) and that the body pro-

duces substances, such as argenine vasopressin, that are naturally antipyretic to prevent fevers from rising to life-threatening levels (Kluger, 1992b).

Maintaining adequate hydration is also a highly important nursing function in the patient who is experiencing FLS, as dehydration can contribute to fever. In addition, it is estimated that fever increases insensible fluid loss by 10% for each 0.5-degree centigrade increase in temperature (Holtzclaw, 1992). If the patient goes through several cycles of fever and defervescence, water loss due to diaphoresis may be considerable. It is important that the patient's intake and output and serum electrolytes be closely monitored during the course of biotherapy. If therapy is administered at home, the patient and family should be instructed regarding increased fluid intake.

Another nursing intervention includes instructing patients in techniques such as relaxation therapy and guided imagery. Since some of the responses to the resetting of the hypothalamic set point are sympathetic and others are behavioral, it is quite possible that techniques such as these can be utilized to control shivering and inhibit vasoconstriction (Rutledge and Holtzclaw, 1988). These methods may also be effective in reducing anxiety and in providing the patient with a sense of control over symptoms and side effects of therapy.

Patient Education. Educating patients and families in the management of FLS is a critical intervention. While an understanding of the pathophysiology of FLS may not relieve symptoms, most patients and families will feel more in control of their treatment and their lives with this knowledge. An understanding of what is happening to their bodies and what symptoms should be expected serves to create this sense of control. The experience of fever and chills is often frightening, but patient education can remove misunderstandings about these symptoms. It is critical that patients be instructed to report extremely elevated temperatures that are not being controlled with antipyretics or fevers that are unrelated to the normal patterns.

RESEARCH

The vast majority of information regarding biotherapy-related FLS has been generated from clinical trials with various BRMs. The same can be said of the various methods that have been utilized to manage these side effects. Since symptom management is an area of professional nursing expertise, it is important that nurses who work with biotherapy patients direct their research skills toward describing the FLS symptom cluster, determining its patterns with the various agents, evaluating tools to quantify symptoms, and organizing clinical studies to develop effective methods of management (Strauman, 1988). In addition, studies to determine the distress associated with these symptoms and the impact of symptoms on quality of life should be given high priority.

Once symptoms are described and patterns adequately defined, clinical measurement is the next logical step. The severity of fever can be measured through temperatures taken from the mouth, rectum, auditory canal, or skin. Headache, myalgias, or arthralgis could be quantified by measurement of associated pain. However, measurement of chills (shivering) is more difficult. The two most common methods found in the literature are electromyographic measurement and observation of shivering stages. Mechanical measurement such as palpation of tremors is less well developed. Systems of visual measurement exist, but there is little standardization among published studies. Abbey *et al.* (1973) developed an ordinal clinical assessment scale that was based on the work of others. This scale evaluated shivering severity by observing stages of muscle involvement. The scale was adapted by Holtzclaw for use with postoperative cardiac patients as follows: 0 = no visible or palpable shivering; 1 = palpable manidular vibration or electrocardiograph ar-

tifact; 2 = visible fasciculation of the head or neck; 3 = visible fasciculation of the pectorals and trunk, and 4 = generalized shaking of the entire body, with or without teeth chattering (Holtzclaw, 1993). For measurement of the biotherapy-related FLS, White (1992) has developed a symptom report form and toxicity scale that can be used to record and manage the side effects of outpatient IL–2 and IFN-α therapies. As she points out, such forms could easily be adapted for use in other settings and with other agents. Toxicity scales utilized in clinical trials to grade the severity of symptoms may also be useful in the clinical setting, but may not be sufficiently discriminatory for research purposes.

Prevention and control of chills is another important area for focus. Although there are no published examples of nursing research in the area of biotherapy-related FLS, there are a few related examples that may offer models for how to proceed on this subject (Morgan, 1990; Caruso *et al.*, 1992; Abbey *et al.*, 1973). Interventions may be grouped into two major areas: pharmacological measures and physical measures. Perhaps the most applicable example of such research is the work by Holtzclaw (1990) on the use of extremity wraps to control shivering caused by the pyrogenic drug amphotericin B. In her carefully crafted study, Holtzclaw compared the experiences of a control group of patients and a treatment group who had their arms and legs wrapped with towels to insulate the dominant skin thermosensors during a standard amphotericin B infusion. The end points that Holtzclaw compared were shivering duration and degree, total meperidine dosage during the amphotericin B infusion, and myocardial oxygen consumption. This study may be used as a model to determine the effectiveness of interventions that attempt to control the shivering component of FLS.

SUMMARY

The advent of the use of biotherapy in the treatment of cancer has been accompanied by an increased awareness of the side effects that occur with its use. The constellation of symptoms known as flu-like syndrome frequently appears during treatment with many BRMs. To some extent, the incidence and patterns of FLS for the various BRMs have been defined in the course of clinical trials with these agents, but additional work needs to be done in this area. To better predict side effects when treating patients with BRMs, nurses who administer biotherapeutic agents should pay attention to their side effects, including FLS, and attempt to achieve a clearer definition of their incidence and patterns.

Research in the area of biotherapy-related FLS remains in its infancy. Although a body of literature is beginning to emerge on the constellation of FLS symptoms in related areas, a tremendous amount of work remains to be done. To date, evaluation and management of shivering has been the most thoroughly researched (Holtzclaw, 1993).

References

Abbey, J., Andrews, C., Avigliano, K. et al. 1973. A pilot study: The control of shivering during hypothermia by a clinical nursing measure. *Journal of Neurosurgical Nursing* 5(2): 78–88.

Atkins, E. 1984. Fever: The old and the new. *Journal of Infectious Diseases* 149(3): 339–348.

Aulitzky, W., Tilg, H., Gastl, G. et al. 1991. Recombinant tumour necrosis factor alpha administered subcutaneously or intramuscularly for treatment of advanced malignant disease: A phase I trial. *European Journal of Cancer* 27(4): 462–467.

Banet, M. 1986. Fever in mammals: Is it beneficial? *Yale Journal of Biology and Medicine* 59(2): 17–124.

Baracos, V., Rodemann, H., Dinarello, C. et al. 1983. Stimulation of muscle protein degradation and prostaglandin E_2 release by leukocytic pyrogen (interleukin–1). *New England Journal of Medicine* 308(10): 553–558.

Bernheim, H. 1986. Is prostaglandin E_2 involved in the pathogenesis of fever? Effects of interleukin–1 on the release of prostaglandins. *Yale Journal of Biology and Medicine* 59(2): 151–158.

Blatteis, C. 1986. Fever: Is it beneficial? *Yale Journal of Biology and Medicine* 59(2): 107–116.

Bligh, J. 1982. Thermoregulation: Its change during infection with endotoxin-producing micro-organisms. In

Milton, A. (ed). *Pyretics and Antipyretics*. New York: Springer-Verlag, pp. 5–24.

Bruce, J., and Grove, S. 1992. Fever: Patholgy and treatment. *Critical Care Nurse* 12(1): 40–49.

Caruso, C., Hadley, B., Shukla, R., et al. 1992. Cooling effects and comfort of four cooling blanket temperatures in humans with fever. *Nursing Research* 41(2):68–72.

Cerami, A. 1992. Inflammatory cytokines. *Clinical Immunology and Immunopathology* 62(1): S3–S10.

Coceani, F., Bishai, I., Lees, J., et al. 1986. Prostaglandin E_2 and fever: A continuing debate. *Yale Journal of Biology and Medicine* 59(2): 169–174.

Dascombe, M. 1986. The pharmacology of fever. *Progress in Neurobiology* 25(4): 327 373.

Dillman, R., Beauregard, J., Halpern, S., et al. 1986. Toxicities and side effects associated with intravenous infusions of murine monoclonal antibodies. *Journal of Biological Response Modifiers* 5(1): 73–84.

Dinarello, C., Cannon, J., and Wolff, S. 1988. New concepts on the pathogenesis of fever. *Reviews of Infectious Diseases* 10(1): 168–189.

Dinarello, C., Conti, P., and Mier, J. 1986. Effects of human interleukin–1 on natural killer cell activity: Is fever a host defense mechanism for tumor killing? *Yale Journal of Biology and Medicine* 59(2): 97–106.

Dinarello, C., Cannon, J., Wolff, S., et al. 1986. Tumor necrosis factor (Cachectin) is an endogenous pyrogen and induces production of interleukin–1. *Journal of Experimental Medicine* 163(6): 1433–1450.

Dinarello, C., Bernheim, H., and Duff, G. 1984. Mechanisms of fever induced by recombinant human interferon. *Journal of Clinical Investigation* 74(3): 906–913.

Eskerud, J., Haftvedt, B., and Laerum, E. 1991. Fever: Knowledge, perception and attitudes: Results from a Norwegian population study. *Family Practice* 8(1): 32–36.

Fletcher, J., and Creten, D. 1986. Perceptions of fever among adults in a family practice setting. *The Journal of Family Practice* 22(5): 427–430.

Gamm, H., Lindemann, A., Mertelsman, R., et al. 1991. Phase I trial of recombinant human tumour necrosis factor alpha in patients with advanced malignancy. *European Journal of Cancer* 27(7): 856–863.

Gietema, J., Postmus, P., Biesma, B. et al. 1992. Acute-phase response in patients given rhIL–3 after chemotherapy (Letter to the Editor). *Lancet* 339: 1616–1617.

Grant, S., and Heel, R. 1992. Recombinant granulocyte-macrophage colony-stimulating factor (rGM-CSF): A review of its pharmacological properties and prospective role in the management of myelosuppression. *Drug Evaluation* 43(4): 516–560.

Haeuber, D. 1989. Recent advances in the management of biotherapy-related side effects: Flu-like syndrome. *Oncology Nursing Forum* 16(6 Suppl): 35–41.

Hashimoto, M., Ishikawa, Y., Yolota, S., *et al.* 1991. Action site of circulating interleukin–1 on the rabbit brain. *Brain Research* 540: 217–223.

Hirano, T. 1992. Interleukin-6 and its relation to inflammation and disease. *Clinical Immunology and Immunopathology* 62(1): S60–S65.

Holtzclaw, B. 1993. The Shivering Response. In Fitzpatrick, J., Stevenson, J., (eds). *Annual Review of Nursing Research*. New York: Springer Publishing Company, pp. 31–55.

Holtzclaw, B. 1992. The febrile response in critical care: State of the science. *Heart & Lung* 21(5): 482–501.

Holtzclaw, B. 1990. Control of febrile shivering during amphotericin B therapy. *Oncology Nursing Forum* 17(4): 521–524.

Isaacs, S., Axelrod, P., and Lorber, B. 1990. Antipyretic orders in a university hospital. *The American Journal of Medicine* 88: 31–35.

Kanz, L., Lindemann, M., Oster, W., *et al.* 1991. Hemopoietins in clinical oncology. *American Journal of Clinical Oncology* 14(Suppl 1): S27–S33.

Karunaweera, N., Grau, G., Gamage, P., *et al.* 1992. Dynamics of fever and serum levels of tumor necrosis factor are closely associated during clinical paroxysms in *Plasmodium vivax* malaria. *Proceedings of the National Academy of Science* 89: 3200–3203.

Khwaja, A., Chopra, R., Goldstone, A., *et al.* 1992 (Letter to the editor). *Lancet* 339: 1617.

Kim, D., Van Arman, C., and Armstrong, D. 1982. The chemistry of the nonsteroidal antipyretic agents: Structure-activity relationships. In Milton, A. (ed). *Pyretics and Antipyretics*. New York: Springer-Verlag, pp. 317–376.

Kintzel, P., and Calis, K. 1991. Recombinant interleukin-2: A biological response modifier. *Clinical Pharmacy* 10: 110–128.

Kluger, M. 1992a. Drugs for childhood fever (Letter to the editor). *Lancet* 339: 70.

Kluger, M. 1992b. Fever revisited. *Pediatrics* 90(6): 846–850.

Kluger, M. 1991. Fever: Role of pyrogens and cryogens. *Physiological Reviews* 71(1): 93–127.

Kluger, M. 1986. Is fever beneficial? *Yale Journal of Biology and Medicine* 59(2): 89–95.

Kurzrock, R., Talpaz, M., Estrov, Z., *et al.* 1991. Phase I study of recombinant human interleukin-3 in patients with bone marrow failure. *Journal of Clinical Oncology* 9(7):1241–1250.

Margolin, K., Rayner, A., Hawkins, M., *et al.* 1989. Interleukin-2 and lymphokine-activated killer cell therapy of solid tumors: Analysis of toxicity and management guidelines. *Journal of Clinical Oncology* 7(4): 486–498.

Meeker, T., Lowder, J., Maloney, D., *et al.* 1985. A clinical trial of anti-idiotype therapy for B cell malignancy. *Blood* 65(6): 1349–1363.

Michie, H., Eberlein, T., Spriggs, D., *et al.* 1988. Interleukin–2 initiates metabolic responses associated with critical illness in humans. *Annals of Surgery* 208(4): 493–503.

Milton, A. 1982. Prostaglandins in fever and the mode of action of antipyretic drugs. In Milton, A. (ed). *Pyretics and Antipyretics*. New York: Springer-Verlag, pp. 257–304.

Morgan, S. 1990. A comparison of three methods of managing fever in the neurologic patient. *Journal of Neuroscience Nursing* 22(1): 19–24.

Murphy, K. 1992. Acetaminophen and ibuprofen: Fever control and overdose. *Pediatric Nursing* 18(4): 428–431, 433.

Quesada, J., Talpaz, M., Rios, A., *et al.* 1986. Clinical toxicity of interferons in cancer patients: A review. *Journal of Clinical Oncology* 4(2): 234–243.

Roberts, N. 1991. Impact of temperature elevation on immunologic defenses. *Reviews of Infectious Diseases* 13: 462–472.

Rosenthal, T., and Silverstein, D. 1988. Fever: What to do and what not to do. *Postgraduate Medicine* 83(8): 75–84.

Rutledge, D., and Holtzclaw, B. 1988. Amphotericin-B-induced shivering in patients with cancer: A nursing approach. *Heart and Lung* 17(4): 432–440.

Sriskandan, K., Garner, P., Watkinson, J., *et al.* 1986. A toxicity study of recombinant interferon-gamma given by intravenous infusion to patients with advanced cancer. *Cancer Chemotherapy and Pharmacology* 18(1): 63–68.

Stettler, N., Schutz, Y., Whitehead, R., *et al.* 1992. Effects of malaria and fever on energy metabolism in Gambian children. *Pediatric Research* 31(2): 101–106.

Strauman, J. 1988. The nurse's role in the biotherapy of cancer: Nursing research of side effects. *Oncology Nursing Forum* 15(6 Suppl): 35–39.

Styrt, B., and Sugarman, B. 1990. Antipyresis and fever. *Archives of Internal Medicine* 150: 1589–1597.

Tabbara, I. 1993. Erythropoietin: Biology and clinical applications. *Archives of Internal Medicine* 153: 298–304.

Thompson, J., Lee, D., Lindgren, C. *et al.*, 1988. Influence of dose and duration of infusion of interleukin–2 on toxicity and immunomodulation. *Journal of Clinical Oncology* 6(4): 669–678.

Vreugdenhil, G., Preyers, F., Croockewit, S. *et al.*, 1992. Fever in neutropenic patients treated with GM-CSF representing enhanced host defense (Letter to the editor). *Lancet* 339: 1118–1119.

White, C. 1992. Symptom assessment and management of outpatients receiving biotherapy: The application of a symptom report form. *Seminars in Oncology Nursing* 8(4 Suppl): 23–28.

CHAPTER 13 | Mental Status Changes

Christina A. Meyers, PHD

Biotherapy is increasingly being used to treat various malignancies and infectious diseases. When cytokines were first introduced it was hoped that they would not be toxic to the nervous system because (1) they were natural products of the body, (2) they were thought to not penetrate the blood-brain barrier, and (3) neurotoxic side effects were not observed in preclinical animal models (Goldstein and Laszlo, 1988). However, clinical trials have since shown that cytokines produce significant toxic effects, and that neurological side effects are at times the major dose-limiting factor (Lenk *et al.*, 1989; Denicoff *et al.*, 1987; Adams *et al.*, 1984).

Although neurotoxic effects are rare after treatment with monoclonal antibodies and hematopoietic growth factors; interferon alpha (IFN-α), interleukin–2 (IL–2), and tumor necrosis factor (TNF) have significant acute, subacute, and chronic toxic effects which have a considerable impact on patients' quality of life. These agents are now known to cause alterations in cognitive functioning and personality, often in the absence of neurological signs. These alterations in mental function are usually acute and reversible (Meyers and Scheibel, 1990), but there is growing concern that some cytokines can produce lasting cognitive deficits (Meyers and Abbruzzese, 1992; Meyers *et al.*, 1991b).

Neurotoxic side effects, even when subtle, may impair patients' ability to function in their usual activities of daily living, impose greater burdens on support systems, lessen the ability to effectively treat other symptoms, and frustrate the attempts of physicians to continue cancer therapy as planned. Often these side effects are so distressing that the patient will discontinue an effective treatment. Quantification of neurotoxic effects associated with biotherapy may aid the development of less toxic but equally efficacious dosing and scheduling, and may even guide the development of agents that can protect the nervous system from the toxic effects of treatment. In addition, assessment, counseling, and intervention strategies may be put into place to enhance the patient's quality of life and ability to function.

Biotherapy-associated neurotoxicity is also of interest because it demonstrates an interaction between the immune system and the brain. Many cytokines, via their role in mounting a host response to infection and inflammation, have profound effects on brain activity when introduced into the systemic circulation (Farkkila *et al.*, 1984; Mattson *et al.*, 1983). This suggests that cytokines can communicate information about immune system functioning to the central nervous system (CNS) (Dafny *et al.*, 1985). Thus, increased understanding of the effect of cytokines on brain function may open a window into the neuro-immune interactions that underlie normal cognitive functioning.

The effects of antineoplastic agents on the nervous system are reflected in altered behavior and personality. Cognitive impairments and personality changes, often in the absence of neurological signs, may be seen in patients who are receiving agents that effect CNS function. This chapter will describe the assessment of cognitive and emotional changes that result from administration of biotherapy, the patterns of both acute and chronic neurotoxic symptoms that are seen with various biotherapy agents, the mechanisms of these effects, and the interventions that can be put into place to help patients cope with these symptoms.

ASSESSMENT OF NEUROBEHAVIORAL FUNCTIONING

Distinguishing cognitive impairment from emotional reactions to illness and stress is very important, but the differential diagnosis of neurobehavioral changes is often difficult. A patient who is apathetic, withdrawn, and lacks motivation may be depressed, or he may

be experiencing treatment-related neurotoxicity. Levine *et al.* (1978) reported that 64% of general cancer patients with delirium (generally from toxic metabolic **encephalopathy**) were misdiagnosed as depressed. Misdiagnosis and subsequent treatment of depression may be inappropriate in a patient who is experiencing alterations of brain function caused by biotherapy.

Impairments of neurobehavioral functioning may also lead to inaccurate judgment on the part of the staff regarding the patient's ability for self-care, his or her reliability in following the therapeutic regimen, and requirements for supervision or special safety measures. Neuropsychological assessment of brain function is often helpful in determining the nature and extent of cognitive impairments that are not detected in routine medical evaluations.

Formal neuropsychological assessment involves the administration of standardized **psychometric tests** that comprehensively evaluate brain function. See Table 13.1 for a list of the cognitive domains assessed. This detailed description of intellectual status and personality characteristics allows for rational planning and management. Conferences held with the patient, family members, and the health care team can utilize this knowledge of the patient's capabilities and limitations to help set realistic goals, to determine his or her capacity for independent self-care, and ability to drive, manage finances, and handle emergencies, and to determine what types of management and compensatory techniques might be most useful.

Of course, not every individual needs or would benefit from an extensive neuropsychological evaluation. The nurse is in an excellent position to assess the patient's mental status and determine if an extended assessment is warranted. A number of standardized, brief mental status examinations are available, such as the Mini-Mental State Examination (Folstein *et al.*, 1975). However, tests of this type only identify patients with severe cognitive problems and do not specify the type of dis-

Table 13.1 Neuropsychological assessment of cognitive functioning

Intellectual Functions
   Attentional abilities
   Abstract reasoning
   Problem solving

Memory
   Verbal learning and recall
   Visual and spatial memory
   Remote memory

Language
   Naming
   Fluency
   Comprehension
   Reading
   Writing

Visual Perception
   Scanning
   Discrimination

Motor Functions
   Strength
   Motor speed
   Coordination and dexterity

Executive (Frontal Lobe) Functions
   Cognitive flexibility (shifting mental set)
   Motivation
   Social judgement
   Planning
   Learning from experience
   Insight and self-awareness

Mood
   Depression
   Anxiety
   Agitation
   Withdrawal

order. For instance, the performances of demented, nondemented, brain-damaged, and control groups significantly overlap on the Mini-Mental State (Auerbach and Faibish, 1989). For the most part, careful evaluation of the patient's general behavior, appearance, ability to maintain a logical conversation, ability to give a concise and accurate history, and ability to paraphrase and comprehend instructions will guide the nurse in evaluating attentiveness, mood, language, and short-term memory (Strub and Black, 1981). These evaluations can then be used to identify individuals who may need a formal examination.

PRESENTATION OF MENTAL STATUS CHANGES

Mental status changes that result from the neurotoxic effects of cytokines have tremendous potential to impact patients' perceived quality of life. Knowledge of which cytokines are most likely to cause neurotoxic effects and the ability to recognize the presentation of mental status changes is the first step toward assisting patients to cope with these effects. This section will focus primarily on cytokines known to cause neurotoxic effects: IFN-α, IL–2, and TNF. See Table 13.2 for an overview of these effects. See Bender (1994) for a concise review of studies of biological response modifier-related cognitive dysfunction. Acute neurotoxicity associated with cytokines resembles the flu-like symptoms and is reviewed in Chapter 12.

Interferon-alpha

Within a week of receiving IFN-α therapy, many patients develop temporary deficits in verbal concept formation, visual-motor skills (i.e., the ability to copy drawings), and mental flexibility (Adams *et al.*, 1984). Adams reported that individuals who received IFN-α developed increasing fatigue, lack of spontaneity, and apathy—symptoms similar to those seen in patients whose frontal lobe function is impaired. Iivanainen and colleagues (1985) also reported cognitive impairments in patients with amyotrophic lateral sclerosis who received IFN-α therapy. Their study of five patients revealed a generalized slowing of behavior and deficits in verbal memory, ability to sequence, motor coordination and visual-motor skills. The symptoms resolved following the discontinuation of treatment. These impairments of motor skills and executive functions were also interpreted as reflecting frontal lobe dysfunction. Intellectual functioning did not appear to decline during treatment, and there were never any impairments in basic language or visual-perceptual skills.

Table 13.2 Neurological side effects associated with biological agents*

Interferon-alpha
  Confusion
  Depression**
  Hypersomnia
  Difficulty concentrating**
  Memory problems**
  Trouble with calculations
  Slowed thinking**
  Impaired motor coordination**
  Impaired visual-motor skills
  Impaired frontal lobe functioning**
  Paraesthesias

Interleukin-2
  Confusion**
  Hypersomnolence**
  Difficulty concentrating**
  Agitation
  Withdrawal from social contact
  Irritability**
  Depression
  Bizarre dreams
  Paranoia
  Delusions
  Hallucinations

Tumor Necrosis Factor
  Confusion
  Somnolence
  Lethargy

---

*The occurrence and severity of side effects tend to increase as the dose is increased. Most side effects are readily reversible when therapy is discontinued. However, some may persist or progress off treatment.

**More frequently seen.

Electrophysiologic studies support the findings of frontal lobe dysfunction during IFN-α therapy. The abnormalities seen on electroencephalography (EEG) typically include background slowing with intermittent, very slow waves in the frontal region (Farkkila et al., 1984; Suter et al., 1984; Rohatiner et al., 1983; Smedley et al., 1983).

A number of investigators have reported that patients who are receiving IFN-α become depressed (Renault et al., 1987; Talpaz et al., 1986), although Adams et al. (1984) did not find that depression was a side effect of IFN-α. Two articles reported on neuropsychiatric symptoms that developed in patients with

chronic active hepatitis who were receiving IFN-α. The incidence of overt symptoms ranged from 7% to 17%, most frequently organic personality syndromes, depression, and frank **delirium** (McDonald et al., 1987; Renault et al., 1987). These side effects usually appeared 1 to 3 months into therapy and improved within 3 to 4 days after decreasing the IFN-α dose. Unfortunately, reports on emotional symptoms associated with IFN-α therapy rely on interviews and other subjective measures of emotional status. Therefore, some symptoms of depression may not be differentiated from the fatigue-asthenia syndrome that is a common side effect of IFN-α.

Chronic Toxicity

Many patients who receive IFN-α over a period of months to years complain of difficulties with mood, memory, and clarity of thinking. A retrospective review reported the neuropsychological test profiles of 16 patients with chronic myelogenous leukemia treated with IFN-α for 5 to 86 months (Meyers et al., 1993). These patients had no history of psychiatric or neurologic problems and were well educated (average of 15 years of education). They performed in the impaired range on tests of verbal memory, information processing speed, and ability to shift mental set (i.e., frontal lobe functioning). Personality testing revealed elevations on measures of depression, somatic concern and denial. In contrast, reasoning skills tended to remain in the normal range. This pattern of slowed thinking, memory difficulty, impaired executive functioning, and mood and personality changes is consistent with the clinical syndrome of **subcortical dementia** (Cummings, 1990). In fact, the type of difficulties that patients on IFN-α experience are very similar to those experienced by patients with multiple sclerosis, a condition that may also be associated with a subcortical dementia.

Interleukin–2

Interleukin–2 also causes alterations in behavior and cognition. In general, as doses are increased, these alterations become more pronounced. In one report, 50% of patients who received IL–2 developed delirium, and over one-third were combative and agitated (Denicoff et al., 1987). These symptoms resolved following discontinuation of treatment. Another study found that mental status changed in 32% of patients with renal cell carcinoma (von der Maase et al., 1991). Many patients who received IL–2 developed depression (Krigel et al., 1988) and tended to withdraw from social contact. Difficulty concentrating or reading (Rieger and Weatherly, 1989) and hypersomnia, in addition to the fatigue-asthenia syndrome were also seen.

Tumor Necrosis Factor

Tumor necrosis factor can be a highly neurotoxic agent; approximately 86% of patients who received high-dose therapy with TNF developed dose-limiting neurotoxic effects in one report (Lenk et al., 1989). In fact, induction of TNF may be one of the mechanisms of IL–2 neurotoxicity (Mier et al., 1990). Elevated TNF levels induced by IL–2 administration have been associated with destruction of brain white matter in animal studies (Ellison and Merchant, 1991). The type of cognitive and emotional changes seen in TNF and IL–2 neurotoxicity are similar. Neuropsychological test findings in patients who experience TNF or combination TNF/IL–2 toxic effects have shown mild to moderate deficits of attentional abilities, verbal memory, motor coordination, and ability to shift mental set (i.e., to think flexibly). Intellectual functions, as in the case of IFN-α toxicity, are preserved. Single photon emission tomography (SPECT), which images regional cerebral perfusion, has been used to further quantify the physiologic changes caused by TNF and IL–2. In one patient, SPECT revealed diminished blood flow in both frontal lobes in the absence of anatomic abnormalities on a computed tomographic (CT) scan (Meyers et al., 1994). The neuropsychological test abnormalities, which also indicated frontal lobe

dysfunction, and the regional cerebral blood flow abnormalities resolved one month after treatment was discontinued.

Irreversible Neurotoxicity

There is increasing evidence that cytokine neurotoxicity does not always resolve following the discontinuation of treatment. A recent report reviewed the neuropsychological evaluations of 46 cancer patients who had received a number of chemotherapeutic and biological agents. These patients were referred for pretreatment assessment before starting a new phase I protocol (Meyers and Abbruzzese, 1992). None of them had a history of neurologic or psychiatric disorder, and all had been off prior therapy for at least three weeks. Cognitive deficits were observed in 18% of individuals who had been treated with chemotherapy only, but in 53% of patients who had also received cytokines. This finding suggests that treatment with cytokines places certain individuals at greater risk for developing neurobehavioral deficits and that these deficits may persist after treatment is discontinued.

Interferon-alpha

Studies of IFN-α neurotoxicity already described have reported prompt resolution of symptoms when treatment was discontinued, usually within several days to two weeks. However, some individuals continue to manifest difficulties with cognition and emotional functioning even years after IFN-α has been discontinued (Meyers et al., 1991b). The impairments of neurobehavioral function, which included memory loss, frontal lobe dysfunction, and outright dementia, could not be attributed to other therapy, changes in disease status, or other medical problems. Although most of the individuals had mild to moderate impairments, a number had very severe cognitive deficits, including progressive dementia, **extrapyramidal motor symptoms,** and florid psychiatric symptoms that necessitated involuntary hospitalization.

Intraventricular IL–2

Treatment with intraventricular IL–2 may also cause progressive deterioration of mental functions. Patients rarely survive long after the diagnosis of leptomeningeal disease, but there is a published case report of a woman who was treated successfully with intraventricular IL–2 (Meyers and Yung, 1993). Following the diagnosis of metastatic melanoma to the leptomeninges, she was treated with 9 MIU of intraventricular IL–2 over one month. She did well following this treatment, with no evidence of tumor recurrence. However, three months after her treatment ended she developed cerebellar signs consisting of a wide-based gait and impaired balance. Neuropsychological testing revealed mild impairments of memory and motor coordination with high average intellectual ability. Four years after therapy with IL–2, the patient had become exceedingly slow, with significant declines in memory and motor coordination. Intellectual function remained unimpaired. Magnetic resonance imaging revealed lesions in the subcortical white matter. This patient was no longer able to work and was confined to a wheelchair as a result of a progressive subcortical dementia.

EFFECTS OF ROUTE OF ADMINISTRATION

Methods of administration and prior treatment with cytokines are factors influencing their neurotoxicity. Intraventricular administration in particular may be associated with more severe neurotoxic side effects, which has limited the use of cytokines in treating leptomeningeal disease. In one study, 7 of 9 patients (78%) treated with intraventricular IFN-α for leptomeningeal disease developed severe neurotoxic effects that did not appear to be dose dependent (Meyers et al., 1991a). These patients became increasingly confused and developed expressive speech difficulty, which finally evolved into **mutism** after cumulative IFN-α doses between 14 and 54 MIU.

The clinical picture was one of a wakeful vegetative state in which the patients could open their eyes to stimulation but would not follow commands and were otherwise completely unresponsive. It took an average of 17 days for the patients to return to their pretreatment level of function, and 2 died before recovering. All of the patients who developed this neurotoxic syndrome had previously received whole brain radiation therapy for their leptomeningeal disease, suggesting a synergism between brain radiation and IFN-α.

A recently completed study using intraventricular IL–2 for leptomeningeal disease revealed less alarming, but significant neurotoxicity. Of 12 patients who received neuropsychological testing before and during therapy, 7 (58%) developed cognitive impairments on treatment. The most common problems were memory, frontal lobe executive function, and generalized slowing of behavior. It is often difficult, however, to sort out the effects of treatment from the effects of progressive disease in these patients.

PATHOPHYSIOLOGY OF MENTAL STATUS CHANGES

Although the CNS is normally protected by the **blood-brain barrier**, the development of cytokine neurotoxicity implies that these substances somehow gain access to the brain. There are two ways that cytokines may bypass this barrier and alter neural activity: (1) by altering vascular permeability, permitting substances normally excluded to enter the brain, or (2) by acting at circumventricular organs where the blood-brain barrier is normally leaky.

Cerebrovascular Alterations

Interleukin–2 is known to alter cerebrovascular permeability, inducing the so-called capillary leak syndrome, which may allow cytokines and other naturally excluded substances into the brain (Ellison et al., 1987) or cerebrospinal fluid (Saris *et al.*, 1988). Although IL–2 also causes vasogenic edema, the amount of cerebral edema does not appear to correlate with the severity of neurotoxic symptoms (Saris *et al.*, 1989). Changes in vascular permeability may also cause acute focal neurologic events that clinically resemble strokes (Bernard *et al.*, 1990). In contrast to IL–2, IFN–α does not appear to cause any changes in blood vessel permeability (Billiau, 1981).

Hypothalamic Actions

There are several lines of evidence suggesting that both IL–2 and IFN–α alter brain activity through actions at circumferential organs associated with the hypothalamus. First, patients who receive cytokines develop fever, anorexia, lethargy, and hypersomnia (Sarna, *et al.*, 1989; Smedley, *et al.*, 1983), symptoms that are similar to those seen following damage to various areas of the hypothalamus (Kupferman, 1981; Ellison *et al.*, 1970; Feldmen and Waller, 1962; Anand and Brobeck, 1951). Second, systemic IFN–α and IL–2 alter electrophysiological activity within the hypothalamus in animal studies. Whereas IFN–α causes neuronal excitability within 5 minutes of systemic administration (Dafny, 1983; Calvet and Gresser, 1979) IL–2 takes somewhat longer to alter neural activity, suggesting that there may be some intermediary steps involved (Bindoni *et al.*, 1988). Systemic administration of TNF also causes an increase in the firing rate of neurons in the circumventricular region of the hypothalamus (Shibata and Blatteis, 1991). Finally, IL–1 has been shown to cause fever and neuroendocrine alterations through an action at the anterior hypothalamus (Tsagarakis *et al.* 1989).

Areas of the hypothalamus have connections with the brainstem, frontal cortex, and all structures of the limbic system (Villalobos and Ferssiwi, 1987a, 1987b; Carpenter and Sutin, 1983; Berk and Finkelstein, 1982; Issacson, 1982). Thus, it is interesting that the electrophysiological and neuropsychological

studies previously cited also suggest brainstem and frontal lobe dysfunction.

Induction of Secondary Cytokines

Interactions among cytokines are complex and include both stimulatory and inhibitory effects. Systemic administration of IL–2, TNF, and IFN–α is thought to increase production of IL–1 (Mier *et al.*, 1988; Herman *et al.*, 1984; Arenzana-Seisdedos and Virelizer, 1983). Interleukin–1 has receptors on neurons within the hypothalamus and causes specific alterations in hypothalamic function (Breder *et al.*, 1988; Kabiersch *et al.*, 1988; Farrar *et al.*, 1987). Interleukin–2 also induces production of TNF (Mier *et al.*, 1990), and TNF and IL–1 are synergistically toxic (Waage and Espevik, 1988).

Neuroendocrine Alterations

Neuroendocrine disturbances occur often during cytokine therapy and may have an effect on brain function. Glucocorticoids can cross the blood-brain barrier (McEwen *et al.*, 1986; McEwen *et al.*, 1968) and have receptors within the CNS (McEwen and Micco, 1980). Glucocorticoid receptors are found within frontal brain regions and neurons of the septo-hippocampal system, a neural network thought to be important for emotion and memory (Squire, 1987; Lynch, 1986; Gray, 1982). In fact, endocrine disturbances are often found in patients with affective disorders (Sachar, 1982). As previously cited, memory and mood alterations are specifically affected by cytokine administration.

Administration of cytokines is known to induce a stress hormone response, elevating cortisol levels (Tracey *et al.*, 1987; Atkins *et al.*, 1986). Corticosterone can potentiate neurotoxic damage within the septo-hippocampal system by enhancing the vulnerability of neurons to other insults, for example, seizure, hypoxia-ischemia, excitatory amino acids, and antimetabolites (Masters *et al.*, 1989; Holsboer, 1988; Sapolsky *et al.*, 1988; Stein and Sapolsky, 1988). These effects have been observed primarily in the hippocampal areas that contain high levels of glucocorticoid receptors (Johnson et al., 1989; Sapolsky et al., 1986; Sapolsky, 1985). In addition to inducing stress hormones, cytokines may behave as neuroendocrine hormones themselves. For instance, IFN-α has structural and functional similarities to adrenocorticotrophic hormone (ACTH) (Blalock and Smith, 1980; Blalock and Stanton, 1980).

Neurotransmitter Alterations

The areas in which IFN has been shown to cause neuronal excitability are also areas with high numbers of opiate receptors (Dafny et al. 1985; Prieto-Gomez et al., 1983). Interferon has been shown to have structural similarities to endorphins and has opiate-like neurotransmitter activity (Dafny et al., 1983; Blalock and Smith, 1981). In fact, many of the effects of IFN can be reversed by the opiate antagonist naloxone. The progressive catatonia observed clinically in patients treated with intraventricular IFN-α are similar to the symptoms seen in animals treated with kappa opiate agonists (Meyers et al., 1991a). This has prompted animal laboratory researchers to determine the opioid-dopamine basis for the behavioral effects of this cytokine.

In one study, rats were trained to discriminate the effects of d-amphetamine from saline. When the rat was given d-amphetamine, it pushed a particular lever for food, and when it was given saline it pushed a different lever. This discrimination response is known to be mediated by the dopamine system. When the dose of amphetamine was cut in half, the animals responded randomly. However, when the dose of amphetamine was halved and the animal also received IFN-α, it responded just as if it had received the full dose of amphetamine; this is called a potentiation response (Ho et al., 1992). Ho and colleagues (1992) also found that the opiate antagonist naloxone suppressed this effect, and that morphine had the same effect as IFN-α. Opiate receptor activity subsequently modu-

lates the release of dopamine, which may be a factor in the extrapyramidal motor abnormalities that are seen in about one-third of patients who receive IFN-α. These data suggesting that IFN-α binds to opiate receptors have guided current interventional drug trials against IFN-α toxicity.

NURSING INTERVENTION STRATEGIES

Mental status changes that result from biotherapy represent a significant nursing challenge. Unless the symptoms experienced are severe and significantly affect patient function, doses are frequently not altered so that the agent's full therapeutic benefit may be realized. Cognizance of common neurotoxic effects related to biotherapy and appropriate interventions will assist the nurse in developing strategies to help patients cope (Bender, 1994; Sparber and Biller-Sparber, 1993).

One of the greatest interventions that can be provided to patients experiencing neurotoxic side effects of biotherapy is knowledge. The potential neurotoxic symptoms of this treatment are frequently not explained to the patient, sometimes because the primary physician does not fully recognize the impact of even subtle symptoms on social and vocational functioning. Not infrequently, patients who experience these symptoms without adequate warning may wonder if they are going "crazy" or will inaccurately attribute their symptoms to other causes. Reassurance that these symptoms are related to therapy can help reduce patient and family anxiety.

In addition, health care providers may not consider subtle neurobehavioral impairments very important in the context of the disease being treated. However, knowing that treatment-related neurobehavioral changes are common and that they can often be managed with a few compensation techniques can help alleviate the patient's anxiety and improve his or her psychosocial functioning. Even simple techniques such as taking intermittent naps, making lists for memory impairment, and taking special care to plan and organize activities may be all that is necessary to effectively cope with these symptoms.

Baseline assessment of individuals who will be treated with biotherapy agents is critical. It is often difficult to determine whether complaints of depression or memory loss are due to the patient's reaction to the diagnosis or concurrent psychosocial problems or are directly attributable to treatment-related neurotoxicity. This assessment will provide the nurse and health care team with knowledge about potential risk factors the patient may bring into the situation (i.e., pre-existing neurobehavioral difficulties related to previous treatment or other neurologic illness, psychosocial stressors, or other medications that can affect mental status) and will help them detect changes in neurobehavioral functioning over time. Because mental status changes associated with biotherapy are often subtle, it is important to request input from the family or significant others. They are often the first to recognize changes in the patient. Ongoing assessment during therapy is paramount. Simple observations such as determining the patient's ability to follow directions, fill out hospital meal menus, answer general orientation questions, and do calculations can provide significant information regarding neurotoxic side effects (Sparber and Biller-Sparber, 1993).

Baseline and interval assessments of the patient's neurocognitive functioning will also guide the implementation of safety measures and compensation techniques. For instance, a patient with memory problems may inaccurately report the type, frequency, or amount of medication he or she has been taking, leading to subtherapeutic or toxic medication levels. A person with poor motivation and apathy caused by frontal lobe dysfunction may appear depressed or uncompliant and may have difficulty initiating and following through personal hygiene routines, performing usual work and leisure activities, and so on. For inpatients experiencing such effects as

confusion or hypersomnia, appropriate safety measures such as fall precautions should be initiated.

Medical management of neurotoxic symptoms is one area of intervention that may be helpful. Low doses of tricyclic antidepressants may be effective in reducing psychological symptomatology, whether organically mediated, reactive, or both. These agents, such as amitriptyline, may also serve as co-analgesics for the diffuse joint pain and body aches frequently associated with cytokine therapy. Development of other agents, many still in the experimental stages, is based on the research on the specific mechanisms of action cytokines have on specific neurotransmitter and neuroendocrine systems in the brain. A preliminary trial to evaluate opiate antagonist therapy in patients complaining of neurotoxic side effects of IFN-α is ongoing (Valentine et al., 1994). Approximately three-quarters of the patients treated so far have had relief from their symptoms on this therapy, although some individuals have experienced intolerable side effects.

RESEARCH

Although there is growing understanding of the neurobehavioral deficits experienced by patients who receive biotherapy, much more research is needed in the area of nursing interventions directed toward specific deficits. To date, few reports of research pertain to mental status changes. Nurses are in a unique position to influence this area, since they coordinate inpatient and outpatient care, directly treat patients' symptoms, and function as researchers (Brophy and Sharp, 1991). It will become increasingly important for nurses and the entire healthcare team to develop and implement proactive programs for their patients, including determination of the cost/benefit ratio and efficacy of such programs, to ensure the best quality of life for patients undergoing these treatments. Interventions designed for patients who are receiving biotherapy will need to include patient education about potential symptoms, psychological support, safety measures, and coordination of adjunct services in neuropsychology, psychiatry, and rehabilitation (Mayer, 1990). Studies that evaluate patterns of neurotoxicity and associated distress will assist with nursing assessment during therapy.

FUTURE DIRECTIONS

The use of cytokines will continue to expand as experience with new agents, such as IL–4 and colony-stimulating factors increases and the number of illnesses that are found to respond to cytokine therapy multiplies. It is increasingly important to consider the long-term impact of these compounds on the social, vocational, and psychological function of the individuals being treated. Early detection and some interventions for neurotoxic side effects are now feasible, and better intervention strategies are being developed. The potential for progressive brain injury and subsequent disability will need to be considered in developing ancillary treatments to improve the risk/benefit ratio of therapy and to enhance the quality of life of patients who receive biotherapy.

References

Adams, F., Quesada, J., and Gutterman, J. 1984. Neuropsychiatric manifestations of human leukocyte interferon therapy in patients with cancer. *Journal of the American Medical Association* 252(7): 938–941.

Anand, B., and Brobeck, J. 1951. Hypothalamic control of food intake in rats and cats. *Yale Journal of Biological Medicine* 24: 123.

Arenzana-Seisdedos, F., and Virelizer, J. 1983. Interferons as macrophage-activating factors. II. Enhanced secretion of interleukin–1 by lipopolysaccharide-stimulated human monocytes. *European Journal of Immunology* 13: 437–440.

Atkins, M., Gould, J., Allegretta, M., et al. 1986. Phase I evaluation of recombinant interleukin–2 in patients with advanced malignant disease. *Journal of Clinical Oncology* 4: 1380–1391.

Auerbach, V., and Faibish, G. 1989. Mini-mental state examination: Diagnostic limitations. *Journal of Clinical and Experimental Neuropsychology* 11: 75 (abstract).

Bender, C. 1994. Cognitive dysfunction associated with biological response modifier therapy. *Oncology Nursing Forum* 21(3): 515–523.

Berk, M., and Finkelstein, J. 1982. Efferent connections of the lateral hypothalamic area of the rat: An autoradiographic investigation. *Brain Research Bulletin* 8: 511–526.

Bernard, J., Ameriso, S., Kempf R., et al. 1990. Transient focal neurologic deficits complicating interleukin–2 therapy. *Neurology* 40: 154–155.

Billiau, A. 1981. Interferon therapy: Pharmacokinetic and pharmacological aspects. *Archives of Virology* 67: 121–133.

Bindoni, M., Perciavalle, V., Berretta, S., et al. 1988. Interleukin-2 modifies the bioelectric activity of some neurosecretory nuclei in the rat hypothalamus. *Brain Research* 462: 10–14.

Blalock, J., and Smith, E. 1981. Human leukocyte interferon (HuIFN-α): Potent endorphin-like opioid activity. *Biochemistry and Biophysics Research Communication* 101: 472–478.

Blalock, J., and Smith, E. 1980. Human leukocyte interferon: Structural and biological relatedness to adrenocorticotropic hormones and endorphins. *Proceedings of the National Academy of Sciences USA* 77: 5972–5974.

Blalock, J., and Stanton, J. 1980. Common pathways of interferon and hormonal action. *Nature* 283: 406–408.

Breder, C., Dinarello, C., and Saper, C. 1988. Interleukin–1 immunoreactive innervation of the human hypothalamus. *Science* 240: 321–324.

Brophy, L., and Sharp, E. 1991. Physical symptoms of combination biotherapy: A quality of life issue. *Oncology Nursing Forum* 18(Suppl): 25–30.

Calvet, M., and Gresser, I. 1979. Interferon enhances the excitability of cultured neurones. *Nature* 278: 558–560.

Carpenter, M., and Sutin, J. 1983. *Human Neuroanatomy*. Baltimore: Williams & Wilkins.

Cummings, J. 1990. *Subcortical Dementia*. New York: Oxford University Press.

Dafny, N. 1983. Interferon modifies EEG and EEG-like activity recorded from sensory, motor, and limbic system structures in freely behaving rats. *Neurotoxicology* 4: 235–240.

Dafny, N., Prieto-Gomez, B., and Reyes-Vasquez, C. 1985. Does the immune system communicate with the central nervous system? Interferon modifies central nervous activity. *Journal of Neuroimmunology* 9: 1–12.

Dafny, N., Zielinnski, M., and Reyes-Vasquez, C. 1983. Alteration of morphine withdrawal to naloxone by interferon. *Neuropeptides* 3: 453–463.

Denicoff, K., Rubinow D., Papa, M., et al. 1987. The neuropsychiatric effects of treatment with interleukin–2 and lymphokine-activated killer cells. *Annals of Internal Medicine* 107: 293–300.

Ellison, M., and Merchant, R. 1991. Appearance of cytokine-associated central nervous system myelin damage coincides temporarily with serum tumor necrosis factor induction after recombinant interleukin–2 infusion in rats. *Journal of Neuroimmunology* 33: 245–251.

Ellison, M., Povlishock, J., Merchant, R. 1987. Blood-brain barrier dysfunction in cats following recombinant interleukin–2 infusion. *Cancer Research* 47: 5765–5770.

Ellison, G., Sorenson, C., and Jacobs, B. 1970. Two feeding syndromes following surgical isolation of the hypothalamus in rats. *Journal of Comparative and Physiological Psychology* 70: 173–188.

Farkkila, M., Iivanainen, M., Roine, R., *et al.* 1984. Neurotoxic and other side effects of high-dose interferon in amyotrophic lateral sclerosis. *Acta Neurologica Scandinavica* 70: 42–46.

Farrar, W., Killian, P., Ruff, M., *et al.* 1987. Visualization and characterization of interleukin 1 receptors in brain. *Journal of Immunology* 139: 459–463.

Feldman, S., and Waller, H. 1962. Dissociation of electrocortical activation and behavioral arousal. *Nature* 196: 1320–1322.

Folstein, M., Folstein, S., and McHugh, P. 1975. "Minimental state": A practical method for grading the cognitive state of patients for the clinicain. *Journal of Psychiatric Research* 12: 189–198.

Goldstein, D., and Laszlo, J. 1988. The role of interferon in cancer therapy: A current perspective. *CA-A Cancer Journal for Clinician* 38(5): 258–277.

Gray, J. 1982. *The Neuropsychology of Anxiety: An Enquiry into the Functions of the Septo-Hippocampal System.* New York: Oxford University Press.

Herman, J., Kew, M., and Rabson, A. 1984. Defective interleukin–1 production by monocytes from patients with malignant disease. *Cancer, Immunology, and Immunotherapy* 16: 182–185.

Ho, B., Huo, Y., Lu, J., *et al.* 1992. Opioid-dopaminergic mechanisms in the potentiation of *d*-amphetamine discrimination by interferon-α. *Pharmacology, Biochemistry and Behavior* 42: 57–60.

Holsboer, F. 1988. Implications of altered limbic-hypothalamic-pituitary-adrenocortical (LHPA)-function for neurobiology of depression. *Acta Psychiatrica Scandinavica* 341(Suppl): 72–111.

Iivanainen, M., Laaksonen, R., Niemi, M., *et al.* 1985. Memory and psychomotor impairment following high-dose interferon treatment in amyotrophic lateral sclerosis. *Acta Neurologica Scandinavica* 72: 475–480.

Issacson, R. 1982. *The Limbic System.* New York: Plenum Press.

Johnson, M., Stone, D., Bush, L., *et al.* 1989. Glucocorticoids and 3,4-methylenedioxymethamphetamine (MDMA)–induced neurotoxicity. *European Journal of Pharmacology* 161: 181–188.

Kabiersch, A., Del Rey, A., Honegger, C., *et al.* 1988. Interleukin–1 produces changes in norepinephrine metabolism in the rat brain. *Brain, Behavior, and Immunity* 2: 267–274.

Krigel, R., Padavic-Shaller, K., Rudolph, A., *et al.* 1988. A phase I study of recombinant interleukin–2 plus recombinant beta interferon. *Cancer Research* 48: 3875–3881.

Kupferman, I. 1981. Hypothalamus and limbic system II: Motivation. In Kandel, E., and Schwartz, J.(eds). *Principles of Neural Science.* New York: Elsevier, pp. 450–460.

Lenk, H., Tanneberger, S., Muller, U., *et al.* 1989. Phase II clinical trial of high-dose recombinant human tumor necrosis factor. *Cancer Chemotherapy and Pharmacology* 24: 391–392.

Levine, P., Silberfarb, P., Kipowski, Z. 1978. Mental disorders in cancer patients: A study of 100 psychiatric referrals. *Cancer* 43: 1385–1391.

Lynch, G. 1986. *Synapses, Circuits, and the Beginnings of Memory.* Cambridge, MA: MIT Press.

Masters, J., Finch, C., and Sapolsky, R. 1989. Glucocorticoid endangerment of hippocampal neurons does not involve deoxyribonucleic acid cleavage. *Endocrinology* 124: 3083–3088.

Mattson, K., Niiranen, A., Iivanainen, M., *et al.* 1983. Neurotoxicity of interferon. *Cancer Treatment Reports* 67: 958–961.

Mayer, D. 1990. Biotherapy: Recent advances and nursing implications. *Nursing Clinics of North America* 25: 291–308.

McDonald, E., Mann, A., and Thomas, H. 1987. Interferons as mediators of psychiatric morbidity: An investigation in a trial of recombinant interferon-alfa in hepatitis B carriers. *Lancet* 2(8569): 1175–1178.

McEwen, B., De Kloet, E., and Rostene, W. 1986. Adrenal steroid receptors and actions in the central nervous system. *Physiological Reviews* 66: 1121–1188.

McEwen, B., and Micco, D. 1980. Toward an understanding of the multiplicity of glucocorticoid actions on brain function and behavior. In De Weid, D., and van Keep, P.(eds). *Hormones and the Brain.* Baltimore: University Park, pp. 11–28.

McEwen, B., Weis, J., and Schwartz, L. 1968. Selective retention of corticosterone by limbic structures in rat brain. *Nature* 220: 911–912.

Meyers, C., Mattis, P., Pavol, M., *et al.* 1993. Pattern of neurobehavioral deficits associated with interferon-α neurotoxicity. *Proceedings of the American Association for Cancer Research* 34: 28 (abstract).

Meyers, C., and Abbruzzese, J. 1992. Cognitive functioning in cancer patients: Effect of previous treatment. *Neurology* 42: 434–436.

Meyers, C., Obbens, E., Scheibel, R., et al. 1991a. Neurotoxicity of intraventricularly administered alpha interferon for leptomeningeal disease. *Cancer* 68: 88–92.

Meyers, C., Scheibel, R., and Forman, A. 1991b. Persistent neurotoxicity of systemically administered interferon-alpha. *Neurology* 41: 672–676.

Meyers, C., and Scheibel, R. 1990. Early detection and diagnosis of neurobehavioral disorders in cancer patients. *Oncology* 4: 115–122.

Meyers, C., Valentine, A., Wong, F., et al. 1994. Reversible neurotoxicity of IL-2 and TNF: Correlation of SPECT with neuropsychological testing. *Journal of Neuropsychiatry and Clinical Neurosciences.* in press.

Meyers, C., and Yung, W. 1993. Delayed neurotoxicity of intraventricular interleukin–2: a case report. *Journal of Neuro-Oncology* 15: 265–267.

Mier, J., Vachino, G., Lempner, M., et al. 1990. Inhibition of interleukin–2-induced tumor necrosis factor release by dexamethasone: Prevention of an acquired neutrophil chemotaxis defect and differential suppression of interleukin–2-associated side effects. *Blood* 76: 1933–1940.

Mier, J., Vachino, G., Van Der Meer, J., et al. 1988. Induction of circulating tumor necrosis factor (TNF-alpha) as the mechanisms for the febrile response to interleukin–2 (IL–1) in cancer patients. *Journal of Clinical Immunology* 8: 426–436.

Prieto-Gomez, B., Reyes-Vazquez, C., and Dafny, N. 1983. Differential effects of interferon on ventromedial hypothalamus and dorsal hippocampus. *Journal of Neuroscience Research* 10: 273–278.

Rieger, P., and Weatherly, B. 1989. Can your nursing skills meet the challenge of a patient receiving IL–2? *Dimensions in Oncology Nursing* 3: 9–19.

Renault, P., Hoofnagle, J., Park, Y., et al. 1987. Psychiatric complications of long-term interferon alfa therapy. *Archives of Internal Medicine* 147: 1577–1580.

Rohatiner, A., Prior, P., Burton, A., et al. 1983. Central nervous system toxicity of interferon. *British Journal of Cancer* 47: 419–422.

Sachar, E. 1982. Endocrine abnormalities in depression. In Paykel, E. (ed). *Handbook of Affective Disorders.* New York: Guilford Press, pp. 191–201.

Sapolsky, R. 1986. Glucocorticoid toxicity in the hippocampus: Reversal by supplementation with brain fuels. *Journal of Neuroscience* 6: 2240–2244.

Sapolsky, R. 1985. A mechanism of glucocorticoid toxicity in the hippocampus: Increased neuronal vulnerability to metabolic insults. *Journal of Neuroscience* 5: 1228–1232.

Sapolsky, R., Pacan, D., and Vale, W. 1988. Glucocorticoid toxicity in the hippocampus: *In vitro* demonstration. *Brain Research* 453: 367–371.

Saris, S., Patronas, N., Rosenberg, S., et al. 1989. The effect of intravenous interleukin–2 on brain water content. *Journal of Neurosurgery* 71: 169–174.

Saris, S., Rosenberg, S., Friedman, R., et al. 1988. Penetration of recombinant interleukin–2 across the blood-cerebrospinal fluid barrier. *Journal of Neurosurgery* 69: 29–34.

Sarna, G., Figlin, R., Pertcheck, M., et al. 1989. Systemic administration of recombinant methionyl human interleukin–2 (Ala 125) to cancer patients: Clinical results. *Journal of Biological Response Modifiers* 8: 16–24.

Shibata, M., and Blatteis, C. 1991. Human recombinant tumor necrosis factor and interferon affect the activity of neurons in the organum vasculosum laminae terminalis. *Brain Research* 562: 323–326.

Smedley, H., Katrak, M., Sikora, K., et al. 1983. Neurological effects of recombinant human interferon. *British Medical Journal* 286: 262–264.

Sparber, A., and Biller-Sparber, K. 1993. Immunotherapy and neuropsychiatric toxicity. *Cancer Nursing* 16(3): 188–192.

Squire, L. 1987. *Memory and Brain.* New York: Oxford University Press.

Stein, B., and Sapolsky, R. 1988. Chemical adrenalectomy reduces hippocampal damage induced by kainic acid. *Brain Research* 473: 175–180.

Strub, R., and Black, F. 1981. *Organic Brain Syndromes.* Philadelphia: F.A. Davis Company.

Suter, C., Westmoreland, B., Sharbrough, F., et al. 1984. Electroencephalographic abnormalities in interferon encephalopathy: A preliminary report. *Mayo Clinic Proceedings* 59: 847–850.

Talpaz, M., Kantarjian, H., McCredie, K., et al. 1986. Hematologic remission and cytogenic improvement induced by recombinant human interferon-alpha in chronic myelogenous leukemia. *New England Journal of Medicine* 314: 1065–1069.

Tracey, K., Lowry, S., Fahey, T. et al. 1987. Cachectin/tumor necrosis factor induces lethal shock and stress hormone responses in the dog. *Surgical Gynecology and Obstetrics* 164: 415–422.

Tsagarakis, S., Gillies, G., Rees, L., et al. 1989. Interleukin–1 directly stimulates the release of corticotropin releasing factor from rat hypothalamus. *Neuroendocrinology* 9: 98–101.

Valentine, A., Meyers, C., and Talpaz, M. In press. Treatment of neurotoxic side effects of Interferon-α with naltrexone. *Cancer Investigation.*

Villalobos, J., and Ferssiwi, A. 1987a. The differential ascending projections from the anterior, central, and posterior regions of the lateral hypothalamic area: An autoradiographic study. *Neuroscience Letters* 81: 89–94.

Villalobos, J., and Ferssiwi, A. 1987b. The differential descending projections from the anterior, central, and posterior regions of the lateral hypothalamic area: An autoradiographic study. *Neuroscience Letters* 81: 95–99.

von der Maase, H., Geertsen, P., Thatcher, C., et al. 1991. Recombinant interleukin–2 in metastatic renal cell carcinoma—a European multicentre phase II study. *European Journal of Cancer* 27: 1583–1589.

Waage, A., and Espevik, T. 1988. Interleukin–1 potentiates the lethal effect of tumor necrosis factor alpha/cachectin in mice. *Journal of Experimental Medicine* 167: 1987–1992.

CHAPTER 14 | Patient Education

Kimberly A. Rumsey, RN, MSN, OCN

Patient education is a vital component of the nurse's role in caring for patients who receive biotherapy. It can also be one of the most challenging and rewarding aspects of caring for these patients. Often, the education provided by nurses may allow patients to receive therapy at home and thereby experience improved quality of life.

Patient education has been defined as "a planned learning experience using a combination of methods such as teaching, counseling, and behavior modification techniques which influence patients' knowledge and health behavior" (Bartlett, 1985). The ultimate goal of patient education is to assist patients and their family members to develop the necessary skills and knowledge for adaptation to the alterations in their health and lifestyle.

In the past several years, there has been an increased emphasis on patient education. Patients today desire information about their health and want to participate in their care. In 1972, the American Hospital Association first published *A Patient's Bill of Rights* (American Hospital Association, 1992) which listed 12 rights of patients. According to this document, patient education is an integral component of the care a patient should expect from health care providers. Explicit in *A Patient's Bill of Rights* is the right to receive information about diagnosis, prognosis, treatment options, and side effects. Published more recently, *The Cancer Survivors' Bill of Rights* (American Cancer Society, 1988) confers on cancer survivors the right to be informed about the future including insurance coverage and employment. Many state and national agencies have required health care professionals to provide patient education. The Joint Commission for the Accreditation of Healthcare Organizations (JCAHO) specifies that "patients receive nursing care based on a documented assessment of their needs," including biophysical, psychosocial, environmental, self-care, educational, and discharge needs (JCAHO, 1993). The Health Care Financing Administration (HCFA) also has specific requirements regarding the education of patients for institutions that participate in Medicare and Medicaid programs (HCFA Code). In addition to JCAHO and HCFA, state nurse practice acts address the role of nursing in patient education, either directly or indirectly. In the *Standards of Oncology Education: Patient/Family and Public* (Oncology Nursing Society, 1989), the Oncology Nursing Society states that nurses at the generalist and advanced practice levels are responsible for patient education related to cancer care. Besides being mandated by state and national organizations, patient education may benefit all who are involved, including patients and family members, health care providers and institutions, and society in general (Fernsler and Cannon, 1991). Educated consumers are better able to participate in their care and facilitate early discharge, lowering health care costs.

Obviously, patient education should be a high priority for nurses in direct contact with patients. According to Close (1988), although patient education is viewed as a role of the nurse, in reality more technical or clinical skills often take priority. Kruger (1991) surveyed staff nurses, nurse administrators, and nurse educators for their attitudes regarding the role of patient educator and perceptions of personal ability to perform this role. Results indicated that all three groups valued the role of patient educator, but did not feel they could satisfactorily perform it. Although some patient education is being successfully conducted, evidence suggests that it is inadequate (Kruger, 1991). Several trends in health care, including early discharge and an increase in the use of ambulatory care facilities, provide new challenges for the nurse implementing the patient education process (Blumberg and Gentry, 1991; Morra, 1991). One of the major obstacles is lack of preparation for the role of patient educator (Rabel, 1992; Close, 1988).

Using the nursing process as a framework, this chapter will describe the process for the education of biotherapy patients and their family members. For the purpose of this chapter, use of the term *patient* will also include family members and significant others.

THE PROCESS OF PATIENT EDUCATION

The role of patient educator can be successfully implemented by the nurse. With planning, the proper tools, and practice, patient education can become a rewarding component of the role of the nurse in all care settings. According to Hicks (1987) an equal partnership between nurses and patients is necessary for successful patient education. With communication, negotiation, and motivation, nurses and patients are able to work together to progress through the process of patient education. The nursing process provides a familiar and practical framework to follow for teaching patients (Anderson, 1990; Kaufman, 1989; Close, 1988; Redman, 1988).

Assessment

Assessment is a key component in the patient education process and forms the basis for the patient teaching plan. The ability to assess patients' learning needs and styles assists the nurse in providing individual instruction, promoting effective use of resources, identifying specific information that is important to patients, and saving valuable time (Volker, 1991; Armstrong, 1989).

The three most important sources of information when assessing the learning needs of patients receiving biotherapy are the patients themselves, the medical record, and other members of the health care team. Formal and informal interviews with patients and family members provide most of the needed information, but a written questionnaire may be helpful and time efficient for the nurse. The medical record provides basic information about health status, including previous learning needs and teaching already completed.

Discussion with other members of the health care team allows nurses to expand and validate their assessments (Volker, 1991; Springhouse, 1987). Often, biotherapy patients have been in the health care system for a considerable length of time and have developed a wealth of knowledge about their disease and its treatment. Adequate learning needs assessment will identify areas that may need reinforcement, areas that require extensive teaching, and areas that need only review.

A comprehensive learning needs assessment includes assessment of the patient's ability, readiness and willingness to learn, and areas of knowledge deficit.

Ability to Learn

Assessment of patients' physical and cognitive status provides information about their ability to learn. Patients should be assessed for physiologic barriers to learning, such as sensory impairment (visual, auditory) or impaired motor ability so that adjustments can be made in the teaching plan to overcome these barriers. For example, a patient with visual disturbance may require written materials with large print and extensive verbal instructions (Anderson, 1991). An assessment of the patient's ability to communicate verbally in English is also very important in planning teaching strategies. It may be necessary to schedule a translator in advance or present a non-English version of a video or written material. In addition, literacy level should be assessed. Nurses tend to use many printed materials as adjuncts to one-to-one teaching. A study of American Cancer Society (ACS) patient education literature showed that this material has an average reading level of grade 11.9 (Meade et al., 1992), even though approximately 23 million adults in the United States tes read at or below a fifth grade level. Meade suggested that patient education materials be developed at the fifth or sixth grade reading level to benefit more individuals. Many patients are hesitant to verbalize their difficulty in reading and may try to conceal it. It is imperative that nurses be able to recognize the nonverbal cues to poor reading skills, including poor attention span, little or no interest in the topic, feelings of frustration, and slow reading speed. Patients also may be unable to answer questions regarding the content of the literature or may request that someone else read the literature (Meade et al., 1992). Low literacy levels can sometimes indicate other limitations to learning such as poor organization of thoughts or impaired ability to learn and synthesize new information. Nurses must be careful not to stereotype patients because of low literacy, but to adapt their teaching strategies appropriately. Furthermore, nurses should always use simple vocabulary and lay terminology during their communications with patients (Barnes, 1992).

The learning style of the patient should be assessed to assure optimal use of teaching time and resources (Arndt and Underwood, 1990). Patient education is more successful when nurses respond to patients' individual learning styles (Villejo and Meyers, 1991; Springhouse, 1987). Numerous learning style theories have been described in the literature, each based on several assumptions. First, each person has a predominant learning style that may be different from that of other people. Second, no one style is superior to another. Third, individuals may process information predominantly by one style, but may also use other styles. It is essential to know patients' preferences prior to initiating the teaching session. The nurse must assess how patients learn best, whether through visual stimuli (reading literature, viewing videos), auditory stimuli (listening to tapes, lecture), or tactile stimuli (handling equipment, return demonstration with critique). Most people prefer a combination of stimuli in their education. Information on learning style and patient preferences provides the rationale for the teaching activities and tools that are chosen for the educational endeavor (Springhouse, 1987). To assess learning syle, nurses can simply ask patients how they best learn.

Readiness and Willingness to Learn

Patients' readiness and willingness to learn are vital components of the learning needs assessment. Several factors should be assessed that may influence patients' readiness and willingness to learn, including social/cultural background, emotional state, and patient/family goals. Patients should be questioned, in a sensitive manner, about their sociocultural background. Responses should be considered in light of current health status and lifestyle (Anderson, 1990; Springhouse, 1987). For example, a male patient from Saudi Arabia may respond negatively to instruction from female nurses. In this situation, having a male nurse do the teaching may provide a more successful educational session. Religious beliefs about treating illness should be considered. If patients' religious beliefs do not allow administration of blood products, nurses may need to emphasize other measures that can be implemented to ensure the safety of thrombocytopenic patients.

The goals of patients help to determine readiness and willingness to learn. For example, if a patient's goal is to be at home for a child's birthday, the nurse's educational sessions on self-injection of interferon would be well received. Nurses should recognize the goals verbalized by patients and assist them in setting realistic goals within the expectations of the health care system. Agreement on the goals by patients and the health care team should help ensure that they are met.

The emotional state of patients influences their ability, as well as their readiness and willingness, to learn and should be included in the learning needs assessment (Anderson, 1990; Springhouse, 1987). Common emotions may have a detrimental effect on teaching and may require that sessions be delayed. A small amount of anxiety, for example, is normal and sometimes can increase patients receptiveness to learning. Too much anxiety, however, can be overwhelming and decrease the ability, readiness, and willingness to learn.

Knowledge Deficits

The patients learning deficits must be assessed during the learning needs assessment. It is vital to assess previous knowledge and experience that may affect current needs. For example, a mother who has been administering insulin subcutaneously to her child should be able to apply the concepts to giving herself subcutaneous interferon. By assessing her previous experience with injections, the nurse can then know to assess the patient's injection technique and teach and reinforce accordingly. It is also important to note topics that patients are most concerned about or interested in. If patients are nervous about actually administering the subcutaneous injection, the nurse may want to plan a demonstration/return demonstration of the injection technique before teaching reconstitution and drawing up the medication. Nurses must also consider specific skills needed by family members to adequately care for patients.

A comprehensive learning needs assessment will assist the nurse in formulating a teaching plan that can be agreed upon by all and will, optimally, meet the needs of the patient within the constraints imposed by the health care system.

Planning

Once the comprehensive learning needs assessment is complete, the nurse should develop a plan for patient education. The teaching plan is an organized document that describes patients' educational needs and how those needs will be met (Springhouse, 1987). Nurses may choose to develop standardized teaching plans for patients who have similar learning needs. See Table 14.1 for the standardized teaching plan used for biotherapy patients at the University of Texas M.D. Anderson Cancer Center. The plan should be formulated in partnership with the patient and other members of the health care team (Hicks, 1987). Components of the plan include goals and objectives of learning, material to be presented, and teaching strategies to be implemented.

Table 14.1 The University of Texas M.D. Anderson Cancer Center—Biotherapy patient teaching plan

Team Member	Objective/Expected Outcome	Content	Teaching Method

MD/Fellow/RN	I. Patients will be able to explain, in their own words, basic immune function, as evidenced by:
	• Expressing comprehension of their immune system, how it functions and the role it plays in their treatment.
	Ia. Patients will be able to explain, in their own words, their treatment plan (including frequency of administration and duration) and its rationale, as evidenced by:
	• Expressing understanding of what type of treatment they will have, for how long, and why it is necessary.
		I. Immune function
		
		Ia. BIOTHERAPY
		A. Definition
		B. Goals of Therapy
		  1. diagnostic
		  2. therapeutic
		  3. supportive
		C. Commercial vs. investigative use
		  1. purpose of treatment
		  2. informed consent
		D. Treatment regimen
		  1. Route of administration
		    a. Frequency of administration
		    b. Duration of therapy
		  2. Location
		    a. Clinic
		    b. Station 19
		    c. Inpatient
		    d. Hometown—referring MD
		  3. When
		    a. scheduled appointments
		    b. Follow-up/evaluation
		E. Laboratory and diagnostic tests
		F. Special requirements (Example: extended hospital admission or need to remain in vicinity for extended period of time.)
			Individual instruction:
			• *Understanding the Immune System,* NCI booklet
			• *Biotherapy: A Patient Guide*
			• Injection Series Videotapes MDA-TV, x27287;
			  IM #82-1-92
			  SC #80-1-92
			  Mixing Meds #81-1-92
			• *What are Clinical Trials all About?* NCI booklet
			• Treatment-specific patient information drug card(s)
			• Other applicable print material (refer to Patient Education Clearinghouse listing and Patient/Family Learning Center) and videotapes (refer to Patient Guide for listings and numbers)
			• Printed calender
			• Question/answer period

Continued

Table 14.1 *Continued*

Team Member	Objective/Expected Outcome	Content	Teaching Method

MD/Fellow/RN	II. Patients will be able to identify potential side effects and appropriate self-management, as evidenced by:
	• Verbalizing understanding of [potential] side effects of their treatment.
		II. Side Effects
		A. Key Areas
		  1. Incidence
		  2. Severity
		  3. Self-management
		B. Potential Side Effects
		  1. Constitutional symptoms
		    a. fever
		    b. chills
		    c. arthralgia
		    d. malaise
		    e. flushing
		  2. Neurological side effects
		  3. Renal toxicity
		  4. Hematologic side effects
		  5. Hepatic side effects
		  6. Dermatologic side effects
		    a. erythema at injection site(s)
		    b. itching
		    c. rash
		    d. dryness
		    e. desquamation (dry or wet)
		  7. GI side effects*
		    a. anorexia
		    b. weight loss
		    c. nauseau/vomiting
		    d. diarrhea
		    e. mucositis
		  8. Cardiovascular/pulmonary side effects
		    a. capillary leak syndrome
		  9. Allergic reactions
			Individual instruction:
			• Treatment-specific patient information drug card(s)
			• Video (MDA-TV x27287):
			  Intro to Interferon #832–1–87
			  (Spanish) #956–1–90

*DIETARY CONSULT FOR NUTRITIONAL PROBLEMS			• *Eating Hints*, NCI Booklet • *Nausea & Vomiting: What You Can Do* (if applicable, e.g., treatment with IL-2) • Other applicable print material (refer to Patient Education Clearinghouse listing) and videos (refer to Patient Education and Guide for listing and numbers)

276

• Describing in their own words the appropriate management of those side effects.	IIa. Reporting of signs and symptoms
	A. Reportable signs and symptoms
	  1. Continuing fever of 40°C
	  2. Weight gain of 5–10 kg over 1 week
	  3. Weight loss of 5–10 kg over several weeks
	  4. Shortness of breath
	  5. Dizziness
	  6. Inability to perform ADL 2° fatigue
	  7. Alteration in mental status
	  8. Inflammation at injection site
	  9. Any other unusual signs/symptoms
		Clinic handout

• Identifying who/where to contact for reportable side effects.	B. Who to contact
	  1. MDACC
	    a. Clinic staff
	    b. RN/fellow/attending MD
	    c. Station 19—after 5pm, weekends, holidays
	  2. Outside MDACC
	    a. Local MD
	    b. Local hospital	

RN/Pharmacist
 	
III. Patients will be able to self-administer IM/SC injection, as evidenced by:
• Accurate return demonstration of drug reconstitution.
• Accurate return demonstration of technique for self-administration of IM/SC injection.
• Describing in their own words the proper storage and disposal of the medication and equipment.
	III. Self administration
	A. Types of equipment
	  1. Medication
	  2. Diluent
	  3. Alcohol swabs
	  4. Syringes
	  5. Needles
	B. Aseptic technique
		Individual instruction:
		
		Demonstration/return demonstration
		
		Injection series videotapes MDA-TV, x27287:
		IM #82–1–92
		SC #80–1–92
		Mixing Meds #81–1–92

Continued

Table 14.1 *Continued*

Team Member	Objective/Expected Outcome	Content	Teaching Method

		1. Definition
		2. Parts of equipment that may be handled
		C. Method of reconstitution
		D. Withdrawing liquid from the vial
		  1. Proper dose
		E. Site selection and rotation
		F. Injection techniques
		G. Storage of the medication
		  1. Stability of medication (single/multiple dose vial)
		H. Disposal of equipment at home
			Patient information cards:
			• Subcutaneous injection
			• Intramuscular injection
			• Drawing up a Liquid Medication
			Dose Preparation Instruction Sheet

RN/Social Worker	IV. Patients will adjust to their altered lifestyle and cope effectively with psychosocial issues related to their diagnosis and treatment, as evidenced by:
	• Identifying problems/issues in need of follow-up.
	• Identifying appropriate strategies and resources for coping with their diagnosis and/or treatment.
	• Seeking information and assistance.
	• Taking actions to promote coping (i.e., participating in discussion/support group)
		IV. Psychosocial Issues
		A. Common problems
		  1. Depression
		  2. Hopelessness
		  3. Decisional conflict
		  4. Financial concerns
		  5. Housing
		  6. Transportation
		B. Support Services
		  1. Social Work
		  2. Discussion/Support groups—hospital & community
		  3. Referrals
		C. How to access community resources
			One-on-One Discussion
			
			Referral/Assistance
			
			Applicable print material (refer to Patient Education Clearinghouse Listing, Patient/Family Learning Center) and videos (refer to Patient Guide for listing and numbers)

| MD/fellow/RN/Pharmacist | V. Patients will be aware of reimbursement issues common to the biotherapy patient, as evidenced by:
 • Verbalizing an understanding of common problems related to reimbursement.
 • Having and referring to written material as needed.
 • Identifying available resources (educational, financial, etc.) as they relate to biotherapy patients. | V. Reimbursement Issues
 A. Common problems
   1. Investigative therapy

   2. Off-label use
   3. Cost of therapy
   4. Lack of insurance coverage for self-administered medications
 B. Support Services
   1. Hospital pharmacy
   2. Pharmaceutical company
   3. Reimbursement programs | One-on-One Discussion

 Referral/Assistance

 Applicable print material |

Source: Reprinted with permission, The University of Texas M.D. Anderson Cancer Center, Department of Patient Education, Houston, Texas.

Goals

The initial step in developing the teaching plan is identifying the goals to be accomplished. Goals give the teaching session direction and act as a guide for evaluation at the completion of the session. For this reason, goals are sometimes referred to as expected outcomes or learning objectives. The goals should directly reflect the learning needs of the patient as determined by the assessment that was previously completed (Smith, 1987).

There are five essential characteristics to an effective goal. First, the goal must be mutually acceptable. Patients should take part in the goal setting (Anderson, 1990; Hicks, 1987) or at least verbalize acceptance of the goal, to promote cooperation and compliance (Springhouse, 1987). The goal should also be realistic, specifying an outcome that can be accomplished. Sometimes it is helpful to set subgoals that will help move learners toward the overall goal while giving them a feeling of accomplishment (Anderson, 1990). For example, the goal of subcutaneous self-injection could be broken down into several smaller goals such as, reconstitution of medication, drawing up the correct dosage, injection technique, and disposal of the equipment at home. An effective goal must also be measurable and patient centered. The goal should be written clearly in behavioral terms. Well-written goals begin with an action verb (e.g., state, discuss, demonstrate), are limited to one task, and specify a time frame in which the goal should be met. Teaching goals are best if they are written in a formal document. Written goals help to communicate what is expected to patients and other health care professionals (Anderson, 1990; Springhouse, 1987), especially if they are always documented in the same manner and kept in an agreed upon location. In summation, to produce the expected result, goals must be mutually agreed upon by all parties involved, be realistic, measurable and patient centered, AND written in an identified, consistent location.

Content

Using the information provided by the learning needs assessment, nurses can determine content areas to be included in the teaching plan. The content chosen should reflect the identified learning needs and meet the outlined goals or objectives. In the *Standards of Oncology Education: Patient/Family and Public* (1989), ONS outlines the knowledge, skills, and attitudes related to the management of human responses to cancer that should be included in patient education. Adams (1991) provides an indepth discussion of the common educational needs of patients across the various phases of cancer care. In prioritizing content, nurses must balance what the patient needs to know with what they want to know. A content outline should be written, beginning with basic ideas and moving toward complex concepts. It is also important to determine which member of the health care team will be responsible for teaching the content. By writing down the content to be taught and indicating the responsible person, nurses can facilitate communication with the patient and other members of the health care team and ensure successful educational endeavors.

Topics to be discussed with patients who are receiving biotherapy include the treatment plan, side effects and management, and self-administration techniques (Rieger and Rumsey, 1992). When discussing the treatment plan, nurses should be sure to include information regarding the goal of the therapy (diagnostic, therapeutic, or supportive). Details about the specific treatment protocol (including how, where and when the agents are to be administered), laboratory and diagnostic tests that are necessary, and any other special requirements of the protocol. Topics that must be covered when educating patients about potential side effects include incidence and severity, self-management, and reportable signs and symptoms. In addition, since many biological agents are given as long-term therapy, it may be necessary for patients to learn to self-administer their treatment.

Teaching Strategies

The final step in developing the teaching plan is to identify the method of teaching and specific teaching aids that will be used. Through careful planning, nurses can choose appropriate teaching techniques and adjuncts that will improve the teaching session.

Principles of adult learning should be considered when selecting teaching strategies. According to Knowles (1980), the approach used when teaching adults is so different from that used with children that a new term, **andragogy** was developed to describe "the art and science of helping adults learn." He puts forth the following four principles that outline the concepts of andragogy:

1. Adults are independent and self-directed learners.
2. The past experiences of adults serve as a resource for learning.
3. Readiness to learn emerges from the need to cope with a developmental task or social role.
4. Adults need to see immediate benefits from learning.

The chosen teaching strategies should not only reflect the learning needs assessment, goals and objectives, and content to be presented, but also should be based on these principles of adult learning, while corresponding to the learning style of the patient or family member. If these factors are all considered when choosing teaching strategies, teaching effectiveness should be improved (Close, 1987).

Several methods are popular for teaching patients. Most patient teaching is done on a one-to-one basis. This provides nurses an opportunity for continuous assessment of the patient and for building a relationship; moreover, the nurse can adapt teaching to individual learning needs (Springhouse, 1987). Usually several teaching methods are employed to improve understanding. It is important to decide which content is to be taught via one-to-one teaching and which is to be taught in a group environment. Group teaching is appro-

priate for groups of patients with similar learning needs. Generally, basic concepts, such as aseptic technique or technique for drawing up medication, are appropriate for group teaching. There are several advantages to group teaching. Many times, patients who share a common need will become supportive of and learn from each other. Teaching a group of patients will also save time for nurses. More individualized content, such as exact dosage to draw up, is appropriate for one-to-one presentation with the learner.

Techniques that can be employed for either individuals or a group include lecture, demonstration/return demonstration, and role playing. Lecture, the traditional teaching strategy, is a formal method of teaching. Content that might be appropriate for this technique include details of the treatment plan and specific goals of therapy. Although lecture is the most frequently used technique, there are several disadvantages to using it. A lecture is usually given in a classroom setting at a specific time each day. Patients must make adjustments in their schedule to be able to attend. Another drawback is that lecture is a passive form of learning. Because adult learners need to actively participate in their learning, lecture may be inappropriate. Lecture would also be unsuitable for patients that have difficulty understanding or are slow in processing the English language. If lecture is used, it may be helpful to use analogies to clarify or illustrate a specific point. For example, the analogy of fertilizer on grass can be used to illustrate the effect of colony-stimulating factors on the hematopoietic stem cells. Demonstration/return demonstration can be extremely helpful when teaching a psychomotor skill such as self-injection. In this technique, nurses can demonstrate step-by-step, so that the patient can imitate exactly what the nurse does. Role playing can provide a nonthreatening environment for the patient to act out new behaviors. For example, the nurses may have patients act out a telephone call in which they are reporting signs and symptoms. This will enable the patient to un-

Table 14.2   Educational resources available from pharmaceutical companies

Amgen

Analogy Book
Calender with laboratory data
Chemotherapy and Neupogen®
Neupogen® (Filgrastim) Patient Fact Sheet
Neupogen® Reimbursement Guide for the Patient
Patient Guide to Therapy with Neupogen (video, handout)
Pediatric Package (includes: Sammy Syringe, Marvin's Marvelous Medicine, Your Body and G-CSF—pamphlets)
Questions & Answers About Therapy with Neupogen® (Filgrastim)
Self-Injection Chart (step-by-step guide)
Self-Injection Video (English & Spanish)
Your Personal Daily Journal

Cetus Corporation

Hospital Based Therapy
Understanding Proleukin® (aldesleukin) for Injection

Immunex

The Cells of the Hematopoietic Cascade (video, monograph)
Hematopoiesis Chart
A Patient Guide to Self-Injection (video)
A Patient Guide to Self-Injection (instruction and site recording chart)
Understanding Your Bone Marrow Transplant: A Videotape for Patients
Understanding Your Bone Marrow Transplant: A Patient Guide (written accompanying BMT videotape)

Ortho-Biotech

Anemia in Cancer. Getting Your Energy Back.
Coping with Fatigue Videotape
Dimensions of Caring: Understanding and Overcoming Fatigue
Patient Diary
Resource Catalogue
RhuEpo and the Anemia of Cancer and Chemotherapy: Two Sides of an Inpatient Story (book and audiocassette)
Self-Injection Starter Kit
Subcutaneous Injection: A Patient Guide to Correct Injection Technique (video, flipchart)
Understanding and Overcoming Fatigue Audiotape
Understanding and Overcoming Fatigue Brochure

Roche Laboratories

Complete home administration kit
Medication travel cooler
Patient Guide
Refrigerator magnet for expiration date
Self-Administration (video)
Syringe disposal container

Schering-Plough

Patient Information Card
Patient kit—home supplies plus brochures on self-administration and side effect management
Self-Injection (video)
Taking Control of Your Therapy (booklet)

---

derstand what information to have on hand when calling the nurse or physician.

Teaching aids should be incorporated with each of these teaching strategies, because they increase the learner's interest and reinforce learning. Numerous resources are available to assist nurses in educating patients who are receiving biotherapy including printed material, posters and flip charts, videotapes, and physical models.

Printed material is routinely used for biotherapy patients. Printed materials are helpful for presenting background information and step-by-step procedures. Another advantage is that patients can read the material at their convenience and refer to it if a question arises.

When choosing printed material nurses must consider the data obtained in the learning needs assessment. All too often, patients who cannot read are expected to have mastered information provided only in the written material. The written material should be evaluated for literacy level. The more pictures in the printed material, the better patients will retain the information (Meade *et al*, 1992; Springhouse, 1987). For agents approved by the Food and Drug Administration (FDA), a good source of written information is the pharmaceutical company that distributes the agent. The American Cancer Society (ACS) and the National Cancer Institute (NCI) have printed materials, some of which are free, for

Table 14.3 Educational resources available from NCI or ACS

National Cancer Institute
1–800–4–CANCER
  Advanced Cancer: Living Each Day
  The Immune System: How It Works
  Managing Interleukin-2 Therapy
  Patient to Patient: Clinical Trials and You
  Taking Time: Support for the People with Cancer
    and the People Who Care About Them
  Understanding the Immune System
  What Are Clinical Trials About?
  When Cancer Recurs: Meeting the Challenge Again

American Cancer Society
Call your local ACS office
  Pamphlets
    Cancer: Your Job, Insurance, and the Law
    Definitions Book
    Finding New/Better Ways to Control Cancer—
    Getting Involved in Clinical Trials
  Videos
    Employment, Insurance, and Cancer Patients
    What Are Clinical Trials About?
  Slide Set
    Cancer: Your Job, Insurance and the Law

Table 14.4 Educational resources available from The University of Texas M.D Anderson Cancer Center

M.D. Anderson Cancer Center
1–713–792–7375
Cards
  Administration of Subcutaneous Injection
  Disposal Tips for Home Health Care
  Erythropoietin
  Granulocyte Colony-Stimulating Factor (G-CSF)
  Human Leukocyte Interferon or Lymphoblastoid
    Interferon (Wellferon)
  Injection Packet
  Interferon
  Intramuscular Injection Instructions
  rGM-CSF (recombinant granulocyte-macrophage
    colony-stimulating factor)
Drug Sheets
  Interleukin-2
  Interleukin-4
  Monoclonal Antibodies (Diagnostic)
  Monoclonal Antibodies (Therapeutic)
  Tumor Necrosis Factor
Videos
  Administration of Intramuscular Injection
  Administration of Subcutaneous Injection
  Coping with Interferon
  Interferon
  Life's Journeys
  Reconstitution of Medication

the biotherapy patient. Some major cancer centers have produced materials that are available for a nominal charge (Tables 14.2, 14.3, and 14.4). If an area has a large population of people who do not speak or read English, it may be necessary to translate materials into other languages. Many of the ACS and NCI booklets are already available in Spanish.

Audiovisual aids such as videos have become more widely accepted in the past few years. Videos allow the patient to learn at their convenience and again have the advantage of easy reference if questions should arise. It is crucial that nurses remember to evaluate and reinforce information that is learned via video. Videos that cover information regarding specific agents, side effects and management, reimbursement, and injection technique are available from pharmaceutical companies and major cancer centers.

The cost of the videos and special equipment required to view them may be prohib-

itive for some health care agencies. In this instance, flip charts and posters may prove helpful. Flipcharts can be useful when teaching step-by-step procedures such as injection. The patient who is learning to reconstitute and draw up the medication can follow along in the flip chart while practicing with the needle and syringe.

Physical models may also prove invaluable when teaching psychomotor skills such as self-injection. Traditionally, patients have practiced injection on oranges and rolled towels. These have served the purpose but are not very lifelike. There are models available that are lifelike and can be actually injected. Other models are available to help patients identify landmarks and proper site selection for their injection (see Figures 14.1 and 14.2).

Figure 14.1   Injection model.

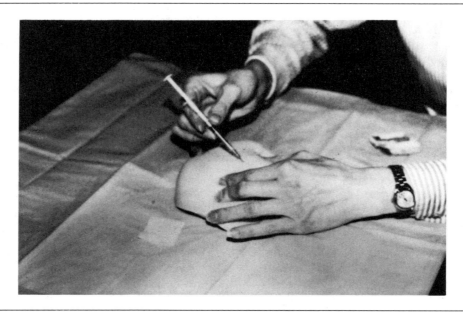

Source: Reprinted with permission from Rieger, P., and Rumsey, K. 1992. Responding to the educational needs of patients receiving biotherapy. In Carroll-Johnson, R. (ed.) *The Biotherapy of Cancer-V* (monograph). Pittsburgh, PA: Oncology Nursing Society and Roche Laboratories, pp. 10–15.

A more technologically advanced teaching aid is computer-assisted instruction (CAI). Computer-assisted instruction has been found to be better than both verbal and written formats for promoting recall and improving performance (Luker and Caress, 1989). The many advantages of CAI include that it allows individuals to work at their own pace and to review or repeat information in a nonthreatening environment. It also has the capability of using graphics to reinforce the message. Patients who are visually impaired or have difficulty reading can use CAI if speaking capability is added to the computer system (Luker and Caress, 1987). One disadvantage of CAI is that many individuals may find computers intimidating. If planning to use this teaching aid, nurses must assess the computer skills of the patient during the learning needs assessment. Even if patients are comfortable with computers, nurses should plan to spend some time orienting patients to the objectives and program.

Because of the amount and complexity of information that biotherapy patients are expected to learn, the nurse should incorporate a variety of teaching strategies and aids into the teaching plan. This will help to provide effective and efficient teaching sessions.

Implementation

Once the plan is complete, it may be implemented. During this stage, nurses must remain creative and flexible in order to accomplish their goals with the materials and time available. If well planned, the implementation should go smoothly.

A frequent obstacle to teaching is time. A definite time must be established with the patient for the teaching session. Most one-to-one teaching sessions are relatively short, usually lasting 10 or 20 minutes. Nurses should keep the patient's schedule and preferences in mind when scheduling teaching time. Some

Figure 14.2   Injection model.

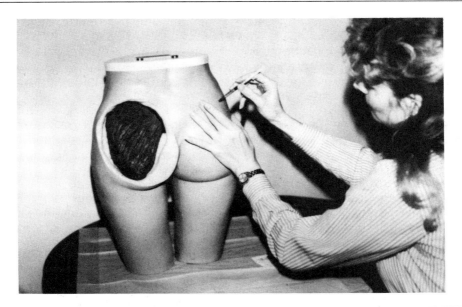

Source: Reprinted with permission from Rieger, P., and Rumsey, K. 1992. Responding to the educational needs of patients receiving biotherapy. In Carroll-Johnson, R. (ed.) *The Biotherapy of Cancer-V* (monograph). Pittsburgh, PA: Oncology Nursing Society and Roche Laboratories, pp. 10–15.

patients may prefer the time after morning care. Others who do not have evening visitors may prefer that teaching be done during that time. Nurses should also consider when family members are available to learn the information. Once the time has been mutually agreed upon, the nurse should make certain that other patient responsibilities will not interfere. Nurses may need to make arrangements so that needs of other patients are taken care of during that time. One way to accomplish this is to trade time with another nurse. Another way to overcome the obstacle of time is to incorporate teaching into patient care. By explaining site selection and injection technique while you are injecting the patient, the nurse is actually teaching or reinforcing teaching that may have been accomplished with written materials or via video.

During the implementation of the teaching plan, the nurse should promote compliance and give feedback to the patient. If the teaching plan has been mutually agreed upon, compliance will be more likely. It is also important to limit the amount of new knowledge at each session. If too much information is provided the patient may become overloaded and confused, which may lead to noncompliance. Keeping the patient actively involved during the implementation phase will also improve compliance. Patients should be apprised of their progress continuously. Positive feedback will enhance self-esteem and motivate patients to continue in their endeavors. Any small success should be praised and difficulties corrected gently. Nurses should be honest in their feedback and be aware of their nonverbal communication, as patients are able to judge genuineness.

Evaluation

Evaluation is the final component of the teaching process. Evaluation should be ongoing during the entire teaching process, not just when teaching is complete. Evaluation and documentation are the most frequently omitted steps in the process (Frank-Stromberg and Cohen, 1991; Close, 1988). This component assists nurses in evaluating their ability and skill in teaching. It helps gives the patients feedback on what they have already learned and may help to motivate them to learn more (Kaufman, 1989). Once the teaching session is over, many nurses consider teaching complete or plan to evaluate learning at a later time. Evaluation should occur at the time of teaching and be reevaluated later as well. In today's climate of liability, accountability, and quality assurance, evaluation and documentation become crucial steps in the process.

Evaluation can be defined as the continuous and systematic review of the patient's progress during and after the teaching session (Springhouse, 1987). It not only determines if the learner learned what was taught but also helps to determine if nursing time was well spent (Kaufman, 1989).

Evaluation should relate to the original goals that were written for the teaching plan. These goals can be used to judge the effectiveness of the teaching and clarify content and method for evaluation. For example, the patient should respond in a verbal manner if the goal required the patient "to state, verbalize, or describe" the goal of the treatment protocol. A return demonstration without coaching may be required for a psychomotor skill, such as self-injection. After evaluating the patient's learning, the nurse might have to revise part or all of the teaching plan and begin again. Nurses should reconsider components of the learning needs assessment, teaching strategies and aids that were used and barriers to teaching/learning, and make the appropriate changes in the plan.

Evaluation of patient teaching should be incorporated into each clinic or hospital visit. Nurses should be ready to correct any misconceptions or bad habits that the patient may have developed. Patients who demonstrated successful self-injection six months ago may have forgotten sterile technique or begun to take "short cuts" when reconstituting medication. It is imperative that nurses remember to periodically evaluate retention of and compliance with learned material.

Patient education is not complete until the teaching has been documented (Kaufman, 1989). As with the nursing process, "if it was not documented, it was not done." The JCAHO (1993) requires that nursing care data related to patient assessments, nursing diagnoses and/or patient needs, nursing interventions, and patient outcomes are permanently integrated into the medical record. Besides proving that the requirement for patient education from JCAHO and other accrediting agencies has been met, documentation serves several other purposes, such as communicating teaching and progress to other members of the health care team and providing a legal record of the teaching that has been completed and the learner's response to the teaching (Anderson, 1990).

Documentation of patient teaching should include several components. All of the learning needs that have been identified should be listed and prioritized with the target date for completion. It is important to indicate if a family member was present during the teaching or was the patient the only one to receive the information. Resources that were used such as a standardized teaching plan or standard of care also should be specified. Teaching aids (written materials, video) that were used should be listed. The outcome of the teaching should be documented. Any unresolved goals must be documented and a plan for follow-up identified. Nurses may also want to consider having the learner sign that the goal was accomplished. A multidisciplinary documentation tool can be helpful to communicate to members of the health care team (see Figure 14.3).

FUTURE DIRECTIONS IN PATIENT EDUCATION

During these times of health care reform, it has become even more important that patients

Figure 14.3 Teaching record.

PATIENT TEACHING RECORD

Directions:

1. Identify learning needs of patient and/or significant other.
2. Indicate, by assigned number, need being instructed and specific topic taught.
3. Indicate readiness to learn (e.g. asking questions, interest in discharge, motivation) and learning barriers (e.g. handicaps, acuity of illness, language).
4. Specify teaching tool(s) utilized, and other written instructions given.
5. Indicate Patient Outcome to teaching.
6. Use Comment section, especially to specify negative outcomes.
7. Obtain signature of patient or significant other taught.

Date	LEARNING NEED IDENTIFIED	Signature, Title	Target Date	✓ When Resolved	Initial When Resolved
	1.				
	2.				
	3.				
	4.				
	5.				
	6.				

Patient demonstrated   Comments:

Readiness to learn   ☐ No ☐ Yes

Barrier to learning   ☐ No ☐ Yes

Instructed on: Significant Other Present ☐ No ☐ Yes
Learning need # _____   Relationship

PATIENT TEACHING OUTCOMES   Demonstrated skills   Verbalized understanding
                             ☐ No ☐ Yes ☐ NA   ☐ No ☐ Yes

Comments:

PATIENT INSTRUCTED ACCORDING TO: (check & specify)
☐ Standard
☐ Teaching Plan
☐ Classes
☐ Other

TEACHING TOOLS UTILIZED: (check & specify)
☐ Video
☐ Written info., cards, pamphlets
☐ Other

Patient/Significant Other Signature

Instructor Signature/Title

Verification Signature/Title

Referrals Initiated	Referral services	Date	Time	Unit/Section
☐ No ☐ Yes	Need			

Source: Reprinted with permission, The University of Texas M.D. Anderson Cancer Center, Division of Nursing, Houston, Texas.

receive adequate and appropriate patient education to be able to care for themselves at home. Over the next few years, according to Morra (1991), at least five trends will influence the methods nurses choose to educate their patients. In the coming years, as our population grows older and lives longer, health care professionals will encounter with greater frequency barriers to learning such as vision and auditory impairment, negative life experi-ences, and chronic diseases. Nurses in particular will have to improve their assessment and teaching skills. As our methods of early detection and treatment of cancer continue to improve, the numbers of cancer patients and cancer survivors will increase. Health care professionals will need to consider the needs of this population and provide more information on survivorship issues. Nurses will have to become astute not only at knowing if patients are receiving accurate and appropriate information, but also at detecting sensory overload (Close, 1987). The needs of the minority population will continue to grow. Members of the health care team will become more sensitive to their cultural differences and will find better ways of communicating with this population. More people will have problems with literacy. Teaching aids will need to become increasingly more visual and auditory. Research is needed on the use of teaching technologies, such as CAI and home video (Smith,1989), that will be implemented to meet the educational needs of the individual. The health care system will be different from what it is today. Changes in the system will influence the methods and content taught to patients and family members, as well as the time frame in which the teaching/learning is to be accomplished.

Nurses will have to examine their own values and attitudes about their role as patient educators over the next few years. They must demonstrate the value they place on education of the patient by advertising their role in patient education through publication in lay journals, prioritizing patient education over non-nursing activities, and implementing research on the economic, physiologic, social, and psychological benefits of patient education (Close, 1987). In these times of health care reform, nurses must be clear about and publicize who they are and what they do that benefits the patient, to ensure themselves an appropriate role in a new health care system.

Education for patients who are receiving biotherapy will continue to provide a challenging opportunity for oncology nurses. Through implementation of the teaching process, nurses can ensure more successful patient education, resulting in patients having a better understanding of their therapy, the ability to manage treatment at home, and call the physician with reportable signs and symptoms. Many issues facing patients, the nation, and the nursing profession will shape the role that nurses play in patient education in the next few years.

References

Adams, M. 1991. Information and education across the phases of cancer care. *Seminars in Oncology Nursing* 7(2): 105–111.

American Hospital Association (AHA). 1992. *A Patient's Bill of Rights*. Chicago: American Hospital Association.

American Cancer Society (ACS). 1988. *Cancer Survivor's Bill of Rights*. Atlanta: American Cancer Society.

Anderson, C. 1990. *Patient Teaching and Communicating in an Information Age*. New York: Delmar Publishers.

Armstrong, M. 1989. Orchestrating the process of patient education. *Nursing Clinics of North America* 24(3): 597–604.

Arndt, M., and Underwood, B. 1990. Learning style theory and patient education. *The Journal of Continuing Education in Nursing* 1(1): 28–31.

Barnes, L. 1992. The illiterate client (editorial). *Maternal and Child Nursing* 17(2): 99.

Bartlett, E. 1985. At last, a definition (editorial). *Patient Education and Counseling* 7(4): 323–324.

Blumberg, B., and Gentry, E. 1991. Selecting a systematic approach for educating hospitalized cancer patients. *Seminars in Oncology Nursing* 7(2): 112–117.

Close, A. 1988. Patient education: A literature review. *Journal of Advanced Nursing* 13(2): 203–213.

Fernsler, J., and Cannon, C. 1991. The whys of patient education. *Seminars in Oncology Nursing* 7(2): 79–86.

Frank-Stromberg, M., and Cohen, R. 1991. Evaluating written patient education materials. *Seminars in Oncology Nursing* 7(2): 125–134.

Health Care Financing Administration. 1988. Code of Federal Regulations, no. 116. *Federal Register* 53: 22506–22513.

Hicks, S. 1987. The nurse and the patient: Partners in education. *Canadian Critical Care Nursing Journal* 4(3): 18–22.

Joint Commission for the Accreditation of Healthcare Organizations (JCAHO). 1993. *Accreditation Manual for Hospitals*. Oakbrook Terrace, IL: Joint Commission.

Kaufman, M. 1989. ABC's of patient education. *Advancing Clinical Care.*, 4(3): 26–28.

Knowles, M. 1980. *The Modern Practice of Adult Education: from Pedagogy to Andragogy*, 2nd ed. New York: Cambridge, The Adult Co.

Kruger, S. 1991. The patient educator role in nursing. *Applied Nursing Research* 4(1): 19–24.

Luker, K., and Caress, A. 1989. Rethinking patient education. *Journal of Advanced Nursing* 14(9): 711–718.

Meade, C., Diekman, J., and Thornhill, D. 1992. Readability of American Cancer Society patient education literature. *Oncology Nursing Forum* 19(1): 51–55.

Morra, M. 1991. Future trends in patient education. *Seminars in Oncology Nursing* 7(2): 143–145.

Nurses Reference Library: Patient Teaching. 1987. Springhouse, PA: Springhouse Corporation.

Oncology Nursing Society. 1989. *Standards of Oncology Nursing Education*. Pittsburgh, PA: Oncology Nursing Press.

Rakel, B. 1992. Interventions related to patient teaching. *Nursing Clinics of North America* 27(2): 397–423.

Redman, B. 1988. *The Process of Patient Education*, 6th ed. St. Louis: C.V. Mosby.

Rieger, P., and Rumsey, K. 1992. Responding to the educational needs of patients receiving biotherapy. In Carroll-Johnson, R. (ed). *The Biotherapy of Cancer* (monograph). Pittsburgh, PA: Oncology Nursing Society and Roche Laboratories, pp. 10–15.

Smith, C. 1989. Overview of patient education: Opportunities and challenges for the twenty-first century. *Nursing Clinics of North America* 24(3): 583-587.

Villejo, L., and Meyers, C. 1991. Brain function, learning styles, and cancer patient education. Seminars in Oncology Nursing 7(2): 97–104.

Volker, D. 1991. Needs assessment and resource identification. *Oncology Nursing Forum* 18(1): 119–123.

CHAPTER 15 | **Reimbursement for Biotherapy**

Mary S. McCabe, RN, BA, BS

Advances in biotechnology are occurring at a dramatic, ever-increasing rate. Their translation into forms of treatment has transformed modern medicine and led to the development of important new biological agents for the treatment of cancer. Beginning with the development of interferon-alpha, approved by the Food and Drug Administration (FDA) in 1986, recombinant engineering techniques have propelled the identification and formulation of a series of oncology related biological agents that could not previously be tested. Recently approved biological agents such as erythropoietin (EPO), granulocyte colony-stimulating factor (G-CSF), granulocyte-macrophage colony-stimulating factor (GM-CSF) and interleukin–2 (IL–2) are part of the armamentarium of successful cancer therapies that are now available for treatment of a variety of clinical indications (Table 15.1). In addition, many promising new biological agents including multiple interleukins, stem-cell fac-

tor, antisense compounds, and retinoids are currently being evaluated.

Accompanying these therapeutic advances has been the increasing focus and concern about the costs of health care. In 1992, the United States Commerce Department reported that the spending for health care accounted for more than 14% of the nation's total economic output, up from 13.2% in 1991. It is estimated that health care spending will account for 16.4% of the nation's total economic output by the year 2000 (Mizrahi *et al.*, 1993). For 1992, the health care bill was $838.5 billion (Pear, 1993). Despite the fact that one in every seven dollars in the U.S. economy was spent on health care in 1992, there are many unresolved and neglected issues in our health care system, such as the growing number of elderly, the increasing number of uninsured and underinsured citizens, and the rapid explosion of expensive medical technology. Daily, one can read reports in both the lay

Table 15.1 Biological response modifiers and their approved oncological indications

Biological Agent	Oncological Indication
aldesleukin, IL-2 (Proleukin®)	Renal tumors
Bacillus Calmette-Guérin	Tumors of the urinary bladder
epoetin-alfa, erythropoietin (Procrit®)	Chronic anemia (Chemotherapy-induced, associated with malignancy)
filgrastim, G-CSF (Neupogen®)	Neutropenia (Chemotherapy-induced, associated with bone marrow transplant)
interferon alfa-2a (Roferon®-A)	Hairy cell leukemia AIDS-related Kaposi's sarcoma
interferon alfa-2b (Intron®-A)	Hairy cell leukemia AIDS-related Kaposi's sarcoma
levamisole (Ergamisol®) octreotide (Sandostatin®)	Colorectal tumors Carcinoid tumors VIP-secreting tumors
sargramostim, GM-CSF (Leukine®)	Neutropenia (Associated with bone marrow transplant)

press and professional journals of a financially burdened health care system that is in crisis. A national debate has ensued within all sectors of society in which plans to restructure the U.S. health care system are being discussed. Central to each perspective is the goal of stabilizing expenditures. Economic considerations have become an integral part of legislative proposals regarding health care planning, clinical research, and patient care. Initial comprehensive efforts at cost containment began with the federal government through the introduction of the Medicare Prospective Payment System (PPS), which categorizes patient admissions into diagnostic-related groups (DRGs). However, the economic focus of clinical decision making now plays a role in all

aspects of health care as evidenced by stringent discharge policies, reductions in health insurance benefits, and the general movement toward managed care. These issues involve all specialties, but they are particularly important in oncology and in the development and use of new biological agents.

The technological explosion that has occurred in medicine in the last ten years has allowed biotherapy to develop into a major component of cancer therapy. Accompanying these advances have been specific economic measures that uniquely affect oncology. Reimbursement denials for oncology treatment and care have been a growing problem nationwide and have a substantial impact on the use of biological agents. There are many reasons that reimbursement issues so strongly affect the use of these therapies. First, state-of-the-art biological cancer therapy often involves an agent that is investigational or is often combined with a technology, such as bone marrow transplant in solid tumors, that is considered investigational. Second, much of standard oncology practice includes the use of approved drugs in treatment regimens or patient populations that are not included in the approved labeling of the drug. Third, biological therapies are relatively costly. All three of these issues contribute to the reimbursement barriers facing cancer clinicians and patients seeking the treatment opportunities biological agents offer.

INVESTIGATIONAL BIOLOGICAL THERAPY

Cancer is a serious, life-threatening group of diseases for which the therapy is less than successful in many cases and is sometimes toxic. For these reasons, clinical investigation constitutes a significant component of cancer treatment, and investigational therapy represents the best available care in cancer patients for whom no standard therapy exists. Many of the drugs within this investigational category are biological agents. As the newest form of cancer treatment, biotherapy is rapidly providing a significant number of promising biological products.

Investigational biological therapy offers patients access to the newest and most promising therapy in the context of a scientific evaluation. By standard definition, a drug or biological agent is listed as investigational when it has not yet been approved by the FDA for any form of treatment. The evaluation of such agents must be conducted as part of a formal, peer-reviewed clinical trial. This distinction between scientifically valid clinical research and the unscrupulous nonresearch use of investigational therapy is an important one. Inappropriate, nonscientific use affects informed patient consent and the agent's potential for benefit. Furthermore, such use adds no scientific information to the effort to identify and evaluate new cancer therapies.

In the formal evaluation of investigational cancer agents, knowledge is accumulated in a step-wise fashion in which the continued evaluation is dependent on positive results. The clinical trials process includes three distinct phases, all of which have therapeutic intent: phase I, identification of the maximum safe dose; phase II, evaluation of efficacy, using outcomes such as response, and phase III, a randomized comparison of the new investigational agent with the standard therapy (See Chapter 1).

The data developed from the clinical trials process provide significant information about the benefits of a new therapy prior to completion of the clinical trials evaluations and FDA approval of the therapy. Because of this continuum of knowledge, the distinction between when a drug should be considered investigational or experimental and when it can be considered "standard" therapy is often blurred (Friedman and McCabe, 1992). Although this distinction is often publicly defined and codified, those definitions are not the best determinants of insurance coverage for life-threatening disease.

Despite the fact that cancer treatment given in the context of a scientifically valid,

peer-reviewed clinical trial represents best available care, many insurers have been reluctant to cover such therapy. In fact, it is likely to be specifically excluded from the contract language of the insurance policy. This lack of insurance coverage for biological agents presents a serious, mounting problem as valuable new products are developed. The colony-stimulating factors (GM-CSF and G-CSF) and IL–2, for example, could never have been evaluated in clinical trials without insurance support for the patients' treatment costs.

Because of this serious obstacle to the availability of the most promising biological agents and their clinical evaluation, the National Cancer Institute (NCI) along with other professional oncology organizations, is working with insurers to ensure patient access to clinical trials both as best available care and as an important research endeavor.

Group C Anticancer Drugs

Recognizing the importance of making new cancer therapies available to patients as soon as possible, the NCI and the FDA established in 1976 a category of drugs called Group C. The purpose in developing this Group C category was to provide a bridge between the identification of drug activity and FDA approval so that patients would not be excluded from access to the newest therapies during the period of regulatory review. This category is specific to cancer and the basis for this special grouping is the acknowledgement that important knowledge about the activity and benefit of a drug becomes evident even while a drug continues to be evaluated. As outlined by the NCI:

> During the evaluation of investigational drugs by the Division of Cancer Treatment, NCI, certain drugs are found to have a role in the treatment of specific tumor types. There is an appreciable time period before these drugs, sponsored by the pharmaceutical industry, receive NDA [New Drug Application] approval. In order to allow

patients with these diseases to have the benefit of this drug therapy, a Group C drug classification has been developed. The purpose of this distribution is to allow access to beneficial therapy and to acquire information on safety in the context in which the drug is likely to be used in clinical practice after marketing. (Drug Master File, NCI).

Early in the history of the Group C program, drugs often remained in this category for an extended period of time if there was no pharmaceutical sponsor. This delay no longer occurs, and the process now operates as was originally intended, with drugs being classified in the Group C category only for a brief period of time. Table 15.2 lists Group C drugs as of July 1994.

For a drug to qualify for Group C status, specific requirements must be met. First, a review of papers, reports, and abstracts must show that it has reproducible efficacy against a specific tumor type. Second, it must alter the pattern of treatment of the disease. Third, it must be able to be administered safely by properly trained physicians, without the need for special supportive care facilities as delineated in criteria from the *Investigator's Handbook* (1993). One exception has been made to this last requirement; when IL–2/lymphokine-activated killer (LAK) cells combination therapy was considered for this category, it required laboratory preparation and intensive care monitoring. It was therefore placed in a Modified Group C category. Drugs included in this category must meet all other Group C criteria, including efficacy.

Despite the strong data and formal review required for a drug to be placed in the Group C category, there are no assurances that the patient care costs associated with the therapy will be covered by third-party payers. (The drugs themselves are distributed free of charge by the NCI as routine policy.) The strongest support in favor of such coverage has come from the Health Care Financing Administration, which administers the federal Medicare pro-

Table 15.2 Current group C drugs as of 7–94

Drug	Approved Group C Use
amsacrine	Refractory adult acute myelogenous leukemia, single-agent use only
azacytidine	Refractory acute myelogenous leukemia, single-agent use only

gram. Both in 1982 and 1988, this agency stated in formal guidelines that "a Group C drug and the related hospital stay are covered by Medicare if all other applicable coverage requirements are satisfied" (Health Care Financing Administration, 1989). This formal statement of coverage is not necessarily supported by other insurers, and many choose not to cover this important group of drugs.

OFF-LABEL USE OF BIOLOGICAL AGENTS

Because of the evolving efforts to improve cancer therapy, new usages are constantly being developed and new combinations are being established for drugs that have already been approved by the FDA. This practice of prescribing cancer drugs to be used in ways not included on the FDA's approved drug label is referred to as "off-label" use. Amendments passed in 1962 to the Federal Food, Drug and Cosmetics Act charged the FDA with evaluating the effectiveness and safety of all new drugs but did not grant the FDA the authority to restrict a physician's use of an oncology drug once it has been approved. The *FDA Drug Bulletin* of April 1982 states: "The FDA act does not limit the manner in which a physician may use an approved drug. Once a product has been approved for marketing, a physician may prescribe it for uses or in treatment regimens or patient populations that are not included in approved labeling" (*FDA Drug Bulletin*, 1982). This publication also stated that off-label drug use may be appropriate and rational in certain circumstances and may include the application of drug therapy results that have been extensively reported in the medical literature. Medicare guidelines also permit wider use of oncology drugs than those indications set out in the labeling, provided the therapy is "medically reasonable and necessary" (*Medicare Carriers Manual*, 1987).

The extent to which off-label use of oncology drugs constitutes standard care in clinical oncology was first documented in 1988 by the Association of Community Cancer Centers (ACCC). In a national survey of oncologists, the ACCC determined that 46% of chemotherapy drugs are used in an off-label manner (Mortenson, 1988). Although it cannot be assumed that all those instances of off-label use constituted state-of-the-art care for cancer patients, the survey demonstrated that a large portion of cancer treatment is developed after the initial marketing of the specific agents (Moertel, 1991).

A more recent survey of off-label use was reported by the United States Government Accounting Office (GAO) in 1991 (U.S. General Accounting Office, 1991). The survey included a randomized sample of oncologist members of the American Society of Clinical Oncology (ASCO). The study found that the prescribing of drugs for off-label use was widespread. One third (33.2%) of the over 5000 drug administrations noted had been given for off-label use. More significantly, over half (56.0%) of the patients received at least one drug in their treatment regimen that was prescribed for off-label use. In general, the rate of off-label use in this study was higher in those cases in which there was no agreement on the best therapy. In addition, off-label drug use for patients being treated with palliative intent was almost twice that for patients being treated with curative intent. In the treatment of colorectal cancer, over 50% of patients received at least one drug off-label. For lung cancer, all patients received at least one drug for off-label use (U.S. General Accounting Office, 1991).

In recent years there has been a national perception of increasing denials for insurance coverage for off-label use of oncology drugs.

These more restrictive policies are part of the insurance industry efforts to curb rising health care costs by limiting coverage for therapies they consider inappropriate and without scientific support for efficacy. Until the GAO study was undertaken, however, only anecdotal reports of such limited coverage of off-label use existed. The study was able to assess the extent of reimbursement denials and the effect of those denials on the treatment of cancer patients (*Federal Register*, 1989). Approximately half of the respondents reported that a third-party payer had denied reimbursement for the cost of a drug when it was used for an off-label indication. Three of four oncologists who reported reimbursement denials for off-label use stated that the rate of denials had increased in recent years. Study results also showed that the policies of third-party payers resulted in 8–11% of oncologists altering their preferred course of treatment for difficult to treat diseases such as metastatic colon cancer, non-small-cell lung cancer, and malignant melanoma (Laetz and Silberman, 1991).

Interferon-alpha, which was approved by the FDA in 1986 for use in treating hairy cell leukemia and AIDS-related Kaposi's sarcoma, was the biological agent that brought insurance denials for off-label use to the forefront. This occurred because IFN-α is expensive, because it is often administered by the patient or in an outpatient setting, and because insurers were initially reluctant to accept data supporting off-label indications (Huber, 1988). Biological agents such as the colony-stimulating factors (CSFs) continue to face reimbursement obstacles because of their cost, route of administration, and widespread use (Xistris, 1992).

REIMBURSEMENT IMPLICATIONS FOR PATIENT CARE

These obstacles to the third-party reimbursement for investigational therapy or for drugs used for off-label indications have the potential to significantly impact clinical cancer research and care.

Historically, there has been a coalition of payers involved in the support of research and the patient care component of clinical trials (Friedman and McCabe, 1992). This coalition has included the federal government, the pharmaceutical industry, third-party insurers, and private institutions such as universities, and has been changing for a number of years as agencies and institutions struggle to limit health care expenditures. Insurance groups, for example, increasingly deny reimbursement for clinical trials in an arbitrary fashion. This increasing lack of support may threaten the future of cancer research, which is such an essential and well-established health care priority. Refusal to reimburse for peer-reviewed, scientifically valid clinical trials such as those sponsored by the NCI, limits the research that can be done and thereby slows the development of new therapies (Pear, 1993). Investigators at the University of Chicago have documented the delayed completion and early closure of studies because of reimbursement problems with biological agents such as IL–2 (Vogelzang and Richards, 1989).

Reimbursement restrictions also have the potential to impact the way medical research is conducted. If the design of clinical trials is determined by third-party payment rather than by the consideration of doses, schedules, and delivery systems that will produce the best possible outcomes, then scientific progress may be limited. The better solution to such an approach is the incorporation of cost-effectiveness and cost-benefit outcomes into the design of clinical trials, which are then supported by reimbursement. Coverage restrictions, as they are now implemented, often limit access to clinical trials. Only patients whose insurance will pay or who can afford the full cost of entering the clinical trial are being enrolled (Antman, 1988). This system is elitist and denies individuals access to promising new therapies. An important example of this situation is studies of bone marrow transplant for solid tumors. These studies address important research questions and include bio-

logical agents, but the success of the studies is dependent on reimbursement issues (Antman, 1988).

Restrictions on off-label use of biological agents are also problematic. Such restrictions also limit patients' options, and cause physicians to alter the preferred course of treatment and setting in which the treatment can be administered (U.S. General Accounting Office, 1991).

COST CONSIDERATIONS

Biological agents, as a group, face reimbursement obstacles because of their relatively high cost. A 10-day course of CSFs costs approximately $1400 and a 1-month supply of interferon at a dose of 10,000 MIU administered three times a week averages $1100 (Xistris, 1992). Insurers are reluctant to approve such expenditures as standard reimbursements because of cost concerns. Thus more focus is being directed toward including cost-effectiveness analysis when considering an expensive biological agent such as CSFs. In the future, clinical trials will include economic end points along with the evaluation of effectiveness.

NATIONAL ATTENTION TO CANCER REIMBURSEMENT ISSUES

Due to the life-threatening nature of many types of cancer, there is a growing national consensus that patients need and should have access to the most promising therapies. This in turn has led to a growing concern over the increasing reimbursement limitations that patients face. A number of national organizations and coalitions have studied this issue and publicly presented statements and recommendations to address it. In 1988, the Institute of Medicine issued a report stating that:

> Third-party payers (government and nongovernment) should pay the necessary and appropriate patient care

costs for beneficiaries enrolled in approved clinical investigational protocols. This requires a clarification in current Medicare regulations involving definitions of medically necessary care. State regulatory agencies should require conforming changes by all other third-party payer policies.

There are diseases for which appropriate and required care involves investigational protocols. Such diseases include certain types of cancer, genetic diseases, and possibly severe, life threatening diseases. In these cases, third party payers (government and non-government) should pay the standard patient care costs while costs related to the investigational conclusions should be borne by the sponsoring agency (Institute of Medicine, 1988).

The American Society of Clinical Oncology, the national association that represents oncologists, has issued position statements addressing off-label use:

Congress should eliminate carrier discretion on drug coverage issues and require coverage of indications in the compendia or otherwise supported in the peer-reviewed medical literature. Further, Congress should explore ways to compel individual private insurance companies—now largely free from federal regulation—to develop fair and rational coverage policies (American Society of Clinical Oncology, 1993).

and addressing clinical trials:

The cost of medical care provided when a patient is entered on a Phase I, II, III, or IV (post-marketing) clinical trial— including hospital, physician, and other health care services as well as the cost of approved agents for labeled or unlabeled uses which might be part of the regimen—should not be denied

coverage and reimbursement when all of the following are demonstrated:

Treatment is provided with a therapeutic intent;

Treatment is being provided pursuant to a clinical trial which has been approved by the National Cancer Institute (NCI), any of its cancer centers, cooperative groups or community clinical oncology programs; the Food and Drug Administration in the form of an investigational new drug exemption; the Department of Veteran Affairs; or a qualified nongovernmental research entity as identified in the guidelines for NCI cancer center support grants;

The proposed therapy has been reviewed and approved by a qualified institutional review board;

The facility and personnel providing the treatment are capable of doing so by virtue of their experience or training;

There is no noninvestigational therapy that is clearly superior to the protocol treatment; and

The available clinical or preclinical data provide a reasonable expectation that the protocol treatment will be at least as efficacious as noninvestigational therapy (American Society of Clinical Oncology, 1993).

The NCI convened a group of health care professionals, attorneys, and administrators to develop a consensus statement advocating that:

Third-party coverage be allowed for patient care costs of all nationally approved (NCI or FDA) cancer treatment research protocols and that third-party coverage should also be allowed for all cancer treatment research protocols not subject to national approval, provided these protocols have been approved by established peer review mechanisms. As in the past, reimbursement should continue for drugs used beyond the labeled indications when such use is based upon sound scientific evidence (McCabe and Friedman, 1989).

The National Committee to Review Current Procedures for the Approval of New Drugs for Cancer and AIDS (the Lasagna Committee) was convened in 1989 and strongly stated the same position by recommending that:

> The cost of investigational drugs and marketed drugs prescribed for unlabeled indications, as well as all ancillary medical care, should be covered by Medicare, Medicaid, and private insurance, if the use has been approved by expert government agencies, in authoritative medical compendia, or by a committee established by the Secretary of Health and Human Services to deal with this matter (National Committee to Review Current Procedures for the Approval of New Drugs for Cancer and AIDS, 1990).

The ACCC has been in the forefront of advocating for reimbursement of off-label use and for coverage of clinical trials (Association of Community Cancer Centers, 1991; Fleetwood, 1993). The Oncology Nursing Society (ONS) has demonstrated its support for both issues by endorsing both the ASCO and the ACCC statements. ONS has also been involved in national lobbying efforts to promote coverage legislation through its membership in the National Coalition for Cancer Research (NCCR).

However, despite the strong, consistent recommendations of these respected national groups, reimbursement problems continue to go unresolved. Efforts are increasing as interested parties work to secure access for cancer patients to the best available treatment. There has been success in passing legislation in states such as California and Illinois to mandate coverage of therapy when it is included in one of the three drug compendia: *The American Medical Association Drug Evaluation; Amer-*

ican Hospital Formulary Service Drug Information; *The United States Pharmacopeia Dispensing Information*. (Young, 1993a; Young, 1993b). Dialogue is ongoing with insurers and members of the NCI to develop consistent coverage for clinical trials (McGivney, 1992; Cova, 1992). The NCCR has been educating Congress about the issue and the acute need to have it resolved. As these efforts continue, patients are still facing practical dilemmas related to their treatment coverage. To deal with these problems, pharmaceutical companies that manufacture biological agents all have national reimbursement programs. These services are available via toll-free telephone numbers to assist nurses and other health professionals (Table 15.3).

NURSING STRATEGIES FOR REIMBURSEMENT

Although the reimbursement debate is taking place within state and national forums, the effect of such restrictions is felt directly by the patients seeking treatment and by the health care professionals providing their care. Therefore, it becomes important and necessary for nurses to become involved both in specific reimbursement cases as patient advocates and in national groups working toward reimbursement policy solutions.

To be informed is one of the principal responsibilities nurses have when interacting with patients seeking information about reimbursement for the therapy that has been recommended. Initially, it is important to have accurate information regarding the reimbursement potential of the therapy. Next, it is important to know the process of working with insurers. In the hospital setting, this may mean assisting and educating patients in the negotiation of their insurance plans with insurer representatives. For nurses in the outpatient setting, this often involves direct communication with insurance companies. Experience has shown that it can be effective to (1) assemble packets of appropriate data (pub-

Table 15.3 Pharmaceutical-company-sponsored reimbursement services

Company	Programs	Biological agents	Telephone
Amgen	Reimbursement Hotline Reimbursement Assistance Program	G-CSF (Neupogen®)	1–800–272–9376 1–800–872–8718
Chiron Therapeutics	Reimbursement Hotline	IL-2 (Proleukin®)	1–800–775–7533
Genentech	Genentech Reimbursement Information Program	Interferon gamma (Actimmune®)	1–800–TRY–GRIP
Hoffmann-La Roche Inc.	Oncoline Indigent Patient Program Cost-assistance Program	Interferon alfa-2a (Roferon®-A)	1–800–443–6676 1–800–526–6367 1–800–227–7448
Immunex Corporation	Reimbursement Hotline Reimbursement Support Program	GM-CSF (Leukine®)	1–800–321–4669
Ortho Biotech	ProCrit® Cost-Sharing Program Procritline™ Financial Assistance Program (FAP™) Reimbursement Assurance Program	Erythropoietin (Procrit®)	1–800–441–1366 1–800–553–3851 1–800–447–3437 1–800–553–3851
Schering	Schering's Commitment to Care *Financial Assistance Programs:* 　　Reimbursement　Assistance Program 　　Patient Assistance Program 　　Indigent Patient Program	Interferon alfa-2b (Intron®-A)	1–800–521–7157

G-CSF, granulocyte colony-stimulating factor; IL-2, interleukin-2; GM-CSF, granulocyte-macrophage colony-stimulating factor.

lished literature demonstrating treatment efficacy) for review by the insurance company's medical director; (2) update local plans about important institutional studies; (3) provide data that demonstrate the standards of excellence of clinical investigators and ongoing clinical trials; and (4) utilize the assistance of pharmaceutical company reimbursement services that are available to provide support in securing reimbursement for patients (Table 15.3). Many cancer centers and community practices have developed good working relationships with insurers in their geographic area. They have cultivated knowledgeable "working groups" of experts, which include physicians, nurses, and pharmacists, to educate and communicate with insurers about the therapy being recommended to the patient as best available care. Insurers see them as "centers of excellence" because of their high quality care and their use of scientifically based

therapies that offer patients potential for real benefit (McCabe, 1992).

In addition to institutionally based reimbursement efforts, nurses can pursue individual and professional activities that address the need to be economically efficient. As outlined in Table 15.4, the following patient care options should be taken into consideration: (1) economic issues when designing equipment and treatment strategies; (2) potential self-care options for the patient; (3) discharge planning strategies that minimize hospital stays and provide for continuity of care at home; and (4) development of an institutional model that balances cost and quality in clinical care.

Nurses should view patient education about the financial issues of treatment as part of the informed consent process. In some clinical trials, such as bone marrow transplant studies, insurance coverage is an eligibility requirement. Patients generally assume that

Table 15.4 Nursing strategies for reimbursement

1. Be informed.
   - Have accurate information regarding the therapy, including knowledge of supportive literature.
   - Be familiar with information sources.
2. Know the process of working with insurers.
   - Develop working relationships with third-party payers (case managers, medical directors).
   - Document the benefits and scientific basis for the treatment planned.
3. Assist patient with financial issues as part of the informed consent process.
   - Educate patients about financial responsibility for specific aspects of treatment. Inform patients of reimbursement issues involving off-label use and investigational therapy when relevant.
   - Facilitate and promote strategies for reimbursement.
   - Access pharmaceutical company reimbursement information services and indigent patient programs.
4. Develop financially efficient plans of care.
   - Include economic considerations in clinical decision making for equipment and treatment strategies.
   - Develop institutional model that balances cost and quality in clinical care.
5. Become involved.
   - Participate in professional organizations that are involved in setting national reimbursement standards in oncology.

their insurance covers such therapy and are frequently shocked to discover that this is not necessarily the case.

As the health care system changes through national and state reform initiatives, oncology reimbursement will certainly be affected. The direction of the discussion and the development of solutions should involve nurses. The most active national groups involved in this public dialogue are discussed in this chapter. Oncology nurses should join with them as active participants in educating and influencing legislators and health care provider groups. The ONS has identified reimbursement for clinical trials and off-label use of drugs as a formal, board-approved priority issue. ONS resources are committed to tracking and supporting reimbursement-related activities and legislation. As part of the largest professional oncology organization, ONS members should be actively involved.

SUMMARY

There is little doubt that the U.S. health care system is in need of reform and that the problems of oncology reimbursement are not easy to resolve. It is hoped, however, that as health care reform programs are proposed, designed, and implemented that the commitment to providing state-of-the-art therapy to cancer patients will continue to be a national health care priority. It is important that ethical, scientific research questions continue to be addressed and that patients continue to receive care of the highest quality. These should be mutual goals of all groups involved in health care. It is only through an honest commitment to communicate and implement change together that progress can continue to be made in the treatment of cancer (McCabe, 1992).

References

American Society of Clinical Oncology, 1993. *Reimbursement position statements* (fact sheet). Washington, D.C.: American Society of Clinical Oncology, Government Relations Office.

Antman, K. 1988. The crisis in clinical cancer research. *New England Journal of Medicine* 319(1): 46–48.

Antman, K., and Gale, R. 1988. Advanced breast cancer: High-dose chemotherapy and bone marrow autotransplants. *Annals of Internal Medicine* 108(4): 570–574.

Association of Community Cancer Centers. 1991. Cancer treatments your insurance should cover (pamphlet). Rockville, MD: ACCC.

Cova, J. 1992. A swift response to a "modest" proposal. *Journal of the National Cancer Institute* 84(10): 744–745.

Drug Master File 2803. 1976. Bethesda, MD: Division of Cancer Treatment, National Cancer Institute.

Federal Register. 1989. January 30. 54: 4302–4316.

Fleetwood, M. 1993. Health care reform: Portrait of change. *Oncology Issues* 8(2): 12–16.

Food and Drug Administration. 1982. Use of approved drugs for unlabeled indications. *FDA Drug Bulletin* 12: 4–5.

Friedman, M. and McCabe, M. 1992. Assigning care costs associated with therapeutics oncology research: A modest proposal. *Journal of the National Cancer Institute* 84(10): 760–763.

Health Care Financing Administration. 1989. Certain drugs distributed by the National Cancer Institute, in *Medicare Coverage Issues Manual*, reprinted in *Medicare and Medicaid Guide* (CCH) 27: 201.

Huber, S. 1988. Reimbursement issues with interferon therapies. *Seminars in Oncology* 15(5): 54–57.

Institute of Medicine. 1988. *Resources for clinical investigation: Report of a study.* Washington, D.C.: Institute of Medicine, pp. 7–8.

Investigator's Handbook. 1993. Bethesda, MD: Cancer Therapy Evaluation Program, National Cancer Institute, pp. 80.

Laetz, T., and Silberman, G. 1991. Reimbursement policies constrain the practice of oncology. *Journal of the American Medical Association* 266(21): 2996–2999.

McCabe, M. 1992. Reimbursement of biotherapy: Present status, future directions: Perspective of the hospital-based oncology nurse. *Seminars in Oncology Nursing* 8(4 Suppl 1): 3–7.

McCabe M., Friedman M . 1989. Impact of third party reimbursement on cancer clinical investigation: A consensus statement coordinated by the National Cancer Institute. *Journal of the National Cancer Institute* 81(20): 1585–1586.

McGivney, W. 1992. Proposal for assuring technology competency and leadership in medicine. *Journal of the National Cancer Institute* 84(10): 742–743.

Medicare Carriers Manual, Part 3—Claims Process. 1987. Coverage and Limitations, HCFA-Pub 14–3 Transmittal no. 1204, August, pp. 2–25.

Mizrahi, T., Fasano, R., and Dooha, S. 1993. Canadian and American health care: Myths and realities. *Health and Social Work* 18(1): 7–12.

Moertel, C. 1991. Off-label drug use for cancer therapy and national health care priorities. *Journal of the American Medical Association* 266(21): 3031–3032.

Mortenson, L. 1988. Audit indicates half of chemotherapy uses lack of FDA approval. *Journal Cancer Program Management* 3(2): 21–25.

National Committee to Review Current Procedures for Approval of New Drugs for Cancer and AIDS. 1990. Final Report.

Pear, R. 1993. Health care costs up sharply again, posing a new threat. *New York Times* 5 January.

U.S. General Accounting Office. 1991. Off-label drugs: Reimbursement policies constrain physicians in their choice of cancer therapies. Washington, D.C.: U.S. General Accounting Office. Publication PEMD 91–14.

Vogelzang, N., and Richards, J. 1989. Third-party reimbursement issues during a phase I trial of interleukin–2. *Journal of the National Cancer Institute* 81(7): 544–545.

Young, J. 1993a. Southern state enacts off-label drug legislation. *Oncology Issues.* 8(2): 6.

Young, J. 1993b. States acting on off-label legislation. *Oncology Issues* 8(1): 8.

Xistris, D. 1992. Reimbursement of biotherapy: Present status, future directions: Perspectives of the office-based oncology nurse. *Seminars in Oncology Nursing* 8(4, suppl 1): 8–12.

CHAPTER 16 | The Future of Biotherapy

Vera Wheeler, RN, MN, OCN

Where will biotherapy be in the year 2000? Will it be a historical event, a bright meteor of the 1980s and 1990s? Or, will it become a full-fledged fourth modality of cancer therapy, used both as a single mode of treatment and in combination with other cancer therapy modalities?

Biotherapy has, in other forms, made two previous attempts to establish itself in cancer therapeutics. First, in the early 1900s, Coley's toxins, crude bacterial extracts were given subcutaneously and intralesionally to patients with sarcoma and other tumors. These extracts were, at that time, the only known systemic treatment for cancer (Balkwill, 1989). Again, in the 1970s, immunotherapy was developed using the bacillus Calmette-Guérin (BCG) vaccine, *C. Parvum* vaccine, and other nonspecific immunomodulators. Although these therapies had some successes in the treatment of melanoma and other cancers, they were not consistently effective in clinical trials (Oldham, 1991a). Now, the age of biological response modifiers (BRMs) or more simply, biotherapy, has arrived. According to Oldham (1991a), this is not immunotherapy revisited but a new therapy: major technological improvements have provided a sound foundation for its development into a useful form of treatment.

Those individuals who are optimistic about the future of biotherapy point out that the following key events in the development of current biological agents have provided a substantial advance from the limitations of immunotherapy. The first important achievement was progress in **molecular biology** and the development of genetic engineering. The ability to identify specific genes responsible for immunologically active molecules such as cytokines has lead to the development of recombinant technology. Recombinant proteins are more purified, specific products than previous nonspecific immunostimulants such as

BCG. This technology has also provided large quantities of these immunological proteins, which has permitted broad-scale testing of these agents in cancer therapy.

A second key development was the hybridoma technique, the fusing of an immortal cell with an antibody-producing cell which yielded very specific antibodies directed at a desired tumor target. These antibodies, known as monoclonal antibodies, have found wide applications in diagnostic use and continue to be explored for therapeutic use in conjugates such as immunotoxins and in other new chimeric forms.

A third development is the ability to culture and expand in number clonally activated lymphocytes, lymphokine-activated killer cells, or tumor-infiltrating lymphocytes (TIL) and return them in large numbers to the patient. This technology has been investigated in combination with existing therapies and has presently formed the basis for gene transduction of TIL with the gene for tumor necrosis factor (TNF) as a means to augment the TIL's tumoricidal capabilities.

Finally, technological advances in instrumentation, computer capabilities, and assay methods have allowed investigators to precisely determine the nature of molecules (Oldham 1991a). Some of these advances have allowed investigators to determine specific nucleotide sequences using an automated method. One example of this novel technology is the polymerase chain reaction (PCR) technique which has become an essential tool in gene research to copy and describe gene sequence.

Because of these technological advances and other continuing discoveries, new possibilities exist for the steady progress of biotherapy over the next decade. Currently, chemotherapy is the primary systemic modality used for cancer treatment. Although effective in treating numerous malignancies, the major problem associated with chemotherapy is its nonspecificity. Both malignant and nonmalignant cells are affected, often resulting in serious adverse effects. Breakthroughs in understanding the transformation of a normal cell to a malignant cell and the identification and refinement of biological proteins has led to the ability to more selectively target the tumor for therapy. As knowledge in these areas continues to grow and as molecular biology becomes increasingly sophisticated, the ability to identify the underlying "defect" in a given malignancy and then "correct it" will become a reality. These new discoveries provide the most reliable evidence of the progress of biotherapy and confirm that it represents a new era in cancer treatment.

This chapter will review developing areas of biotherapy that represent opportunities for the continued advancement of cancer treatment. The ongoing discovery of novel biological proteins, such as interleukins, as well as the production of genetically engineered molecules will be reviewed and methods for increasing the therapeutic index of drugs through innovative dosing and delivery will be examined. And lastly, gene therapy and new methods for increasing the selectivity of therapy will also be discussed. Several published studies will be reviewed to illustrate key points.

DISCOVERY OF NEW AGENTS

Progress with established treatment strategies and the introduction of new approaches in biotherapy continue at rapid rates. Discoveries of new biological proteins that may have therapeutic benefit has steadily added to the armamentarium available for investigation in clinical trials. Furthermore, the melding of molecular biology and immunology has led to the creation of a variety of novel biological agents through the use of recombinant DNA technology to genetically engineer proteins (Borden and Schlom, 1993).

New Developments in Interleukins

Cytokines known as interleukins (ILs) continue to be an active area of research. Newly discovered molecules are assigned successive

Table 16.1   Interleukins in development

Name	Other Name	Major Functions
Interleukin 6 (Weber 1993; Weber *et al.*, 1993)	IL-6, B-cell stimulatory factor, hepatocyte stimulating factor, thrombopoietin.	Stimulates synthesis of acute phase proteins in liver; stimulates cytotoxic T-cell growth; increases platelet count.
Interleukin 7 (Henny, 1989)	IL-7, lymphopoietin-1	Growth factor for early lymphoid B and T cells
Interleukin 8 (Takahashi *et al.*, 1993)	IL-8, neutrophil activating peptide	Neutrophil chemotactic factor.
Interleukin 9 (Quesniaux, 1992)	IL-9, P40	T-cell growth factor for T_H clones, T_C clones; mast cell growth-promoting factor; stimulates erythroid burst formation (BFU-E) with erythropoietin.
Interleukin 10 (Quesniaux, 1992)	IL-10, cytokine synthesis inhibitory factor	Inhibits synthesis of IL-2, IL-3, TNF, IFN-γ by TH1 cells; downregulation of major histocompatibility complex class II antigens on monocytes; stimulates IL-2 dependent CD8 T cell growth and cytolytic activity.
Interleukin 11 (Hangoc *et al.*, 1993; Neben *et al.*, 1993; Quesniaux, 1992)	IL-11, adipogenesis inhibitory factor	Enhances early hematopoietic progenitor cells and megakaryocytopoiesis with IL-3; inhibits lipoprotein lipase activity.
Interleukin 12 (Quesniaux, 1992)	IL-12, natural killer cell stimulatory factor, cytotoxic lymphocyte maturation factor	Activates NK-mediated cytotoxicity; synergizes with IL-2 to activate cytotoxic lymphocytes and lymphokine-activated killer cells.

IL numbers as their gene sequence is described. Not all interleukins are studied in cancer clinical trials, as their primary function may not appear applicable to cancer therapy. An example of such a cytokine is IL–5.

There are two areas of interleukin functions presently being explored for potential use in cancer therapy. One involves their use as hematopoietic growth factors. Currently, IL–1, IL–3, and IL–6 are being investigated in phase I and II clinical trials; IL–7, IL–8, and IL–11 also appear to have promising effects on specific hematopoietic or early progenitor cells that develop into platelets, granulocytes, monocytes, and red blood cells. Table 16.1 outlines some key characteristics of these promising interleukins. This field is progressing rapidly and interleukins have promising potential as supportive therapy with high-dose chemotherapy, radiation therapy, and bone marrow transplant.

A second area of interleukin development focuses on interleukins as anticancer agents. Clinical investigation of IL–2, for example, led to its approval by the Food and Drug Administration (FDA) in 1992 for treatment of renal cell cancer. Another interleukin, IL–6, has shown preclinical evidence of potential as an anticancer agent as well as a hematopoietic growth factor. It is currently being investigated in phase I and II clinical trials, which will be described shortly. Interleukins that are utilized as single tumoricidal agents may have limited clinical applications until their biology and multiple overlapping functions with other interleukins are better understood. It is more likely that the combination of these agents and other forms of therapy, such as chemotherapy, may provide the most effective tumoricidal therapy. Combination therapy is a complex aspect of biotherapy, however, and progress in this field may be slower than for other applications of biological agents (Lindemann, 1992).

Interleukin–6

Interleukin–6 was discovered in 1980 and originally named interferon-β–2. Other researchers called this factor "B-cell stimulating factor II" and "T-cell differentiation factor" based on observed T- and B-cell effects. Overall, IL–6 is a pleiotropic interleukin with wide-ranging effects on hematopoiesis, T and B lymphocytes, and the liver and the endocrine systems as they relate to the immune response.

Interleukin–6 is a growth factor for activated cytotoxic T cells and works synergistically with IL–1 for stimulation of T cells (Weber, 1993). It stimulates T cells to enter the cell cycle, moving them from phase G_0 to phase G_1. For the cell to complete its cycle and proliferate, IL–2 is then required. Interleukin–6 may, therefore, act as a co-factor with IL–2 in stimulating tumor-specific cytolytic T cells.

Interleukin–6 has also demonstrated promising hematopoietic effects in both preclinical and clinical studies. It appears to stimulate dormant hematopoietic stem cells into entering the cell cycle and induces a multi-lineage response in mice following radiation. In particular, IL–6 enhances platelet production, possibly by acting as a megakaryocyte colony-stimulating factor or as a thrombopoietin. It may also work synergistically with other factors such as IL–3 to shorten chemotherapy-induced thrombocytopenia (Weber, 1993).

As part of the immune response, IL–6 has wide-ranging systemic effects. Primarily, it increases the production of acute phase proteins in the liver and also increases plasma cortisol levels. These are inherent responses to infection and trauma, and may serve to regulate and prevent an over response of the immune system (Weber, 1993).

Phase I clinical trial of IL–6.   Weber and colleagues (1993) at the Surgery Branch of the National Cancer Institute recently published results of a phase I study of IL–6. The agent was administered subcutaneously once a day for 7 days, followed by a week's rest. An additional week of therapy was then administered according to the same schedule. At least 3 patients were entered at each of 3 dose levels: 3, 10, or 30 μg/kg/day of IL–6. The maximum tolerated dose was not defined in this study because of limitations in the agent's formulation, i.e., the volume of IL–6 administered at the highest dose (30 μg/kg) was greater than 2 cc.

The results of this study demonstrated that IL–6 could be safely administered at the dose levels and schedule utilized, and was generally well tolerated. Two-fold increases were seen in platelet counts at the two higher dose levels after IL–6 treatment was completed. No antitumor effects were noted in the study. The most common toxic effects experienced were fever and chills, transient anemia, and hyperglycemia. Fever with mild to moderate chills, along with headache and moderate fatigue occurred within 1 hour or less of administration. No tachyphylaxis to the fever was reported. Acetaminophen and indomethacin with ranitidine were useful in controlling these symptoms. Transient anemia returned to baseline within one week of stopping therapy. Transient hyperglycemia was seen at all dose levels, and for some patients blood glucose monitoring was required. Other changes in laboratory values included increases in levels of creatinine, alkaline phosphatase, and transaminase. Hepatotoxicity and atrial fibrillation occurred in one patient each and were cited as dose-limiting toxicities. There were no reports of hypotension or vascular leak syndrome with resultant weight gain in this study.

New Developments in Genetically Engineered Molecules

The creation of novel molecules through genetic engineering or through the linking of toxic substances to biological agents (specifi cally to monoclonal antibodies) will continue to advance the introduction of new biological agents over the next decade. Several areas of focus include the development of cytokine molecules that have enhanced biological properties, vaccines that contain a gene coding for unique tumor-associated antigens, and monoclonal antibodies with altered pharmacokinetics, binding properties, and immunogenicity. The use of monoclonal antibodies to selectively deliver chemotherapy, radiotherapy, or toxin molecules to the tumor cell is also being developed.

There has long been interest in the use of vaccines to either treat or prevent the recurrence of cancer. The success of this approach hinges on the existence of tumor specific antigens that can be targeted by the immune system. However, it has been difficult to find antigens that are selectively expressed by tumor cells. Most tumor cells express surface antigens that also are expressed on the surface of normal cells. These antigens, known as tumor-associated antigens, are generally expressed in greater concentrations on the surface of the tumor cells than on the surface of normal cells. A current area of investigation involves the use of recombinant vaccines developed by inserting the gene coding for a tumor-associated antigen into a virus (Borden and Schlom, 1993).

Several avenues exist for the use of biological agents to selectively deliver toxic agents to tumor cells. Monoclonal antibody immunoconjugates, as reviewed in Chapter 7, represent one avenue and will remain an area of focus. A second area involves the use of genetically engineered molecules. One example is the DAB_{486} IL–2 molecule, in which the native binding domain of diphtheria toxin has been replaced with human IL–2 (see Figure 16.1). This molecule has been investigated as a treatment for hematologic malignancies and inflammatory conditions such as rheumatoid arthritis (Dutcher and Wiernik, 1993; Cobb *et al.*, 1991). Cells expressing the IL–2 receptor would bind to the toxin, and cell death would ensue. Another example of using genetically engineered molecules to treat tumors is the use of bifunctional monoclonal antibodies. Through genetic engineering techniques, antibodies have been designed in which one arm of the antibody binds to the tumor and the second arm binds to a drug, toxin, or effector cell (Murray, 1991).

New Developments in Understanding the Biology of Cancer

It is currently believed that the development of tumors is caused by activation of oncogenes and inactivation of tumor suppressor genes. Further progress in understanding the molecular mechanisms responsible for carcinogenesis and cancer metastases will lead to the development of treatments that selectively target the cellular defects of tumor cells or decrease the cancer cell's ability to survive once it metastasizes. Although such molecular treatment approaches are at a very early stage (see section on gene therapy), they do represent future uses of biotherapy in the treatment of cancer (Weinberg, 1994; Yarbro, 1993; Aggarwal, 1991).

Metastases from the primary tumor ultimately cause the death of the host. An understanding of the biology of the metastatic process, however, is only beginning. Researchers have begun to define the process of metastasis and subsequent invasion and to characterize this process into sequential steps. Elucidation of the cellular processes and interactions responsible for each step will provide future avenues for impeding these processes. Potential antimetastasis therapies include prevention of tumor invasion, antiadhesive therapy, modulation of tumor vascularization, anticoagulation therapy, and genetic manipulation (Groenwald, 1993).

Antisense Therapy

As mentioned above, cancer results from the "turning on" of certain genes and the "turning off" of others. The ability to synthesize natural **oligodeoxynucleotides** through auto-

Figure 16.1   Interleukin-2 fusion toxin. DAB_{486} is a genetically engineered ligand toxin created by replacing the binding domain of diptheria toxin with sequences for human IL-2.

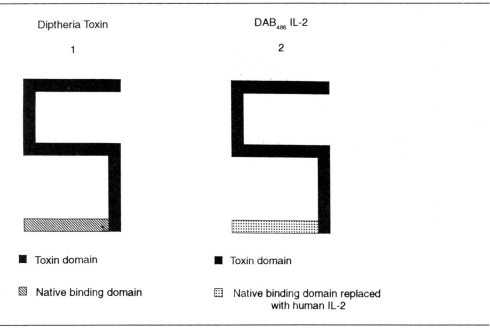

Source: Reprinted with permission from Cobb, P., LeMaistre, C., and Jackson, L. 1991. Clinical evaluation of immunotoxins. *The Cancer Bulletin* 43(3): 233–239. Copyright 1991 Medical Arts Publishing Foundation; Houston, Texas.

mation presents the possibility of selectively modifying the activity of any given gene. Antisense RNA and DNA are small synthetic oligodeoxynucleotide chains (oligos) that bind with specific messenger RNAs and can turn off the gene. The principle of this therapy, therefore, involves interference in the process by which the cell expresses its genetic information. The information transfer from DNA to RNA, known as **transcription,** and from RNA to protein, known as **translation,** is disrupted. Theoretically, one could design an antisense oligo to block the function of a proto-oncogene. Although this approach remains at a very early stage, the ability may one day exist to treat certain cancers with antisense oligos that affect genes involved in the formation and progression of tumors and in the

metastasis to and invasion of other organs (Aggarwal, 1991; Cohen, 1991).

Anti-Angiogenic Drugs

Tumor neovascularization is established through secretion of angiogenic molecules. Therefore, it appears plausible that inhibition of this process could be a potential anticancer therapy. At least two obvious methods exist for inhibition of pathological angiogenesis. One involves blocking the expression or production of angiogenic factors or neutralizing their activity. A second is blocking capillary endothelial cells from responding to angiogenic factors (Folkman, 1991). Clinical studies evaluating a new class of angiostatic agents termed angioinhibins are now in progress. One example of these angioinhibins is TNP–

470, an analogue of fumagillin, an antibiotic derived from the fungus *Aspergillus fumigatus fresenius*. This compound has demonstrated potent inhibition of endothelial cell growth (Kusaka *et al.*, 1991). Phase I trials evaluating its use in a variety of advanced malignancies are now in progress.

NEW ADVANCES IN DOSING AND DELIVERY

In Chapter 3, issues surrounding dosing and scheduling of biologicals were reviewed. Once the appropriate dose for a given biological agent in a specific situation is identified, how can this dose be achieved? Several methods such as regional perfusion therapy, the use of lipid vesicles as novel drug delivery systems, combination therapies, and monoclonal antibody (MAB) immunoconjugate therapy are currently being investigated.

Regional Perfusion of Biological Agents

Regional or isolated limb perfusion was introduced in the late 1950s by Creech as a technique to administer high-dose chemotherapy to an isolated site of melanoma or sarcoma. Later, moderate hyperthermia was added to the regimen through the use of heated perfusion circuits to improve the tumor-killing effect of the chemotherapy (Muchmore *et al.* 1985). Presently, this combination is being adapted to biological agents with promising results.

One biological agent being investigated in limb perfusion studies is tumor necrosis factor-alpha (TNF-α) which has direct antitumor effects. First, it acts by damaging the neovascular circulation surrounding tumors without destroying normal tissue. Second, it liberates highly reactive molecules and enzymes, which leads to cell death (Old, 1988). In preclinical trials, TNF-α was shown to be effective in the treatment of murine tumors

(Asher *et al.*, 1987). However, in phase I and II studies in humans, the maximum dose of TNF-α tolerated by humans, 8–10µg/kg, is substantially less than the dose used in murine studies (Fraker and Alexander, 1993; Rosenberg, 1992c). Severe toxic effects that resemble septic shock have limited the use of TNF-α as a systemic agent.

A group of investigators from the Jules Bordet Institute in Belgium have successfully adapted administration of TNF-α to the isolated limb perfusion technique. Thus, the dose of TNF-α administered at the tumor site can be increased without excessive systemic toxic effects. This protocol included treatment with interferon-gamma (IFN-γ), which has been shown to increase the number of TNF-α receptors on malignant cells; melphalan, which has synergistic effects as an alkylating agent with TNF-α; and moderate hyperthermia, which enhances the cytolytic activity of TNF-α (Lienard *et al.*, 1992; Watanabe *et al.*, 1988). The following is a report of their phase I and II study.

Phase II Study of TNF-α and IFN-γ in Isolated Limb Perfusions

Lienard *et al.* (1992) studied 23 patients with stage III melanoma or sarcoma to test the toxicity and efficacy of the triple combination of chemotherapy, hyperthermia, and biological agents. Tumor necrosis factor-α was given at a dose of 2–4 mg/kg, IFN-γ at 0.2 mg, and melphalan at 10–13 mg/liter volume of the limb, as measured by water displacement. The circulation to the limb was isolated, perfused for 90 minutes with these agents, and then normal circulation was restored.

After treatment with perfusions, Lienard *et al.* (1992) reported spectacular changes in the tumors of all patients: large, bulky tumors became blackened and soft, with no viable tumor cells at biopsy. In this study, 89% of patients achieved a complete response. Two patients had a partial response, and no treatment failures were reported. Most of the complete responses occurred with the bulkier tumors. The overall survival rate was 70% to 76% at 12 months.

Side effects of the isolated limb perfusion with TNF-α included fever and chills, skin changes and hematologic toxic effects. Fever and chills, with temperatures up to 40°C, and moderate hypotension, were noted up to 4–6 hours after surgery. Dopamine was administered as needed. Grade II skin toxic effects were present in all patients, grade III effects in two. Patients typically had reddened, swollen limbs, with occasional areas of skin breakdown immediately after treatment. There was some permanent residual swelling and tanning of the skin after recovery from the procedure. Hematologic toxic effects occurred in 11 patients. Grade IV toxicity was documented in one patient who experienced a 31% leak from the perfusion circuit into the systemic circulation. Other effects included postoperative infections, thrombophlebitis, arterial thrombosis, and acute hemorrhage. The investigators concluded that the combination of TNF-α, IFN-γ, and melphalan which achieved dramatic tumor responses could be safely administered with no more severe or frequent toxic effects than perfusions of melphalan alone.

Ongoing preclinical and phase I clinical studies at the National Institutes of Health are investigating the application of this isolated perfusion of biological agents and hyperthermia to isolate and perfuse organs, such as the lung or liver, that have isolated tumors that have metastasized from melanoma or other malignancies. There are no published reports of their progress at present, however, published results should be available in the near future.

Liposomes as Novel Drug Delivery Systems

Liposomes are lipid vesicles composed of single or multiple concentric phospholipid bilayers. These vesicles are formed spontaneously when an aqueous solution is added to a dried lipid film (Bangham *et al.*, 1974). Over the past decade, the potential use of liposomes as drug carriers has been recognized. Their unique ability to encapsulate both **hydrophilic** and **hydrophobic** drugs has led to numerous investigations evaluating their use in the administration of antimicrobial agents (Lopez-Berestein, 1987), antifungal agents (Lopez-Berestein *et al.*, 1989), chemotherapeutic agents (Lautersztain *et al.*, 1986) , and biological response modifiers. The primary objective in using liposomes as drug carriers is to enhance the therapeutic index of drugs. This can be accomplished by maintaining or amplifying the therapeutic activity of a drug, decreasing toxicity, or both. Liposomes are appealing as drug carriers because they are easy to prepare, are biodegradable, and lack toxicity. An additional feature, the natural targeting of liposomes to organs rich in reticuloendothelial cells (liver, spleen, and bone marrow), provides further opportunities for investigation (Leyland-Jones, 1993; Lopez-Berestein, 1985).

Liposomal Muramyl Tripeptide (MTP-PE)

Because liposomes are rapidly cleared from the circulation by the reticuloendothelial system (phagocytic cells primarily located in the liver and spleen) (Fidler, 1992), liposomes are potentially useful as delivery agents for immunomodulators that increase the tumoricidal activity of monocytes and macrophages. One such immunomodulator, muramyl dipeptide (MDP) is a component of bacterial cell walls that is capable of activating an immune response. However, it has an extremely short half-life in the bloodstream (Fidler, 1992), thus limiting its clinical usefulness. The agent MTP-PE is a synthetic analogue of MDP that has been investigated in clinical phase I studies to evaluate its toxicity and potential efficacy as an anticancer agent. The trials involved parenteral administration of liposomal MTP-PE for 1 hour twice weekly for 4 to 9 weeks. Patients experienced moderate toxic effects, primarily chills and fever, nausea and vomiting, fatigue, and both hypotension or hypertension. Toxic effects were most severe after the first dose but were not cumulative (Murray *et al.*, 1989; Creaven *et al.*, 1990). The maximum tolerated dose was 6 mg/m^2, and the optimal biological dose to produce activation of blood monocytes was 2–4 mg/m^2. Only one patient, with renal cell carcinoma, had an objective response to treatment with MTP-PE. Thus, liposomal MTP-PE can target and activate cytotoxic properties of monocytes and macrophages and is generally well tolerated. Phase II studies may help to clarify what role it may take in other malignancies or in conjunction with other biological agents or treatment modalities.

Combination Therapies

The development of biological agents in many ways parallels that of chemotherapy. After the efficacy of a single agent has been established, greater response rates may be achieved by combining this agent with others in a variety of schedules. As reviewed in Chapter 3, combination therapy can have several goals. An agent such as a hematopoietic growth factor can be used to decrease the toxicity of other agents such as chemotherapy or radiation. An example is the use of G-CSF to abrogate toxic hematologic effects following treatment with high-dose, myelosuppressive chemotherapy. Another goal would be to combine biological agents with each other or with chemotherapy to achieve a synergistic or additive therapeutic effect. This type of therapy is often termed chemoimmunotherapy and there are several promising regimens (Snzol and Longo, 1993; Gilewski and Golomb, 1990; Mitchell, 1988). For example, interferon-α and 5-fluorouracil and calcium leucovorin are being investigated as treatment for gastrointestinal cancers. A study by Richards *et al.* (1993) in patients with renal cell cancer evaluated the combination of dacarbazine, BCNU, cisplatin, and tamoxifen followed by interferon-α and IL–2. The reported response rate of 57%, including both complete and partial remissions, was greater than that achieved with chemotherapy or bio-

logical agents alone. Biological agents can be given in combination to achieve a greater therapeutic effect than either agent alone (Gilewski and Golomb, 1990). One of the most promising examples is the administration of interferon-α and IL–2 in renal cell carcinoma and melanoma. Although the response rate in some studies is greater than that seen for each agent alone, toxic effects can also be increased, particularly neurotoxicity (Rosenberg *et al.*, 1989).

The research discussed here only begins to solve the problem of finding the optimal dose and schedule of biological agents to maximize the potential antitumor effects of each agent while not increasing toxicity to the patient. Not all of these potential combinations will prove valuable, but they may offer insights into newer, more effective combinations.

SELECTIVITY

One of the greatest assets of certain biological agents is the ability to selectively target therapy to the tumor cell. This represents a major advance in the treatment of cancer over nonselective therapies such as chemotherapy. Numerous avenues exist by which this goal may be achieved. One involves the delivery of toxic agents such as chemotherapy or toxins through the use of monoclonal antibodies (MABs) or genetically engineered molecules, as reviewed previously. Another approach capitalizes on the natural biology of the tumor. Receptors expressed on the surface of tumor cells may serve as potential targets for therapy; thus, receptor-based therapy is an emerging strategy. The examples reviewed below illustrate this strategy.

Receptor-Based Therapy

Clinical trials evaluating the use of receptor-based therapy are beginning to emerge. Human epithelial tumors frequently express high levels of epidermal growth factor (EGF) receptor and of its **ligand**, transforming growth factor-alpha (TGF-α). It has been suggested that an autocrine pathway constituted by the EGF receptor and TGF-α may have an important role in human tumors (Derynck *et al.*, 1987). In some tumors, expression of high levels of the EGF receptor and its ligand TGF-α are associated with a poor prognosis. The use of monoclonal antibodies that block the binding of TGF-α or activation of the EGF receptor may inhibit proliferation of tumor cells expressing this receptor. Clinical trials with an anti-EGF receptor MAB are in progress.

The biological therapy of sepsis provides a very different example of receptor-based therapy. The role of IL–1 as a mediator during severe bacterial infection or septic shock (see Chapter 5) has been supported by numerous studies. A naturally occurring IL–1 receptor antagonist was discovered in 1985. This protein binds to the IL–1 receptor with similar affinity as IL–1, but does not have **agonist** activity when coupled to that receptor. Clinical trials are in progress evaluating its use in modulating the deleterious effects of IL–1 (Fraker *et al.*, 1992).

HUMAN GENE THERAPY IN CANCER

Biological agents may not always be administered as they are now, using recombinant proteins given subcutaneously or parenterally like a drug. The gene for these products may eventually be placed in a cell within the body or in a tumor to create an anticancer response, possibly in a specific target area.

Gene therapy is a technique in which a functioning gene is inserted into a patient's cells to reverse an acquired gene defect or add a new function to the cell (Rosenberg, 1992a). Cancer therapy is only one field beginning to explore these techniques for use in patient care (Morgan and Anderson, 1993; Anderson, 1992). At present, gene therapy has two possible applications. First, it can be used to correct a deficiency such as the lack of an important enzyme that is critical to cell function. An example of this is the adenosine deaminase

enzyme (ADA). In Severe Combined Immune Deficiency (SCID) syndrome, the absence of this enzyme leads to T-cell destruction and the breakdown of the immune system. Second, gene therapy may add a novel function to a cell or enhance the amount of a substance, such as TNF in lymphocytes, that is already present. A protocol utilizing this technique will be described later.

A gene can also be inserted into cells to mark or label them for future identification. This marking technique is call **gene transfer**, and it is presently being utilized in experimental protocols such as bone marrow transplant to label certain cell populations before and after treatment (Deisseroth 1993). What gene therapy cannot do at present is to remove a dysfunctional gene or limit the overproduction of an enzyme that has damaging effects. Future technologies may soon provide answers for these problems.

How then is the process of gene therapy actually accomplished in a clinical protocol? Gene therapy can be delivered by either an *in vivo* or *ex vivo* method. The *in vivo* method delivers the gene directly to the desired target cell in the body. One innovative method for *in vivo* gene delivery is via liposomal complexes. Nabel *et al.* (1992) are investigating the feasibility of delivering the desired gene to the target cell using liposomes complexed to plasmid DNA. This approach avoids the need to use a viral carrier and to culture the target cells outside the host. It may also increase the gene expression at a specific site (Nabel *et al.*, 1992).

In contrast, the *ex vivo* method takes the target cells out of the body and utilizes a vector such as a **retrovirus** to insert the desired gene. A **vector** is simply the vehicle that carries the gene into the target cell, getting it through the cell wall into the cell's cytoplasm and usually into the chromosome. When retroviruses, which have a special ability to enter cells, are used as vectors the viral DNA is removed, thus eliminating the possibility of retroviral reproduction. In place of the viral DNA, the desired marking or therapeutic gene is inserted. The retroviral vector then carries this gene into the cell as if it were its own DNA and inserts it into the chromosome at random in dividing cells. This random placement has the potential to affect the gene's expression and may cause mutagenesis. However, there have been no reports of malignancies in any of the gene therapy trials presently underway (Jenks 1993b).

Once the target cells are exposed to the retroviral vector in a process called **transduction**, the cells are then grown in culture to increase the total number of cells containing the transduced gene. During this time, checks can be made on the cell's expression of the gene. With present technology, retroviral transfer is not an efficient process and gene expression can be quite variable. Before the cells are returned to the patient, gene expression must to be at an adequate level.

The final step is to return the modified cells to the patient and observe the patient for the desired effects and for any potential problems. The transduced cells may be administered as an intravenous infusion, however, other methods such as direct injection into a tumor are possible.

Special safety precautions have been taken with the construction of the retroviral vector to prevent it from reacquiring replication genes from other viruses and creating a viral infection of its own. Figure 16.2 is a schematic of a retroviral vector containing TNF. Several sequences in the original retrovirus were altered or deleted to reduce the possibility of retroviral infection. Also, as Miller (1992) points out, the retrovirus vector is a complex mixture of proteins and nucleic acids, and thus cannot be purified to homogeneity. Therefore, there must be extensive testing of the vector cell culture for possible contamination by microorganisms or replication-competent retroviruses.

The first gene therapy protocol with therapeutic intent was performed in a child with SCID. The therapeutic gene was the adenosine deaminase gene and the target cell was T lymphocytes. The infusion of gene-modified cells

Table 16.2 Potential for gene transfer

Somatic Cell Therapy	Insertion of a gene into a non-germ cell. Alteration lasts only for individual's lifespan.
Germ Line Therapy	Insertion of a gene into human egg or sperm cell. Alteration becomes part of inheritable genome.
Enhancement Genetic Engineering	Gene for favorable traits such as height is inserted to produce desired human trait in offspring. Also has been called the ultimate cosmetic surgery.
Eugenics	An attempt to improve the human genome by eliminating what is believed to be undesirable traits.

was well-tolerated by the child, with the only side effects being mild chills and fevers. The two children treated in this protocol have shown significant improvement in their immune defense, but have required repeated infusions of the ADA-transduced lymphocytes (Culver et al., 1992). At present, no retroviral infections or mutagenesis have been observed in this child or any clinical protocol using retroviral vectors (Anderson et al., 1993; Jenks, 1993b).

Controversy about the use of gene therapy can result from confusion about the specific type of gene transfer being used. Table 16.2 lists the four major potential applications of gene transfer technology. Current gene therapy protocols focus on the insertion of a new gene into various somatic cells such as bone marrow stem cells, hepatocyte stem cells, or lymphocytes. These genes cannot be carried to future human generations, but may survive for a long period of time in the patient receiving the altered cells. Although technically feasible at present, germ line gene therapy, in which a desired gene would be inser-

Figure 16.2   Retroviral vector used to transduce tumor-infiltrating lymphocytes and tumor cells with the genes for neomycin phosphotransferase (Neo®) and tumor necrosis factor (TNF). LTR indicates long terminal repeat, and SV, simian virus. Titer equals 100,000 colony-forming units per milliliter, and TNF, 128 units per milliliter in an L929 cytotoxicity assay.

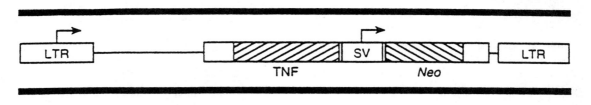

Source: Reprinted with permission from: *JAMA,* 268: 2418–2419, 1992.

ted into reproductive cells is a source of considerable debate (Neel, 1993; Juengst, 1992). As the benefits of somatic therapy are realized, there will be increased debate on how and when germ line gene therapy be used (Carmen, 1993).

Other challenges for the future will include the development of a regulatory framework by the FDA and the Recombinant DNA Advisory Committee of the National Institutes of Health that will keep pace with the growing number of protocols and complexity of scientific developments in gene therapy (Jenks, 1993c; Kessler *et al.*, 1993).

Clinical Protocols in Cancer Therapy

In May 1989, the first gene transfer study was successfully begun by the introduction of a marker gene for Neo®, a neomycin resistance gene, to identify a specific population of lymphocytes. With the successful completion of that study, the feasibility and safety of gene transfer to lymphocytes using a retroviral vector was established (Platsoucas and Freedman, 1993). The first therapeutic clinical trial using gene transfer techniques in cancer patients was begun in 1991. This protocol involved the transfer of the gene coding for tumor necrosis factor (TNF) into TIL. Rosenberg (1992b) has reported on six patients who have received TNF-modified TIL. Three patients received TNF-TIL in escalating doses biweekly without interleukin–2 (IL–2) starting with 1.1×10^8 (approximately 100 million cells) up to 5.4×10^9 cells. No TNF-related side effects were reported. The FDA, which monitored the trial, then gave approval to treat patients with 1.0×10^{10} gene modified cells along with IL–2. Three additional patients received up to a maximum of 1.0×10^{11} TIL cells and 180,000 IU/kg of IL–2 every 8 hours. The number of TIL varied according to their ability to grow in culture. One patient who received TNF-TIL, in whom conventional TIL therapy had previously failed, had a substantial objective response lasting greater than one year.

Several gene therapy protocols have begun that will attempt to modify tumors by increasing immunogenicity and recognition by the immune system. The majority of these protocols will insert the gene for cytokines such as IL–2, IL–4 or TNF, however one protocol will transfer a human major histocompatibility complex (MHC) class 1 gene, HLA-B7, normally used in cell recognition. Rosenberg (1992b) has reported on the first three patients in his protocol. These patients had a small amount of tumor removed and transduced with the gene for TNF along with the NEO® marker gene using a retroviral vector. The altered tumor cells are then returned to the patient in intradermal or subcutaneous injections in the thigh. Three weeks later the thigh is widely excised to remove the implanted tumor along with the draining lymph nodes. Lymphocytes from the lymph nodes are then grown in culture similar to that for TIL cells and later re-infused in the patient. Dr. Rosenberg has noted that one of the three patients with advanced melanoma treated with this regimen exhibited a partial response.

Another new area for gene therapy in cancer is a clinical protocol utilizing the retroviral vector carrying the herpes simplex-thymidine kinase (HSV-TK) gene. When the HSV-TK gene is injected into brain tumors, the tumor takes on characteristics of a herpes virus. The patient is then given the antiviral drug, ganciclovir and the tumor cells are killed. There is also a little understood "bystander" effect. Nearby tumor cells that were not altered by the HSV-TK gene are also killed when ganciclovir is administered. (Deisseroth, 1993; Jenks, 1992).

Finally, one new protocol seeks to use gene therapy to support current cancer therapy using high-dose chemotherapy. The gene for multi-drug resistance (*mdr*–1) is known to be responsible for the development of tumor cell resistance to the lethal effects of chemotherapy (Bielder, 1992). The proposed protocol will insert the *mdr*–1 gene into normal hematopoietic cells of patients with ovarian and breast cancer in order to protect them from the myelosuppressive effects of high-dose chemotherapy (Deisseroth, 1993).

These protocols are the first steps in exploring the use of gene transfer techniques in treating cancer. At present, only a limited number of patients have been treated with these altered cells. Despite many concerns about the toxicities associated with the expression of the TNF gene in TIL, no significant toxicity has yet occurred. Also, no untoward effects related to retroviral replication in these patients have been reported (Jenks, 1993). More work is presently underway at a variety of medical centers using both the *in vivo* and *ex vivo* vector methods of gene transfer.

Future research in human gene therapy in cancer will be directed toward developing new vectors with increased carrying capacity;

increasing expression of the transduced gene; developing new methods of direct gene transfer; targeting tumor cells to reintroduce tumor suppressor genes such as NM23 or P53, that are apparently lost in the development of invasive carcinoma; and targeting progenitor or stem cells to achieve a longer life span (Vanchieri, 1993). These first gene transfer studies have shown that it is feasible and safe to administer gene-altered cells to cancer patients. However, there is considerable research yet to be done before it is clear how gene therapy may be best utilized in cancer therapy.

SUMMARY

Advances in molecular biology have essentially made the human genome available as a source of potentially therapeutic biological agents (Oldham, 1991b). Constant discovery of new agents and the refinement of molecules through genetic engineering techniques will continue to provide new therapeutic avenues. A more complete understanding of the biology of cancer will lead to increasingly selective therapy and ultimately to repair of underlying cellular defects. Gene therapy is one aspect of this potential that continues to grow, with the number of new strategies and protocols increasing at an exponential rate.

Yet despite this promising growth, there are reasons for concern about the future of these therapies. One of the primary concerns is that of costs for development and the dilemma of who will pay these costs. Longstreet (1993) estimates that it costs a pharmaceutical company over $230 million to bring a new agent from development to market, and only three of every ten new agents successfully recover their development costs. What roles should the government, pharmaceutical companies, and the consumer play in realizing the usefulness of this new technology?

Another concern is the time-consuming product development process. (See Chapter 3.) Oldham (1991b) points out the need to develop a new paradigm for the development and licensing of new biological agents.

He argues that because biotherapy works through the body's physiologic mechanisms and cellular receptors in a manner that is different from that of chemotherapeutic agents, different evaluative methods are required. Biological agents such as interferon, believed in the 1970s to be the "magic bullet" for curing cancer, are now beginning to be used in a more rational manner. For example, after two decades of clinical research, there now appears to be a better understanding of interferon's effects and of how to combine interferon with other treatment modalities for an improved therapeutic outcome (Jenks, 1993a). The cost of discovering these optimal therapeutic strategies for other biological agents could be prohibitive unless new methods for development of biotherapy are created. Presently, as Longstreet (1993) states, it takes from seven to ten years from the time of discovery of a product to its commercial approval. Thus, in the future, there may be more potentially valuable biological agents than there are the means to develop them into approved treatments, so priorities will have to be created. Finding a balance between the cost of development, the potential treatment value of an agent, and the needs of the patient will be the challenge for the next decade.

The next ten years will represent one of the most exciting eras in the treatment of cancer as the secrets of the cause of cancer are unlocked. The ability to determine the cellular defect for a given cancer (Sandberg, 1994) and then design effective therapy may one day become reality. Biotherapy has the potential to be a part of this revolution. Nurses caring for patients receiving biotherapy will be continually challenged to remain abreast of changes in a rapidly expanding field and to chart new territory in developing strategies of care for these patients.

References

Aggarwal, B. 1991. Development of new biologics: Views of the future. *Cancer Bulletin* 43(2): 163–168.

Anderson, W. 1993. End-of-the-year potpourri—1993. *Human Gene Therapy* 4: 701–702.

Anderson, W., McGarrity, G., and Moen, R. 1993. Report to the NIH recombinant DNA advisory committee on murine replication-competent retrovirus (RCR) assays (February 17 1993). *Human Gene Therapy* 4: 311–321.

Asher, A., Mulé, J., Reichert, C., *et al.* 1987. Studies of the anti-tumor efficacy of systemically administered recombinant tumor necrosis factor against several murine tumors in vivo. *Journal of Immunology* 138: 963–974.

Balkwill, F. 1989. *Cytokines in Cancer Therapy* New York: Oxford University Press.

Bangham, A., Hill, M., and Miller, N. 1974. Preparation and use of liposomes as models of biological membranes. In Korn, E. (ed). *Methods in Membrane Biology.* New York: Plenum Publishing Corporation vol. 1, pp. 1–68.

Biedler, J. 1992. Genetic aspects of multidrug resistance. *Cancer Supplement* 70: 1799–1809.

Borden, E., and Schlom, J. 1993. Williamsburg conference on biological and immunological treatments for cancer, 1992. *Journal of the National Cancer Institute* 85(16): 1288–1293.

Carmen, I. 1993. Human gene therapy: A biopolitical overview and analysis. *Human Gene Therapy* 4: 187–193.

Cobb, P., LeMaistre, C., and Jackson, L. 1991. Clinical evaluation of immunotoxins. *Cancer Bulletin* 43(3): 233–239.

Cohen, J. 1991. Biochemical therapy: Antisense compounds. In DeVita, V., Hellman, S., Rosenberg, S. (eds). *Biologic Therapy of Cancer.* Philadelphia: J.B. Lippincott, pp. 763–775.

Creaven, P., Cowens, J., Brenner, D., *et al.* 1990. Initial clinical trial of the macrophage activator muramyl tripeptide-phosphatidylethanolamine encapsulated in liposomes in patients with advanced cancer. *Journal of Biological Response Modifiers* 9(5): 429–498.

Culver, K., Berger, M., Miller, A., *et al.* 1992. Lymphocyte gene therapy for adenosine deaminase deficiency. *Pediatric Research* 31: 149(abstract).

Deisseroth, A. 1993. Current trends and future directions in the genetic therapy of human neoplastic disease. *Cancer* 72: 2069–2074.

Deisseroth, A., Kantarjian, H., Talpaz, M., *et al.* 1993. Clinical protocol: Use of two retroviral markers to test relative contribution of marrow and peripheral blood autologous cells to recovery after preparative therapy. *Human Gene Therapy* 4: 71–85.

Derynck, R., Goeddel, D., Ullrich, A., *et al.* 1987. Synthesis of messenger RNAs for transforming growth factors α and β and the epidermal growth factor receptor by human tumors. *Cancer Research* 47: 707–712.

Dutcher, J., and Wiernik, P. 1993. The role of recombinant interleukin-2 in therapy for hematologic malignancies. *Seminars in Oncology* 20(6 Suppl 9): 33–40.

Fidler, I. 1992. Therapy of disseminated melanoma by liposome-activated macrophages. *World Journal Surgery* 16: 270–276.

Folkman, M. 1991. Antiangiogenesis. In DeVita, V., Hellman, S., Rosenberg, S. (eds). *Biologic Therapy of Cancer.* Philadelphia: J.B. Lippincott, pp. 743–753.

Fraker, D., and Alexander, H. 1993. The use of tumor necrosis factor in isolated limb perfusions for melanoma and sarcoma. *Principles and Practice of Oncology Updates.* Philadelphia: J.B. Lippincott, vol. 7, pp. 1–10.

Fraker, D., Alexander, H., and Norton, J. 1992. Biologic therapy of sepsis: The role of antibodies to endotoxin and tumor necrosis factor and the interleukin–1 receptor antagonist. *Biologic Therapy of Cancer Updates.* Philadelphia: J.B. Lippincott, vol. 2, pp. 1–12.

Gilewski, T., and Golomb, H. 1990. Design of combination biotherapy studies: Future goals and challenges. *Seminars in Oncology* 17(1): 3–10.

Groenwald, S. 1993. Invasion and metastasis. In Groenwald, S., Hansen-Frogge, M., Goodman, M., Yarbro, C. (eds). *Cancer Nursing: Principles and Practice,* 3rd ed. Boston: Jones and Bartlett, pp. 58–69.

Hangoc, G., Vin, T., Cooper, S., *et al* 1993. In vivo effects of recombinant interleukin–11 on myelopoiesis in mice. *Blood* 81(4): 965–972.

Henney, C. 1989. Interleukin-7: Effects on early events in lymphopoiesis. *Immunology Today* 10(5): 170–173.

Jenks, S. 1993a. After the early hype, interferons spark interest. *Journal of National Cancer Institute* 85: 773–774.

Jenks, S. 1993b. Gene therapy review finds few complications. *Journal of National Cancer Institute* 85: 1188–1190.

Jenks, S. 1993c. RAC ponders its purpose: To be or not to be. *Journal of National Cancer Institute* 85: 1544–1546.

Jenks, S. 1992. Dramatic new strategies for brain tumors emerge. *Journal of National Cancer Institute* 84: 662–663.

Juengst, E. 1992. Germ-line gene therapy: Back to basics. *Human Gene Therapy* 3: 45–49.

Kessler, D., Siegel, J., Noguchi, P., *et al.* 1993. Regulation of somatic-cell therapy and gene therapy by the Food and Drug Administration. *New England Journal of Medicine* 329(16): 1169–1173.

Kusaka, M., Sudo, K., Fujita, T., *et al.* 1991. Potent anti-angiogenic action of AGM–1470: Comparison to the fumafillin parent. *Biochemistry and Biophysics Research Communication* 174: 1070–1076.

Lautersztain, J., Perez-Soler, R., Khokhar, A., *et al.* 1986. Pharmacokinetics and tissue distribution of liposome-encapsulated *cis*-bis-N-decyliminodiacetato–1, 2-diaminocyclohexane-platinum (II). *Cancer Chemotherapy and Pharmacology* 18: 93–97.

Leyland-Jones, B. 1993. Targeted drug delivery. *Seminars in Oncology* 20: 12–17.

Lienard, D., Ewalenko, P., Delmolte, J., *et al* 1992. High-dose recombinant tumor necrosis factor alpha in combination with interferon-gamma and melphalan in isolation perfusion of the limbs for melanoma and sarcoma. *Journal of Clinical Oncology* 10(1): 52–60.

Lindemann, A. 1992. Introduction and overview. In Mertelsmann, R. (ed). *Lymphohaematopoietic Growth Factors* in Cancer Therapy II. Monograph European School of Oncology. Berlin: Springer-Verlag, pp. 1–2.

Longstreet, D. 1993. Biotechnology and Oncology. *Cope* 9: 50.

Lopez-Berestein, G., Bodey, G., Fainstein, V., *et al.* 1989. Treatment of systemic fungal infections with liposomal amphotericin B. *Archives of Internal Medicine* 149: 2533–2536.

Lopez-Berestein, G. 1987. Liposomes as carriers of antimicrobial agents. *Antimicrobial Agents and Chemotherapy* 31(5): 675–678.

Lopez-Berestein, G. 1985. Prospects for liposomes as a novel drug delivery system. *Cancer Bulletin* 37(4): 203–206.

Mitchell, M. 1988. Combining chemotherapy with biological response modifiers in treatment of cancer. *Journal of National Cancer Institute* 80(18): 1445–1450.

Miller, A. 1992. Human gene therapy comes of age. *Nature* 357: 455–460.

Morgan, R., and Anderson, W. 1993. Human Gene Therapy. *Annual Review of Biochemistry* 62: 191–217.

Muchmore, J., Carter, R., and Krementz, E. 1985. Regional perfusion for malignant melanoma and soft tissue sarcoma: A review. *Cancer Investigation* 3: 129–143.

Murray, J. 1991. Current clinical applications of monoclonal antibodies. *Cancer Bulletin* 43(2): 152–162.

Murray, J., Kleinerman, E., Tatom, J., *et al.* 1989. Phase I trial of liposomal muramyl tripeptide phosphatidylethanolamine in cancer patients. *Journal of Clinical Oncology* 7(12): 1915–1925.

Nabel, G., Chang, A., Nabel, E., *et al.* 1992. Clinical Protocol: Immunotherapy of malignancy by *in vivo* gene transfer into tumors. *Human Gene Therapy* 3: 399–410.

Neben, T., Loebelenz, J., Hayes, L., *et al.* 1993. Recombinant human interleukin–11 stimulates megakaryocytopoiesis and increases peripheral platelets in normal and splenectomized mice. *Blood* 81(4):901–908.

Neel, J. 1993. Germ-line gene therapy: Another view. *Human Gene Therapy* 4: 127–128.

Old, L. 1988. Tumor necrosis factor. *Scientific American* 258: 59–75.

Oldham, R. 1991a. Cancer biotherapy: General principles. In Oldham, R. (ed). *Principles of Cancer Biotherapy,* 2nd ed. New York: Marcel Dekker, Inc., pp. 1–21.

Oldham, R. 1991b. Speculations for the 1990s. In Oldham, R. (ed). *Principles of Cancer Biotherapy,* 2nd ed. New York: Marcel Dekker, Inc., pp. 667–674.

Platsoucas, C., and Freedman, R. 1993. Tumor infiltrating lymphocytes in gene therapy. *Cancer Bulletin* 45: 118–124.

Quesniaux, V. 1992. Interleukins 9, 10, 11 and 12 and kit ligand: A brief overview. *Research in Immunology* 143: 385–400.

Richards, J., Mehta, N., Ramming, K., *et al.* 1993. Sequential chemoimmunotherapy in the treatment of metastatic melanoma. *Journal of Clinical Oncology* 10: 1338–1343.

Rosenberg, S. 1992a. Gene therapy of cancer. In DeVita, V., Hellman, S., Rosenberg, S. (eds). *Important Advances in Oncology*. Philadelphia: J.B. Lippincott, pp. 17–37.

Rosenberg, S. 1992b. Gene therapy for cancer. *Journal of the American Medical Association* 268: 2416–2419.

Rosenberg, S. 1992c. The immunotherapy and gene therapy of cancer. *Journal of Clinical Oncology* 10: 180–199.

Rosenberg, S., Lotze, M., and Yang, J. 1989. Combination therapy with interleukin–2 and alpha interferon for the treatment of patients with advanced cancer. *Journal of Clinical Oncology* 7: 1863–1874.

Sandburg, A. 1994. Cancer cytogenetics for clinicians. *CA: A Journal for Clinicians* 44(3): 136–159.

Sznol, M., and Longo, D. 1993. Chemotherapy drug interactions with biological agents. *Seminars in Oncology* 20(1): 80–93.

Takahashi, G., Andrews, F., Lilly, M., *et al.* 1993. Effects of granulocyte-macrophage colony stimulating factor and interleukin-3 on interleukin-8 production by human neutrophils and monocytes. *Blood* 81(2): 357–364.

Vanchieri, C. 1993. Opportunities "opening up" for gene therapy. *Journal of the National Cancer Institute* 85: 90–91.

Watanabe, N., Niitsu, Y., Umeno, H., *et al* 1988. Synergistic, cytotoxic, and antitumor effects of recombinant tumor necrosis factor and hyperthermia. *Cancer Research* 48(3): 650–653.

Weber, J. 1993. Interleukin–6: Multifunctional cytokine. In *Biologic Therapy of Cancer Updates*. Philadelphia: J.P. Lippincott, vol. 3, pp. 1–5.

Weber, J., Yang, J., Topalian, S., *et al.* 1993. Phase I trial of subcutaneous interleukin–6 in patients with advanced malignancies. *Journal of Clinical Oncology* 11(3): 499–506.

Weinburg, R. 1994. Oncogenes and tumor suppressor genes. *CA: A Journal for Clinicians* 44(3): 160–170.

Yarbro, J. 1993. Milestones in our understanding of the causes of cancer. In Groenwald, S., Hansen-Frogge, M., Goodman, M., Yarbro, C. (eds.). *Cancer Nursing: Principles and Practice*, 3rd ed. Boston: Jones and Bartlett, pp. 28–46.

Glossary

Absorption The rate at which a drug leaves the site of administration and the extent to which this occurs.

Adaptive immunity Immunity generated in response to a specific antigen. Hallmarks are memory and specificity.

ADCC (Antibody-dependent, cell mediated cytotoxicity) A phenomenon in which target cells, coated with antibody, are destroyed by specialized killer cells which bear receptors for the Fc portion of the coating antibody. These receptors allow the killer cells to bind to the antibody-coated target.

Additive The relationship between two or more components such that their combined effect is the algebraic sum of their individual effects.

Adoptive cellular therapy Therapy that involves the transfer to the tumor-bearing host of immune cells with antitumor activity.

Agonist A drug capable of combining with receptors to initiate drug actions.

Alleles Variants of genes at a locus.

Alloantigens Molecules that distinguish one individual from another individual of the same species. An example is the ABO blood type molecule.

Anamnestic Memory response; a powerful antibody response (of secondary immune response type) following what is assumed to be initial exposure to an antigen.

Andragogy The art and science of helping adults to learn.

Antagonistic A substance that neutralizes or impedes the action or effect of another.

Antibody Proteins whose function it is to bind antigen.

Antigen Any substance, that, as a result of coming in contact with appropriate tissues, induces a state of sensitivity. Traditionally, an antigen is thought of as something foreign that when introduced to the immune system will generate an immune response. Antigens are also molecules which react with antibodies or primed T-cells regardless of their ability to generate a response (e.g., histocompatibility antigens, differentiation antigens).

Antigen processing cells Non-lymphocyte cells that carry antigen and present it to lymphocytes, resulting in induction of an immune response.

Antigenic determinant The particular chemical group of a molecule that determines immunological specificity (dominant epitope clusters). This is the part that binds directly with the immunoglobulin or T-cell receptor.

Anthelmintic Of or pertaining to a substance capable of destroying or eliminating parasitic worms.

Antigen modulation The process by which the surface antigen on the cell is internalized or shed into the circulation after binding with antibody.

Anti-idiotype An antibody targeted to the idiotype found on antibodies.

Apoptosis Programmed cell death.

Arthralgias Joint pain.

Attenuate To lessen the amount, force, or magnitude; weaken.

AUC (Area under the curve) The area under a pharmacology curve that defines the exposure of the target cell to a drug.

Autocrine Binding and activation of a cell by a substance produced by the same cell.

Autoimmunity A state in which the immune system reacts against self antigens.

B lymphocyte Lymphocytes derived from the bone marrow that develop into plasma cells and are responsible for the production of antibodies.

Biotherapy The use of agents derived from biological sources or of agents that affect biological responses.

Biotransformation Enzymatic alteration of a drug.

Blood-brain barrier The ability of brain capillaries to restrict the diffusion of substances from the blood supply into the brain because of their unique structure. Brain capillaries have no pores and are tightly wrapped in a sheath of astrocytes.

BRMs (biological response modifiers) Agents or approaches that modify the relationship between tumor and host by modifying the host's biologic response to tumor cells with a resultant therapeutic effect.

C1q One of the serum proteins involved in the immune response, the first component of complement.

Catalysis The effect that a catalyst exerts on a chemical reaction.

Catalyst A substance that accelerates a chemical reaction but is not consumed or changed during the reaction.

Chemoimmunoconjugate Linking of a drug to an antibody; usually an antineoplastic drug such as doxorubicin or methotrexate.

Chills A sensation of cold.

Chimeric Composed of parts of different origin.

Chromosomes One of the bodies in the cell nucleus that is the bearer of genes, normally 46 in humans. Chromosomes consist of DNA associated with RNA and proteins known as histones.

Clearance A measure of the speed at which the drug leaves the system.

Clonal anergy A theory for immunological unresponsiveness (tolerance) in which antigen-reactive lymphocytes are present but are functionally inactive.

Colony assays WBC colonies formed in the petri dish when nutrients and bone marrow stem cells are combined and incubated. The colonies are identified and counted for the assay.

Complement A series of serum proteins involved in the mediation of immune reactions. The complement cascade is triggered classically by the interaction of antibody with specific antigen.

Complementarity-determining regions The hypervariable region of the antibody that binds to an antigen.

Conjugate The process of attaching a drug, toxin, or radioactive substance to a biological molecule such as an antibody.

Cytogenetics   The study of cytology in relation to genetics.

Cytokines   A generic term for proteins released by cells on contact with a specific antigen that affect the functions of other cells. Cytokines affect the growth and differentiation of white blood cells and regulate immune and inflammatory responses.

Cytokine cascade   Network of interactions which occur through mutual cytokine induction, through transmodulation of cell surface receptors and by synergistic, additive, or antagonistic interactions that affect the function of a target cell.

Cytotoxic T cell   Effector T lymphocyte subset which directly lyses target cells.

Delirium   A type of organic mental disturbance characterized by confusion, decreased ability to attend and process information, and occasionally hallucinations or delusions. Agitation is a common feature. This state generally develops over a short period of time, fluctuates during the day, and is usually reversible when the underlying etiology is corrected. Delirium is often caused by metabolic disturbance or medication effects. This disturbance is also referred to as an acute confusional state, and is one of the conditions included under the term encephalopathy.

(DNA) Deoxyribonucleic acid   The type of nucleic acid found principally in the nucleus of animal and vegetable cells. The repository of hereditary characteristics (genetic information).

Differentiation antigens   Antigens (proteins) expressed during different stages of development. For example, different cell surface antigens are expressed on T cells as they mature.

Distribution   Movement of a drug from the site of administration to the site of action.

Encapsulated   The surrounding of one substance or compound with a thin coat of another.

Encephalopathy   A term used to describe a number of organic mental disturbances including delirium, post-traumatic confusional states, etc. These are distinguished from more gradual, progressive dementias by their relatively abrupt onset. Depending upon the specific entity, an encephalopathy may be reversible (i.e., toxic-metabolic encephalopathy) or permanent (i.e., severe anoxia).

Endocrine   An action that occurs when a substance is secreted by a cell and binds to distant cells in the body.

Endogenous   Originating or produced within an organism.

Endotoxin   A complex phospholipid-polysaccharide macromolecule which forms part of the cell wall of a variety of gram negative bacteria.

(Epo) erythropoietin   Hematopoietic growth factor produced in response to decreased oxygen saturation in the blood circulating through the kidneys; stimulates erythroblast differentiation, and recruits immature progenitors.

Exogenous   Originating or produced outside of the body.

Extrapyramidal motor symptoms   A symptom constellation that may include rigidity, tremor, slowness of movement, poor coordination, and difficulty maintaining balance. These symptoms are due to dysfunction of subcortical brain regions.

FAB   Fragment of antibody containing the antigen-binding site, generated by cleavage of the antibody with the enzyme papain, which cuts at the hinge region.

Fc   Fragment of antibody without antigen-binding sites, generated by cleavage with papain the Fc fragment contains the C terminal domains of the heavy immunoglobulin chains.

FDA   Food and Drug Administration.

Feeder layers   Semisolid medium used for clonal assays that contain medium, nutrients, accessory cells, cell extracts or medium conditioned by tissues.

Freund's complete adjuvant   A vehicle used to increase antigenicity. A water-in-oil emulsion of antigen, to which killed mycobacterium are added.

Gene therapy The use of therapy in which a gene is inserted into a patient's cells to reverse an acquired gene defect or to add a new function to the cell.

Gene transfer The insertion of genetic material into a patient's cells.

Genetics The branch of science concerned with heredity.

Graft-versus-host disease Reaction of a graft rich in immunologically competent cells against the tissue of a genetically nonidentical recipient.

(G-CSF) Granulocyte colony-stimulating factor Hematopoietic growth factor that stimulates neutrophil production and maturation and enhances the function of mature neutrophils.

(GM-CSF) Granulocyte-macrophage colony stimulating factor Hematopoietic growth factor that preferentially supports neutrophil, eosinophil, and macrophage development and interacts with early progenitors; inhibits neutrophil migration.

HACA (Human anti-chimeric antibody) The immune response generated by the infusion of a chimeric antibody into an immunocompetent individual. The response is targeted to the mouse portion of the antibody.

HAHA (Human anti-human antibody) The immune response generated by the infusion of a human antibody into an immunocompetent individual.

HAMA (Human anti-mouse antibody) The immune response generated by the infusion of a murine antibody into an immunocompetent individual.

Haplotype Half of a genotype, refers to the complete set of MHC loci inherited from one parent.

Hapten An incomplete or partial antigen, incapable of causing antibody production alone, but capable of binding to antibody.

Haptenated An abbreviated form.

Helper/inducer T cell A subset of T lymphocytes (CD4) whose presence is required by B cells for normal antibody production.

HGF (hematopoietic growth factors) A family of glycosylated proteins that interact with specific cell surface receptors to regulate the reproduction, maturation, and functional activity of blood cells.

Histologic examination The examination of stained sections of tissue under the microscope.

HLA complex (human leukocyte antigen complex) A complex group of antigens that define human tissue histocompatibility.

Hybridoma A hybrid cell that results from the fusion of an antibody-secreting cell with a malignant cell; the progeny secrete antibody without stimulation and proliferate continuously both *in vivo* and *in vitro*.

Hydrolytic enzymes An enzyme that breaks down a molecule into its constituent parts with incorporation of the elements of water.

Hydrophobic Water hating, the tendency to repel water.

Hydrophilic Water loving, the tendency to attract and hold water.

Idiotype The combined antigenic determinants (idiotypes) found on antibodies of an individual that are directed at a particular antigen; such antigenic determinants are found only in the variable region.

INDA Investigational new drug application.

Immune surveillance The concept that immunological mechanisms "recognize" and remove malignant cells as they arise.

Immunoconjugate A generic term to describe the linking of a toxic substance such as chemotherapy or plant or bacterial toxins to a cell-binding substance (often a monoclonal antibody).

Immunogenic "Antigenic," having the properties of an antigen. An immunogen is a molecule capable of inducing an immune response.

Immunoglobulin Protein molecules composed of four polypeptide chains that function as antibodies. There are five classes of immunoglobulins IgG, M, A, D and E.

Immunomodulation Alteration of immune responses through inhibition or stimulation.

Immunophenotyping The observed immunological characteristics of an organ or cell.

Immunoregulation Having the biological property of regulating immune responses.

Innate immunity Nonspecific immunity that does not involve the specific recognition of antigen.

Interleukin Literally, "between leukocytes." This term refers to the protein molecules responsible for the signaling and communication that occur between cells in the immune system.

Interleukin–3 (IL–3) Hematopoietic growth factor that causes stem cells to differentiate into granulocytes, macrophages, megakaryocytes, erythrocytes, and lymphocytes.

Lectins Protein mitogens.

Ligand Something which binds, especially molecules that bind to cells or other molecules.

Locus The position on the chromosome where the gene is positioned.

Lymphokines Protein molecules secreted by lymphocytes that serves as messengers between cells of the immune system.

Lymphokine activated killer (LAK) cells Peripheral blood lymphocytes capable of lysing a variety of tumor cell lines after exposure to IL–2.

Macrophage An immune cell that serves as a phagocyte, an antigen-presenting cell, and an important source of immune secretions. Macrophages are fully mature monocytes found in the tissues.

Macrophage colony-stimulating factor (M-CSF) Hematopoietic growth factor that activates monocytes, prompting macrophage production and stimulates enhanced cytotoxicity against fungi.

Major histocompatibility (MHC) complex The collection of genes coding for cell surface compatibility antigens.

Malaise A feeling of general discomfort, often the first indication of infection or disease.

Margination A process that occurs during early phases of inflammation, when leukocytes adhere to the endothelial cells lining blood vessel walls.

Marker Characteristic or factor by which a cell or molecule can be recognized or identified.

Meiosis The process of cell division that results in the production of gametes, each containing one-half the normal number of chromosomes.

Memory response The capacity of the immune system to respond much faster and more powerfully to subsequent antigen exposure than the first time.

Mitogen A molecule that can induce nonspecific division and activation of lymphocytes.

Mitosis The process of cell division that results in the production of two daughter cells.

Molecular biology Knowledge of how the cell expresses its information from DNA to RNA to protein.

Monoclonal antibody Literally, an antibody from a single clone. A clone is the progeny of a single cell. The antibody is homogeneous.

Monokines Regulatory proteins produced by monocytes.

Mutism The absence of speech in a conscious person who does not have a primary disturbance of language (aphasia) or of motor function (paralysis of voice musculature).

Myalgias Muscle aches.

Natural killer cells Lymphocytes (non B or T) which kill a range of tumor cell targets without antigen specificity; sometimes known as "large granular lymphocytes".

NDA New drug application.

Nude mouse Hairless mouse with congenital absence of the thymus, hence thymus dependent areas are depleted of T lymphocytes.

Null cells Lymphocytes that lack both T- or B-cell markers.

OBD Optimal biological dose may be defined as the minimum dose at which biological activity is maximally stimulated.

Oligodeoxynucleotides Short segments of deoxyribonucleic acid (DNA) synthesized primarily in an automatic synthesizer or "gene machine."

Oncofetal Products that are normally present during embryonic and fetal development but that are either not present or present at very low levels in normal adult tissue. Examples include carcinoembryonic antigen (CEA) and alpha-fetal protein (AFP).

Oncogene   A gene associated with carcinogenesis.

Paracrine   Binding of a substance and activation of nearby cells.

Passive antibody therapy   Administration of serum containing antibody.

Phagocytosis   The process of ingestion of microbes, other cells, and foreign particles by phagocytes. Neutrophils and macrophages function as phagocytes.

Phagosome   An intracellular vesicle in a phagocyte formed by invagination of the cell membrane during phagocytosis. It contains phagocytized material. Digestion generally occurs by lysosomal enzymes.

Pharmacodynamics   Defined simply, what the drug does to the body.

Pharmacokinetics   Defined simply, what the body does to a drug.

Phenotype   The observed characteristics of an organism that result from interaction of genes and the environment.

Philadelphia chromosome Ph¹   An abnormal chromosome formed as a result of translocation between the arms of chromosome 9 and 22. Found in patients diagnosed with chronic myelogenous leukemia.

Piloerection   Erection of the hair.

Plasma concentration   The amount of both free and bound drug in the plasma.

Pleiotropic   Characterized by the production of multiple effects.

Pluripotent stem cells (PPSC)   An uncommitted cell that produces two daughter cells, one enters a differentiation pathway and the other returns to a resting pool of cells.

Polyclonal   Proteins from more than a single clone of cells.

Polymerase chain reaction (PCR)   A technique to amplify specific genes, for example those that code for the variable region of the mouse antibody. The two strands of DNA are separated and the separated strands serve as a template for a complementary strand of DNA.

Repetitions of the process can result in more than two million copies of the desired gene in a matter of hours .

PPD   Abbreviation for purified protein derivative, substance used in intradermal test for tuberculosis.

Precursors   Immature forms of blood cells.

Progenitors   Earliest committed cells in each lineage.

Promoter   A DNA sequence at which RNA polymerase binds and initiates transcription.

Proto-oncogenes   A gene present in the normal genome that appears to have a role in regulation of normal cell growth, that is converted into an oncogene through somatic mutation.

Psychometric testing   The administration of standardized psychological tests with known validity and reliability.

Pyrogens   An agent that causes a rise in temperature.

Racemic   The state of being optically inactive and separable into two other substances of the same chemical composition as the original substance, one of which is dextrorotatory and the other levorotatory.

RAID   (Radioimmunodetection)   External imaging to disclose foci of increased radioactivity after injection of radioactive antibodies.

Redundant   Repetitive.

Reticulocyte   Immature red blood cells larger than mature erythrocytes yet nonnucleated. They circulate in the blood for one to two days while maturing.

Retrovirus   A virus from the family retroviridae. These viruses possess the enzyme RNA dependent DNA polymerase (reverse transcriptase).

Rigors   A feeling of cold with severe shivering and pallor, accompanied by an elevation of temperature.

SIDs (Shared anti-idiotypes)   Anti-idiotype antibodies that share an idiotypic determining site with another anti-idiotype.

Stem cell factor (SCF)   Hematopoietic growth factor that works at the earliest level of commitment and possibly effects the PPSC.

Synergistic   The coordinated action of two or more substances such that the combined action is greater than that of each acting separately.

Subcortical dementia   A clinical syndrome characterized by behavioral slowing, loss of memory, frontal lobe dysfunction, and mood and personality changes. Cortical functions such as speech and language tend to be preserved. This syndrome can be due to dysfunction of subcortical brain regions or of the connections between the subcortical and frontal lobe regions. Typical examples of subcortical dementia are Parkinson's disease and Huntington's disease.

Super antigens   Very potent T-cell mitogens that stimulate T-helper cells.

Suppressor T cell   A subset of T lymphocytes responsible for suppression of the immune response.

Tachyphylaxis   A progressive decrease in response following repetitive administration of a physiologically or pharmacologically active substance.

Tolergens   Molecules that induce a state of immunologic unresponsiveness.

Transcription   Information transfer from DNA to RNA.

Transduction   Transfer of genetic material from one cell to another by viral infection.

Transformation   A permanent genetic change induced in a cell following incorporation of new DNA.

Translation   Information transfer from RNA to protein.

Translocation   Transposition of two segments between nonhomologous chromosomes as a result of abnormal breakage.

Tumor-associated antigens   Antigens expressed to a greater degree on tumor cells than on normal cells. There are four basic types: oncofetal, unique, antigens from unrelated tissue, antigens from the same tissue.

Tumor infiltrating lymphocytes (TIL)   Lymphocytes obtained from tumor specimens.

Upregulate   Increased expression of receptors or cell surface proteins.

Vector   The vehicle that carries a gene into the target cell, getting it through the cell wall into the nucleus and then the chromosome. A "carrier" that is used to introduce foreign genetic material into a host.

Xenograft   A graft transferred from an animal of one species to an animal of another.

Index

DATE DUE

DEMCO 38-297